Insurance Coding and Electronic Claims for the Medical Office

Shelley C. Safian, MAOM/HSM, CCS-P, CHA, NCICS

Herzing College
Orlando, Florida

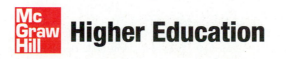 **Higher Education**

Boston Burr Ridge, IL Dubuque, IA Madison, WI New York San Francisco St. Louis
Bangkok Bogotá Caracas Kuala Lumpur Lisbon London Madrid Mexico City
Milan Montreal New Delhi Santiago Seoul Singapore Sydney Taipei Toronto

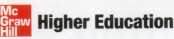

The McGraw·Hill Companies

Higher Education

INSURANCE CODING AND ELECTRONIC CLAIMS FOR THE MEDICAL OFFICE

Published by McGraw-Hill, a business unit of The McGraw-Hill Companies, Inc., 1221 Avenue of the Americas, New York, NY 10020. Copyright © 2006 by The McGraw-Hill Companies, Inc. All rights reserved. No part of this publication may be reproduced or distributed in any form or by any means, or stored in a database or retrieval system, without the prior written consent of The McGraw-Hill Companies, Inc., including, but not limited to, in any network or other electronic storage or transmission, or broadcast for distance learning.

Some ancillaries, including electronic and print components, may not be available to customers outside the United States.

This book is printed on recycled, acid-free paper containing 10% postconsumer waste.

3 4 5 6 7 8 9 0 QPD/QPD 0 9 8

ISBN 978-0-07-304099-8
MHID 0-07-304099-1

Publisher, Career Education: *David T. Culverwell*
Senior Sponsoring Editor: *Roxan Kinsey*
Managing Developmental Editor: *Patricia Hesse*
Editorial Coordinator: *Connie Kuhl*
Outside Developmental Services: *Kim Wyatt*
Senior Marketing Manager: *James F. Connely*
Project Manager: *Peggy S. Lucas*
Senior Production Supervisor: *Kara Kudronowicz*
Lead Media Project Manager: *Audrey A. Reiter*
Media Technology Producer: *Janna Martin*
Designer: *Laurie B. Janssen*
Cover/Interior Designer: *Rokusek Design, Inc.*
Senior Photo Research Coordinator: *Lori Hancock*
Supplement Producer: *Tracy L. Konrardy*
Compositor: *The GTS Companies/York, PA Campus*
Typeface: *11.5/13.5 Berkeley*
Printer: *Quebecor World Dubuque, IA*

Front Matter: © PhotoDisc and Corbis Royalty Free.
Figure 1.1 © Vol. 2/Corbis; 1.2: Vol. 1/Corbis; 2.1: © Royalty Free/Corbis; 2.2: © Vol. 59/PhotoDisc; 2.3: © Vol. 69/PhotoDisc; 2.5: © Vol. 83/PhotoDisc, Page 33: © Vol. 124/PhotoDisc.

CPT five-digit codes, nomenclature, and other data are copyright 2005, American Medical Association. All Rights Reserved. No fee schedules, basic units, relative values or related listings are included in CPT. The AMA assumes no liability for the data contained herein.

CPT codes are based on CPT 2005
ICD-9-CM codes are based on ICD-9-CM 2005

Library of Congress Cataloging-in-Publication Data

Safian, Shelley C.
    Insurance coding and electronic claims for the medical office / Shelley C. Safian.—1st ed.
        p.   cm.
    Includes index.
        ISBN 0–07–304099–1
        1. Medical offices—Management. 2. Health insurance claims—Data processing. 3. Medicine—Practice—Finance. 4. Medical fees. I. Title.

R728.5.S244   2006   2005043769
651'961—dc22   CIP

www.mhhe.com

Brief Contents

Contents

CHAPTER 7

Coding Procedures: CPT   132

CHAPTER 8

Coding Procedures: ICD-9-CM Volume 3 and ICD-10-PCS   165

CHAPTER 9

Complete Coding Practice: ICD-9-CM and CPT   182

CHAPTER 10

Health Insurance Claim Form CMS-1500   192

CHAPTER 11

Electronic Claims Management: Using Patient Accounting Software   218

About the Author

Shelley C. Safian is an assistant professor and chair of the allied health department at Herzing College in Winter Park, Florida. She began teaching at the college level in 2000. Prior to that time, Shelley launched a successful career in advertising, marketing, and business planning. The only person in her family not working in some aspect of the health care industry, Shelley was thrilled when asked to investigate the requirements of a coding and billing specialist for a special project. The results of that research led her to go back to school to study and become a nationally certified coding specialist. When asked about going back to school more than 25 years after getting her bachelor's degree, she says, "You are never too old to learn something new and get excited about it!"

Shelley is an enthusiastic, passionate, and knowledgeable educator who uses humor, real-world experiences, and current events to make learning enjoyable for her students.

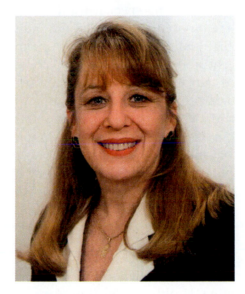

Preface

The health care industry is growing at an incredible rate. Think about it. Not only are people living longer, but we are more health conscious. There is more emphasis placed on preventive medicine and early screenings. We, as a society, desire a healthy, productive population, and ideally everyone should be covered by some form of insurance.

For every encounter or visit between an individual and a health care professional, there must be a record. In almost every circumstance, a claim or an invoice is created, so that the health care professionals can be paid for the services they have provided. Opportunities for health information management professionals continue to rise, particularly insurance coding and billing professionals. According to the Bureau of Labor Statistics, the demand for health information management professionals will increase 40%–50% by the year 2012. This is a fabulous time to join the profession.

The intent of this text is to prepare students to work in the health information management field. Reflecting a typical "day in the life" of a coding specialist, this book combines all of the concepts into one, user-friendly text. It is important for students to learn the individual concepts and recognize how they fit together. This is something that I could not find in any one text. In the past, my students needed three chapters from one book, two chapters from another, and additional information supplemented in handouts and lectures. I also noticed that my students studying NDCMedisoft™ Advanced, for example, did much better when they could understand how the information they entered would be used to create the health insurance claim form. My students excelled in reimbursement procedures when they understood the coding processes involved in creating the initial claim form. These observations motivated me to create a new text that met my needs and the needs of my students. I created a text that connects the critical processes and procedures for insurance coding and electronic claims in the medical office that can be used as a learning tool, guidebook, and reference book.

The Audience

The level of this textbook is geared toward students in a one-semester, entry level program such as Medical Billing and/or Insurance Coding, Health Information Management, and Medical Assisting.

This book speaks directly to the reader and enables them to see themselves in the situations presented with immediate application of the concepts. Theory and hands-on practice reflect a typical "day in the life" of a coding specialist.

What Makes this Book Special?

The author is a classroom instructor who wants to see her students succeed in their chosen allied health careers. She discovered that students learning about reimbursement procedures and policies pulled all the pieces together more quickly when they understood what insurance carriers needed to know to approve a claim.

Responding to the comments and recommendations of over 50 classroom instructors, the author has created a student-friendly text presenting current insurance coding and billing content.

- Content is presented in a logical sequence from the patient walking through the door of the health care facility until the claim is paid.
- Pedagogical elements such as key terms, memory tips, case studies, and review questions are integrated throughout all chapters. This provides a solid learning system for the student and saves the instructor time by providing useful examples.
- Current coding and billing information is presented using CPT, ICD-9-CM, ICD-9-CM Volume 3, and ICD-10-CM.
- The text outlines what is acceptable as well as what is not acceptable to insurance carriers and offers practical solutions in dealing with denials.
- The text can be used for both the entry level worker and as a review for an experienced health professional.
- Students are given the opportunity for real-world, hands-on practice using NCDMedisoft™ Advanced Version 9.
- The writing style is conversational and understandable with basic explanation of new terminology.

Overview

This textbook is structured to reflect a day in the life of an insurance coding and billing specialist. Using a "layered learning" concept, the student will move through the book in a logical progression, building upon each element learned at each stage. The student begins with establishing a firm foundation of understanding their soon-to-be partner in the reimbursement process—the insurance carrier. Once that foundation is laid, the student is better equipped to understand important concepts for successful claims processing and reimbursement. For example, issues of medical necessity, documentation, and accurate coding are critical to health information management professionals.

Layer 1—The Foundation: Insurance, HIPAA, and Documentation

- **Chapter 1** presents the different types of insurance that a coding and billing specialist might come across in a health care facility as well as the various ways they might receive payment.
- **Chapter 2** explains the responsibilities and obligations that each specialist must understand as directed by the Privacy Rule portion of the Health Insurance Portability and Accountability Act (HIPAA).
- **Chapter 3** provides examples of a typical health care facility's documentation—the watchword for every health information professional.

Layer 2—Coding

- **Chapters 4 through 9** are the heart of the textbook, carefully explaining each aspect of health care coding, the process of translating diagnoses and procedures into ICD-9-CM, CPT, ICD-9-CM Vol. 3, ICD-10-CM, and ICD-10-PCS codes. Chapter 4 begins with a review of the guidelines. Then, using case studies and examples of patient scenarios, the process of coding diagnoses and procedures is examined, one step at a time. This section culminates with a coding review chapter. Here, students will find physicians' notes for several patient encounters. They will need to simulate a day in the life of a professional by reading the notes, abstracting the key words, and finding the best, most appropriate codes for the diagnoses and procedures mentioned.

Layer 3—Billing and Receiving Payments

- **Chapters 10 through 13** move into the billing portion of our "day" by teaching students how to enter patients' data into a patient accounting software program in order to create the health insurance claim form and send it to the third-party payer. Once the claims are sent, students must then track them, prepare to deal with denied claims, and, of course, enter payments into the computer to document monies received (either by check or electronic funds transfer).

Layer 4—Review

- **Chapter 14** provides a recap of the entire process. Registration forms and physicians' notes are included to code and create claims forms for new patients. These are followed by notifications from the third-party payers responding to those claims—some paid, some denied. This chapter offers a rehearsal of the full scope of responsibilities of a coding and billing specialist in a health care facility.

This textbook speaks to students one-on-one and presents a real-world connection to the profession of insurance coding. In addition, the book's examples, case studies, memory tips, and highlighted important notes help connect the dots, so to speak, and facilitate the students' understanding of complex concepts.

Teaching and Learning Supplements

INSTRUCTOR'S MANUAL includes the answers to the end-of-chapter review exercises, chapter outlines, discussion activities, Teaching Tips, correlation guides to certification competencies, website resources, and additional quizzes.

INSTRUCTORS PRODUCTIVITY CENTER CD-ROM contains PowerPoint® presentations for each chapter, and exam questions using the EZ-Test format. McGraw-Hill's EZ-Test is a flexible and easy-to-use electronic testing program. The program allows instructors to create tests from book specific items. It accommodates a wide range of question types and instructors may add their own questions. Multiple versions of the test can be created and any test can be exported for use with course management systems such as WebCT, BlackBoard or PageOut. EZ-Test Online is a new service and gives you a place to easily administer your EZ-Test created exams and quizzes online. The program is available for Windows and Macintosh environments.

ONLINE LEARNING CENTER www.mhhe.com/icec-safian offers an extensive array of learning and teaching tools. The site includes quizzes for each chapter, links to websites, crossword puzzles, concentration games, and flashcards for vocabulary reinforcement. Instructor resources on this site include PowerPoints®, links to professional associations, NDCMedisoft™ information, and the instructor's manual.

SOFTWARE NDCMedisoft™ Advanced, Version 9 is recommended for use in Chapter 11. Please contact your McGraw-Hill Higher Education sales representative for a Medisoft demo disk.

Acknowledgments

Any textbook is the result of hard work by a large team. The editorial, marketing, production, and media departments of McGraw-Hill Publishing have coordinated the development and presentation of this text to provide students with a valuable resource in health information management.

In addition to the skills of these publishing professionals, and the guidance of reviewers, I wish to thank my students for their help in developing this book. They provided me with ideas, direction, and insight into the content creation for this text. My students inspired me to create a text that meets their professional needs and learning styles.

Reviewers

I would also like to thank the many instructors who provided detailed recommendations for improving chapter content throughout the review process.

Jannie R. Adams, PhD, RN, MS-HSA, BSN
Clayton College & State University
Morrow, GA

Teresa Barbour, CPC, AST
Pittsburgh Technical Institute
Oakdale, PA

Katie Barton, LPN, BA
Kerr Business College
Augusta, GA

Nenna L. Bayes, AAB, BBA, MA
Ashland Community and Technical College
Ashland, KY

Maxine Bazán
Northland Pioneer College
Winslow, AZ

Marsha L. Benedict, MSA, CMA-A, CPC
Baker College of Flint
Flint, MI

Dorine Bennett, MBA, RHIA, FAHIMA
Dakota State University
Madison, SD

Norma Bird, M.Ed., CMA
Idaho State University College of Technology
Pocatello, ID

Kathryn A. Booth, RN, MS
Wildwood Medical Clinic
Henrico, NC

Lisa L. Campbell, MHA, CCS-P, CPC, CPC-H, CMA
South Suburban College
South Holland, IL

Naomi E. W. Carrol, PhD, RN, Board Certified-Nursing Administration, Advanced; Professor, HIT
Austin Community College, Highland Business Center
Austin, TX

Kyusuk Chung, Ph.D.
Governors State University
University Park, IL

Barbara S. Desch, LVN, AHI
San Joaquin Valley College
Visalia, CA

Shirley Eittreim
Northland Pioneer College
Holbrook, AZ

Jennifer M. Evans, Coordinator/Instructor
South Seattle Community College
Seattle, WA

Herbert J. Feitelberg, BS, DPM
Kings College
Charlotte, NC

Jan C. Fuller, MBA, RHIA
Louisiana Tech University
Ruston, LA

Carolyn H. Greene
Virginia College at Birmingham
Birmingham, AL

Dr. Joyce A. Hahn
ECPI College of Technology
Manassas, VA

Stephanie Hales, ADN, BA
Parks College
Aurora, CO

Barbara Hammond
Tri-County Technical College
Pendleton, SC

Joyce Havlik, BS, MSIS, RHIA
Dakota State University
Madison, SD

Janet Hunter
Northland Pioneer College
Holbrook, AZ

Melody S. Irvine, CCS-P, CPC, CMBS
Institute of Business & Medical Careers
Ft Collins, CO

Deborah M. Jones, BS, MA
High Tech Institute
Phoenix, AZ

Ray Dumlao Johns, PT, MSHSA
Medical Careers Institute
Virginia Beach, VA

Jean Jurek, MS, RHIA, CPC
Erie Community College
Williamsville, NY

Naomi Kupfer, CMA, CMBS
Heritage College
Las Vegas, NV

Amy Lee
Valencia Community College
Altamonte Springs, FL

Norma Mercado, BS, MAHS, RHIA
Austin Community College
Austin, TX

Sharon McCaughrin
Ross Medical Education Centers
Southfield, MI

Wilsetta L. McClain
Dorsey Schools
Roseville, MI

Joyce A. Minton, BS, CMA, RMA
Wilkes Community College
Wilkesboro, NC

James J. Mizner Jr. RPh, BS, MBA
ACT College
Arlington, VA

Deborah M. Mullen, CPC
Sanford Brown Institute
Atlanta, GA

Kathy Newsom. CMA
Idaho State University
Pocatello, ID

Emily A. Noel
Vatterott College
Des Moines, IA

Linda Oliver, Instructor
Vista Adult School
Vista, CA

Linda Oprean
Applied Career Training, Manassas Campus
Director
Manassas, VA

Julie Orloff CPC, RMA, CMA, CPT
Career Education Corp.
Miami, FL

Kristina L. Perry, BFA
Heritage College
Las Vegas, NV

Alice Marie Reybitz, BA, CPC
EduTech Centers
Clearwater, FL

Melanie Schmidt, Program Manager HIS/HIT
Arizona College of Allied Health
Glendale, AZ

Ona Schulz, CMA, ATA
Lake Washington Technical College
Kirkland, VA

Janet I. B. Seggern, MS, M.ED.
Lehigh Carbon Community College
Schnecksville, PA

Nona K. Stinemetz
Vatternott College
Des Moines, IA

Jim Wallace, MHSA
Maric College
Los Angeles, CA

Danny Webb, RMA (AMT), AS
Golden State College
Visalia, CA

Jan West-Baogni
American Career College
Anaheim, CA

Lessa G. Whicker
Central Piedmont Community College
Charlotte, NC

Terri D. Wyman, CMRS, MBCS
Sanford Brown Institute
Springfield, MA

The Learning System

This text takes a unique approach to the learning process by presenting material to reflect a day in the life of an insurance coding and billing specialist. Each chapter provides **consistent learning devices.** No matter what the topic of a chapter, this system enables you to develop a solid learning strategy.

Objectives provide a road map to important chapter topics.

Key Terms and Definitions anchor your understanding of key concepts and build a solid insurance and coding vocabulary.

Case Studies and Coding Examples help you apply concepts to "real-life."

Forms Common to Most Health Care Facilities give you the chance to practice working with documentation.

"The abundance of examples and case studies is excellent and helpful to the students. I think the chapter format leads to picking out important points easily without being overwhelming or distracting."

Terri D. Wyman, CMRS, MBCS
Sanford Brown Institute
Springfield, MA

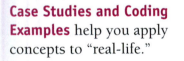

Coding Diagnoses: ICD-9-CM — 5

OBJECTIVES

- Explain the foundation of diagnosis codes using ICD-9-CM.
- Identify the best way to determine the key words located in physician's notes as they relate to the diagnoses for a specific encounter.
- Describe the rules regarding the determination of choosing the best, most appropriate code.
- Use the determined diagnosis codes for establishing medical

KEY TERMS

Alphabetic Index to Diseases
adverse reaction
anatomical site
causal condition
condition
eponyms
E (External cause) code

GETTING READY TO CODE

First, let's discuss the parts of the ICD-9-CM book, so you can understand where to look to find the best, most appropriate code. There are three sections in the book, referred to as volumes.

Volume 1, the **Tabular List of Diseases**, is the section of the book that lists all of the ICD-9-CM codes, in numerical order from 001 to ___ des V01–V84.8, and then E codes E800–E999.1. ___ and E codes, in the pages to come.)

__ **Alphabetic Index to Diseases**, the alphabetical __ that lists all of the diagnoses in alphabetical order.

___ (such as history)

___ lume 2 is Section 2, which contains the

___ Chemicals
__ Causes, the alphabetical listing for the causes of

Key Terms

Tabular List of Diseases: The portion of the ICD-9-CM book listed in numerical order.

Alphabetic Index to Diseases: The portion of the ICD-9-CM book listed in alphabetical order from A to Z.

Condition: The situation, such as infection, fracture, or wound.

Anatomical site: The place in the body, such as the knee or heart.

Eponyms: A condition named after a person, such as Epstein-Barr syndrome or Cushing's disease.

Three Categories of ICD-9-CM Diagnostic Codes   87

V16 Family history of malignant neoplasm
V16.0 Gastrointestinal tract
   Family history of condition classifiable to 140-159
   AHA: 10,'99,4
V16.1 Trachea, bronchus, and lung
   Family history of condition classifiable to 162
V16.2 Other respiratory and intrathoracic organs
   Family history of condition classifiable to 160-161, 163-165
V16.3 Breast
   Family history of condition classifiable to 174
   AHA: 20,'03, 4; 20,'00, 8; 10,'92,11

FIGURE 5-1
V Code for family history of malignant neoplasm.

Example

Harriet, a 22-year-old female, goes to her physician's office for a mammogram because she has a family history of malignant neoplasm of the female breast (breast cancer). The appropriate code would *not* be:

174 Malignant neoplasm of female breast

Using this code would indicate that Harriet has been confirmed to have a diagnosis of breast cancer, but she does not. The physician's notes do state that she has a family history of malignant neoplasm of the breast. Therefore, the correct code (Figure 5-1) is

V16.3 Family history of malignant neoplasm, breast

Take a few minutes to look through the V code section in the tabular listing of the ICD-9-CM book. Get a feeling for the category headlines and sections. The descriptions for all V codes are included in Volume 2, the Alphabetic Index to Diseases, so the ICD-9-CM book will guide you as to when to use them.

Example

V codes cover screenings, such as a mammogram or a colonoscopy; preventive medicines, such as vaccinations; fertility testing and treatments; prenatal checkups; and well-baby exams.

Memory
V in V code stands for preVentive.

CASE STUDY

Drew just found out that his son's best friend has come down with a case of rubella. His son was over at his house, playing, just two days ago. So, Drew takes his son to his pediatrician to get checked. Dr. Morgan writes in his notes that the reason for the visit was Exposure to Rubella. What is the best ICD-9-CM code to use on the claim form?

The correct code is: V01.4 Exposure to Rubella.

---

194   Chapter 10 Health Insurance Claim Form CMS-1500

FIGURE 10-1
CMS-1500 health insurance claim form.

Important Notes highlight and rephrase important concepts and issues from the narrative.

Memory Tips assist you in remembering key concepts or terms.

Memory Tip
Subjective
Objective
Assessment
Plan

Subjective (impressions and patient observations) is the first section and will include the patient's reason for the visit today: the chief complaint in his or her own words; status regarding current medications and/or treatments; history (family history; problem-focused history [of the current condition] and/or social history e.g., personal habits affecting health such as smoking, drinking); and an itemization of the reported symptoms.

Physician's Notes document a patient's health care encounter. Various formats of notes used by physicians are shown and discussed.

PROGRESS NOTE

PT NAME:	ROBBINS, ARLENE	DATE: 03/03/06
DOB:	05/27/88	
MRN:	05003579	

S: This pt is an 18-year-old white female, g 0, LMP 2/18, not sexually active, not on any birth control who presents today with two main complaints. The first complaint is she feels a lump in her right groin. The second complaint is a vaginal discharge, no odor or itching, just feels irritated.

O: Pelvic exam revealed the external genitalia to be within normal limits. The vagina was without lesions. Scant discharge seen. Wet mount neg for Trichomonas, clue cells or hyphae. Increased bacteria in the background noted. Inspection of the rt groin revealed no abnormality. The pt was asked to point out the area of abnormality and this felt to be dilated areas within one of the vessels in the groin. These were less than the size of a pea and did not feel like lymphadenopathy. Similar areas were felt on the lt side as well. The patient was reassured.

A: Possible nonspecific vaginitis

P:
1. Cleocin vaginal cream qhs times seven nights.
2. Follow up in one month for reinspection of the rt groin.
3. Otherwise follow up with us prn. She verbalized understanding.
4. All questions were answered. She will follow up with us prn or for her yearly Pap smear.

Harold Doctor, M.D.

D: 03/03/06
T: 03/08/06 nk

FIGURE 3-5
Example of SOAP notes.

CHAPTER SUMMARY

E codes, V codes, three digits, four digits, five digits, major complications, underlying diseases, and so on—don't worry; as you look back over this chapter, you should notice one very important thing—the ICD-9-CM book will almost always guide you to the correct code. The book will tell you when you need a fourth or a fifth digit. The alphabetic listing will guide you to the correct page in the numerical (tabular) listings, so you can find the best, most appropriate code. And, if the code's description doesn't match the physician's notes, just go back and keep looking.

The ICD-9-CM process with its notat direction toward the

Chapter Summaries briefly restate the key points of the chapter.

Chapter Review

Find the best diagnosis code(s) for the following patients.

1. A 35-year-old female comes into the physician's office for an elective sterilization (to have her tubes tied). _____

2. A 27-year-old female is seen in the physician's office for a checkup. Her pregnancy has been complicated by a case of gonorrhea. _____

3. A 5-year-old male is seen by the physician for a Rubella screening. _____

4. A 65-year-old male is seen in the physician's office. The diagnosis is type I uncontrolled diabetes with circulatory problems. _____

5. A 47-year-old male is seen in the physician's office for stomach pains. The diagnosis is confirmed for a sigmoid colon carcinoma. _____

6. A 3-year-old male is seen by the physician because he has gotten a jelly bean stuck up his nose. _____

7. A 29-year-old female is brought into the emergency room diagnosed with anaphylactic shock caused by eating peanuts. _____

8. A 43-year-old female is seen by the physician and diagnosed with an endometrial ovarian cyst. _____

9. A 32-year-old male is seen by the physician, complaining that he cannot stay awake. The diagnosis of narcolepsy is confirmed. _____

Chapter Reviews challenge you to test your mastery of a concept before moving on to another topic.

"The content is presented at a level appropriate for its audience. Also, it does a great job of following Bloom's Taxonomy, with regard to the knowledge, comprehension, application, and analysis."

Lisa L. Campbell,
MHA, CCS-P, CPC, CPC-H, CMA
South Suburban College
South Holland, IL

To the Student

Your Career

This class introduces you to skills you will need in order to work in the health information management profession. A fundamental part of an insurance coding and medical billing specialist's job is to work with the insurance companies that will reimburse your health care facility for the services and treatments you provide to your patients. You may be employed by a hospital, clinic, doctor's office, health maintenance organization, mental health care facility, insurance company, government agency, or long term care facility. This career is challenging, interesting, and one of the ten fastest growing allied health occupations.

How can I succeed in this class?

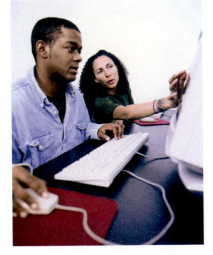

If you're reading this, you're on the right track.

> "You are the same today that you are going to be five years from now except for two things: the people with whom you associate and the books you read."   Charles Jones

Right now, you're probably leafing through this book feeling just a little overwhelmed. You're trying to juggle several other classes (which probably are equally as intimidating), possibly a job, and on top of it all, a life.

These helpful hints have been designed specifically to help you focus. They're here to help you learn how to manage your time and your studies to succeed.

➡ Start here.

It's true—you are what you put into your studies. You have a lot of time and money invested in your education. Don't blow it now by putting in only half of the effort this class requires. Succeeding in this class (and life) requires

- Making a commitment—of time and perseverance
- Knowing and motivating yourself
- Getting organized
- Managing your time

This text will help you learn how to be effective in these areas, as well as offer guidance in

- Getting the most out of your lecture
- Thinking through—and applying—the material
- Getting the most out of your textbook
- Finding extra help when you need it

Making a Commitment—of Time and Perseverance

Learning—and mastering—takes time, and patience. Nothing worthwhile comes easily. Be committed to your studies and you will reap the benefits in the long run.

Consider this: Your college education is building the foundation for your future—a future in your chosen profession. Sloppy and hurried craftsmanship now will only lead to ruin later.

Side note: A good rule of thumb is to allow two hours of study time for every hour you spend in lecture.

For instance, a three-hour lecture deserves six hours of study time. If you commit time for this course daily, you're investing a little less than one hour per day, including the weekend. Study time includes writing reports, completing practice problems, reading textual material, and reviewing notes.

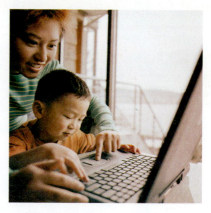

Knowing and Motivating Yourself

What type of a learner are you? When are you most productive? Know yourself and your limits and work within them. Know how to motivate yourself to give your all to your studies and achieve your goals. Quite bluntly, you are the one who benefits most from your success. If you lack self-motivation and drive, you are the first person that suffers.

Knowing yourself—there are many types of learners and no right or wrong way of learning. Which category do you fall into?

Visual learner—you respond best to "seeing" processes and information. Particularly focus on text illustrations and charts and course handouts, and check to see if there are animations on the course or text website to help you. Also, consider drawing diagrams in your notes to illustrate concepts.

Auditory learner—you work best by listening to—and possibly tape recording—the lecture and by talking through information with a study partner.

Tactile/kinesthetic learner—you learn best by being "hands on." You'll benefit by applying what you've learned during lab time. Think of ways to apply your critical thinking skills in application ways.

Identify your personal preferences for learning and seek out the resources that will best help you with your studies. Also, learn by recognizing your weaknesses and try to compensate/work to improve them.

Getting Organized

It's simple, yet it's fundamental. It seems, the more organized you are, the easier things come. Take the time before your course begins to look around and analyze your life and your study habits. Get organized now and you'll find you have a little more time—and a lot less stress.

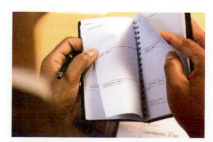

- **Find a calendar system that works for you.** The best kind is one that you can take with you everywhere. To be truly organized, you should integrate all aspects of your life into this one calendar—school, work, leisure. Some people also find it helpful to have an additional monthly calendar posted by their desk for "at a glance" dates and to have a visual of what's to come. If you do this, be sure you are consistently synchronizing both calendars so as not to miss anything. *More tips for organizing your calendar can be found in the time management discussion.*

- By the same token, **keep everything for your course or courses in one place**—and at your fingertips. A three-ring binder works well because it allows you to add or organize handouts and notes from class in any order you prefer. Incorporating your own custom tabs helps you flip to exactly what you need at a moments notice.

- **Find your space.** Find a place that helps you be organized and focused. If it's your desk in your dorm room or in your home, keep it clean. Clutter adds confusion and stress and wastes time. Or perhaps your "space" is at the library. If that's the case, keep a backpack or bag that's fully stocked with what you might need—your text, binder or notes, pens, highlighters, Post-its, phone numbers of study partners (a good place to keep phone numbers is in your "one place for everything calendar").

A helpful hint—add extra "padding" into your deadlines for yourself. If you have a report due on Friday, set a goal for yourself to have it done on Wednesday. Then, take time on Thursday to look over your project again, with a fresh eye. Make any corrections or enhancements and have it ready to turn in on Friday.

Managing Your Time

Managing your time is the single most important thing you can do to help yourself. And it's probably one of the most difficult tasks to master.

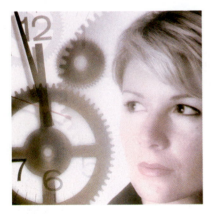

You are in college taking this course because you want to succeed in life. You are preparing for a career. In college, you are expected to work much harder and to learn much more than you ever have before. To be successful, you need to invest in your education with a commitment of time.

We all lead busy lives. But we all make choices as to how we spend our time. Choose wisely and make the most of every minute you have by implementing these tips:

- **Know yourself and when you'll be able to study most efficiently.** When are you most productive? Are you a late nighter? Or an early bird? Plan to study when you are most alert and can have uninterrupted segments. This could include a quick, five-minute review before class or a one-hour problem-solving study session with a friend.

- **Create a set study time for yourself daily.** Having a set schedule for yourself helps you commit to studying and helps you plan instead of cram. Find—and use—a planner that is small enough that you can take it with you—everywhere. This can be a $2.50 paper calendar or a more expensive electronic version. They all work on the same premise—**organize *all* of your activities in one place.**

- Less is more. **Schedule study time using shorter, focused blocks with small breaks.** Doing this offers two benefits:
  1. You will be less fatigued and gain more from your effort.
  2. Studying will seem less overwhelming and you will be less likely to procrastinate.
- **Plan time for leisure, friends, exercise, and sleep.** Studying should be your main focus, but you need to balance your time—and your life.
- Make sure you **log your projects and homework deadlines** in your personal calendar.
- **"Plot" your assignments on your calendar or task list.** If you have a large report, for instance, break down the assignment into smaller targets. Set a goal for a first draft, second draft, and final copy.
- Try to **complete tasks ahead of schedule.** This will give you a chance to review your work carefully before you hand it in (instead of at 1 A.M., when you are half awake). You'll feel less stressed in the end.
- **Prioritize!** In your calendar or planner, highlight or number key projects; do them first, and then cross them off when you've completed them. Give yourself a pat on the back for getting them done!
- **Review your calendar and reprioritize** *daily*.
- Try to **resist distractions by setting and sticking to a designated study time** (remember your commitment and perseverance!). Distractions include friends and surfing the Internet.
- **Multitask when possible.** You may find a lot of extra time you didn't think you had. Review material or organize your term paper in your head while walking to class or doing laundry.

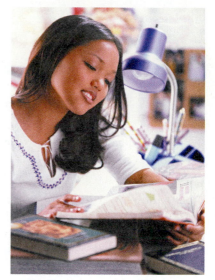

Side note: Plan to study and plan for leisure. Being well balanced will help you focus when it is time to study.

Tip: Try combining social time with studying or social time with mealtime or exercise. Being a good student doesn't mean you have to be a hermit. It does mean you need to know how to budget your time smartly.

- **Learn to manage or avoid time wasters.**

  <u>Don't</u>

  - **Let friends manage your time.**
    Tip: Kindly ask, "Can we talk later?" when you are trying to study; this will keep you in control of your time without alienating your friends.

  - **Get sucked into the Internet.**
    It's easy to lose hours in front of the computer surfing the web. Set a time limit for yourself and stick to it.

  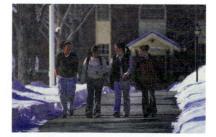

  <u>Do</u>

  - **Use small bits of time to your advantage.**
    Example: Arrive to class five minutes early and review notes. Review your personal calendar for upcoming due dates and events while eating meals or waiting for appointments.

  - **Balance your life.**
    Sleep, study, and leisure are all important. Keep each in balance.

Getting the Most Out of Lectures

Believe it or not, instructors want you to succeed. They put a lot of effort into helping you learn and preparing their lectures. Attending class is one of the simplest, most valuable things you can do to help yourself. But it doesn't end there—getting the most out of your lectures means being organized. Here's how:

Prepare Before You Go to Class

You'll be amazed at how much more comprehensible the material will be when you preview the chapter before you go to class. Don't feel overwhelmed by this already. One tip that may help you is to plan to arrive to class 5–15 minutes before the lecture. Take your text with you and skim the chapter before lecture begins. At the very least, this will give you an overview of what may be discussed.

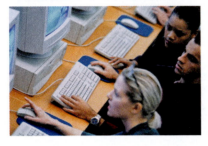

Be a Good Listener

Most people think they are good listeners, but few really are. Are you? Following are obvious but important points to remember:

- You can't listen if you're talking.
- You aren't listening if you're daydreaming.
- Listening and comprehending are two different things. If you don't understand something your instructor is saying, ask a question or jot a note and visit the instructor after hours. Don't feel dumb or intimidated; you probably aren't the only person who "doesn't get it."

Take Good Notes

- Use a standard-size notebook or, better yet, a three-ring binder with loose-leaf notepaper. The binder will allow you to organize and integrate your notes and handouts, integrate easy-to-reference tabs, and so on.
- Use a standard black or blue ink pen to take your initial notes. You can annotate later using a pencil, which can be erased if need be.
- Start a new page with each lecture or note-taking session (yes—you can and should also take notes from your textbook).
- Label each page with the date and a heading for each day.
- Focus on main points and try to use an outline format to take notes to capture key ideas and organize subpoints.
- Review and edit your notes shortly after class—at least within 24 hours—to make sure they make sense and that you've recorded core thoughts. You may also want to compare your notes with a study partner's later to make sure neither of you has missed anything.

Get a Study Partner

Having a study partner has so many benefits. First, he or she can help you keep your commitment to this class. By having set study dates, you can combine study and social time, and maybe even make it fun! In addition, you now have two sets of eyes and ears and two minds to help digest the information from the lecture and the text. Talk through concepts, compare notes, and quiz each other.

An obvious note: Don't take advantage of your study partner by skipping class or skipping study dates. You obviously won't have a study partner—or a friend—very long if it's not a mutually beneficial arrangement!

Helpful hint: Take your text to lecture, and keep it open to the topics being discussed. You can take brief notes in your textbook margin or reference textbook pages in your notebook to help you study later.

How to Study for an Exam

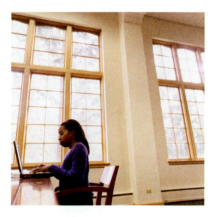

- Study, don't simply reread material.
- Be an active learner.
- Finish reading all material—text, notes, handouts—at least three days prior to the exam.
- Be an active participant in class; ask questions.
- Apply what you've learned; think through scenarios rather than memorize your notes.
- Three days prior to the exam, set aside time each day to do self-testing, to practice problems, and to review notes.
- Create an "I don't know this yet" list. Focus on strengthening these areas and narrow your list as your study.
- Create your own study tools, such as index card flash cards and checklists, and practice writing short essays if this is how your instructor tests.

Very important: Be sure to sleep and eat well before the exam.

Getting the Most Out of Your Textbook

McGraw-Hill and the author of this book have invested their time, research, and talents to help you succeed, as well. The goal is to make learning—for you—easier.

Here's how:

- Use the chapter objectives to guide you through the material presented.
- Review the key terms and definitions, and make certain you understand them.
- Read and jot down the important notes.
- Use the memory tips.
- Practice critical thinking skills.
- Practice coding using the sample cases and examples.
- Read chapter summaries.
- Complete chapter reviews.
- Explore the online learning center activities.

Insurance Overview

1

OBJECTIVES

- Define the role of health insurance and managed care plans in the delivery of health care services.
- Identify and define the types of health insurance plans.
- Identify the type of insurance plan responsible for payment of patient charges.
- Describe the methods of payment to a health care facility.

A health insurance policy is a contractual agreement between an insurance carrier (company) and an individual with regard to health care issues. However, this contract is about risk. Insurance is just like gambling in Las Vegas. Basically, the insurance company is betting that a certain event will *not* happen to you, such as your getting sick. If that happens, it would have to pay your medical bills. On the other side of the table, you are betting (by paying an **insurance premium**) that you *will* have a major illness or health catastrophe. Think about it—if you knew for a fact that you would never get ill or have any injury, and would only have to go to the doctor for your annual checkups, would you pay all that money every month for insurance premiums? Of course not. You are betting that you will, at some point, get all that money back, when you need it to pay for some type of treatment.

KEY TERMS

automobile insurance

capitation plans

Centers for Medicare & Medicaid Services (CMS)

dependents

disability compensation

discounted FFS

episodic care

fee-for-service (FFS) plans

gatekeeper

health care

health maintenance organization (HMO)

insurance premium

liability insurance

managed care

point-of-service (POS)

preferred provider organization (PPO)

third-party payer

TriCare/CHAMPUS/CHAMPVA

usual, customary, and reasonable (UCR)

workers' compensation

Key Terms

Insurance premium: The amount of money, often paid monthly, by a policyholder or insured, to an insurance company to obtain coverage.

Managed care: A type of health insurance coverage that controls the care of each subscriber (or insured person) by using a primary care provider as a central health care supervisor.

Health care: The total management of an individual's well-being by a health care professional.

When **managed care** was developed, the health insurance industry realized that it could lower its risk (and save money) if it could keep people healthy by encouraging them to go to the doctor for regular checkups, tests, and so forth. This thinking created a major change in the health insurance industry and in the medical care industry.

Medical care is the identification and treatment of illnesses and injuries—in other words, whatever a health care provider does to help you with a health problem or concern that you have (Figure 1-1).

Preventive care is the ability of the medical industry to identify and take care of the possibility or early stages of illness or injury in order to prevent the problem from getting worse. Preventive care includes well-baby visits (Figure 1-2), screenings, diagnostics, and routine checkups.

The term **health care** refers to a combination of these two types of services.

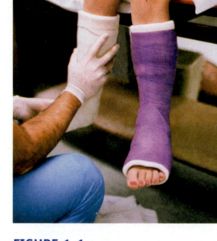

FIGURE 1-1
Treatment of a broken leg is an example of medical care.

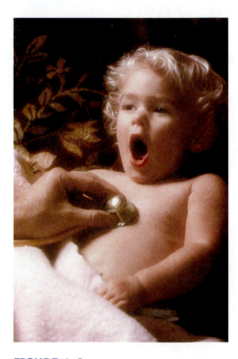

FIGURE 1-2
Well-baby visits are an example of preventive care.

Examples

The physician examines you and gives you a shot of antibiotics to help you get rid of an infection. The doctor has identified your illness and is treating your illness. This is medical care.

The physician knows you work at a day care center and gives you a flu shot to help you avoid getting the flu. The doctor is preventing your illness. This is preventive care.

Memory Tip

MEDICAL CARE
+ PREVENTIVE CARE
= HEALTH CARE

THE PARTICIPANTS

Essentially, there are three participants in each health care encounter, or visit:

1. The physician or health care provider
2. The patient—the person seeking services
3. The insurance carrier covering the costs of health care activities for the patient

Some people get their health insurance policies through a program at their place of employment, some through the government, and others directly with the insurance carriers as individual policyholders. It doesn't matter very much to the health care facility where you work. In any case, a **third-party payer** will pay, in part, the patient's bills for services that your facility will provide. Health insurance carriers are often referred to as third-party payers. This means that someone not directly involved in the health care relationship is paying for the service. The health care provider is party #1, the patient is party #2, and the insurance carrier is party #3—the third party. Therefore, the insurance company is the third-party payer.

Key Term

Third-party payer: An individual or organization that is not directly involved in an encounter but has a connection because of its obligation to pay, in full or part, for that encounter.

Memory Tip

Party #1: The health care provider
Party #2: The patient
Party #3: The insurance carrier

KEY TYPES OF INSURANCE PLANS

There are many types of health plans that people may purchase, or contract for, with companies that specialize in these matters.

Health Maintenance Organization (HMO)

In a **health maintenance organization** (HMO), members, also called enrollees, prepay for health care services. The members are encouraged to get preventive treatment to promote wellness (and keep medical costs down). In addition, each member has a primary care physician (PCP), also known as a **gatekeeper**. The PCP is responsible for monitoring the individual's well-being and making all decisions regarding care. It is the PCP who determines if a specialist is required for a certain evaluation or procedure. When this occurs, it is the PCP who is responsible for completing the patient referral form and getting approval from the HMO for the patient to visit the specialist. Generally, HMOs do not require a patient to satisfy a deductible before benefits begin. (See the section "Individual Insurance Contributions" later in this chapter.)

Key Terms

Health maintenance organization (HMO): A type of health insurance that uses a primary care physician, also known as a gatekeeper, to manage all health care services for an individual.

Gatekeeper: A physician, typically a family practitioner or an internist, who serves as the primary care physician for an individual. This physician is responsible for evaluating and determining the course of treatment or services, as well as for deciding whether or not a specialist should be involved in care.

Memory Tip

HMOs use a "home base" concept, with a primary care physician (PCP), also known as the gatekeeper, serving as the central base to supervise each individual's health care.

Preferred Provider Organization (PPO)

In a **preferred provider organization (PPO)**, physicians, hospitals, and other health care providers join together and agree to offer services to members of a group (often called subscribers) at a lower cost or discount. These plans usually permit the individual subscriber (the patient) to choose the physician or specialist to see, with a discount for staying in the network by using a physician who is a member of the plan. If the individual chooses a physician who does not belong to the network, or is not participating with that PPO, the individual will pay a penalty or receive less of a discount in the cost of those services. This can give the individual more control over his or her health care. It can save time and money, as well.

Some PPO plans require the patient to satisfy a deductible first before benefits begin. (See the section "Individual Insurance Contributions" later in this chapter.) Typically, a higher deductible will translate into a lower monthly premium for this type of insurance coverage.

Example

If a person covered under a PPO plan, is having problems sneezing and knows the problem is his or her allergies, the individual can choose an allergist—a provider who specializes in the treatment of allergies—from the PPO network without having to go to his or her primary care physician for a referral. If the plan were an HMO, the person would have to make an appointment with the PCP first, in order to get the referral to the allergist. Then the person could make an appointment to see the allergist.

Point-of-Service (POS) Plan

Giving individuals a little more flexibility, a **point-of-service (POS)** plan is almost a combination of an HMO and a PPO. Each insured person has a primary care physician (PCP) and a list of providers that participate in the HMO. When health care providers within the HMO network are used, the insured pays only a regular co-payment amount or a small charge. There is no deductible or co-insurance payment involved. However, this plan may also include a self-referral option, in which the individual insured can choose to go to an out-of-network provider. In that case, the individual may be responsible for paying both a deductible and a co-insurance payment.

Centers for Medicare & Medicaid Services (CMS)

In 1977, the Health Care Financing Administration (HCFA, pronounced hic-fah) was created to coordinate federal health services programs. On July 1, 2001, HCFA became the **Centers for Medicare & Medicaid Services (CMS)**. Many health care professionals still refer to this agency as "HicFah" and to the CMS-1500 claim form as the "HicFah 1500." Old habits take a while to change. At least you now understand that these two acronyms refer to the same federal organization.

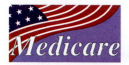

Medicare is a national health insurance program that pays, or reimburses, for health care services provided to those over the age of 65. In addition, this plan may cover individuals who are under the age of 65 and are permanently disabled (such as the blind), as well as those with end-stage renal disease (ESRD) who are suffering from permanent kidney failure and require either dialysis or a kidney transplant.

Medicaid is a plan that pays, or reimburses, for medical assistance and health care services for people who are indigent (low-income). Medicaid is funded by the federal government in cooperation with, and administered by, each state government. This means that each state determines who is eligible and what services are covered. It is important to know that each state has its own requirements, in case you have a patient that has just moved to your state. Each state may even have a unique name or term for its program. For example, in California the program is called Medi-Cal.

TriCare/CHAMPUS/CHAMPVA

TriCare (formerly CHAMPUS) and CHAMPVA are the most common health care policies you will encounter when caring for individuals in the military and their families.

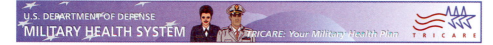

TriCare was created to help the following individuals receive better access to improved health care services:

- The **dependents** of those who are on active duty in the military
- CHAMPUS-eligible retirees and their dependents
- The dependents of active military who are now deceased

The <u>C</u>ivilian <u>H</u>ealth <u>A</u>nd <u>M</u>edical <u>P</u>rogram of the <u>U</u>niformed <u>S</u>ervices (**CHAMPUS**) was created to provide health care benefits for the dependents of those serving in the uniformed services and retirees. TriCare replaced CHAMPUS in 1998; however, many people who have been covered by this plan for a long time may still call it CHAMPUS. *Uniformed services* include the U.S. military (the Army, Navy, Air Force, Marines, and Coast Guard), as well as those serving in the Public Health Service, the National Oceanic and Atmospheric Administration (NOAA), and the North Atlantic Treaty Organization (NATO).

The <u>C</u>ivilian <u>H</u>ealth <u>A</u>nd <u>M</u>edical <u>P</u>rogram of the Department of <u>V</u>eterans <u>A</u>ffairs (**CHAMPVA**) was created to provide health care benefits for the dependents of veterans with total and permanent disabilities and the dependents of those who have died from service-connected conditions, as well as the survivors of veterans who have died in the line of duty.

Key Terms

Workers' compensation: An insurance program that covers medical care for those injured or for those who become ill as a consequence of their employment.

Disability compensation: A plan that reimburses a covered individual a portion of his or her income that is lost as a result of being unable to work due to illness or injury.

Other Insurance Plans

Workers' compensation is an insurance program designed to pay the medical costs for treating those injured or made ill at their place of work or by their job. This includes injuries resulting from a fall off a ladder while performing a job-related task, getting hurt in an accident while driving a company car on a business trip, or developing a lung disorder caused by toxic fumes in the office. Generally, a workers' compensation plan covers only specific medical bills, such as laboratory bills, physicians' fees, and other medical services. Lost income is not covered by this policy. Generally, each state oversees the workers' compensation contracts with particular insurance carriers.

Disability compensation is an insurance plan that reimburses disabled individuals for a percentage of what they used to earn each month. This plan does not pay physicians' bills or for therapy treatments. A disability plan only provides the insured with money to replace a portion of their lost paycheck because they are unable to work. Disability payments might come through a federal government agency such as the Social Security Administration, or patients may have a private insurance plan (such as AFLAC).

CASE STUDY

Joe Hines works as an electrician for a small company. One day, he falls off a ladder at work and injures his back severely. He is taken to the emergency room by ambulance, and the attending physician orders X-rays and a CT scan. The tests confirm that Joe's spine is broken in two places and a cast is applied around Joe's entire torso. After a week in the hospital, Joe is discharged. The physician's discharge orders state that Joe is to stay in bed for seven months, in traction, while the fracture heals. A home health agency is contracted to provide a trained health care professional to go to Joe's house to care for him and attend to his needs around the clock.

In this scenario, what type of insurance will be responsible for the payment of each of Joe's expenses due to this accident?

_____

_____

Joe Hines will have two companies helping him through this very difficult time:

- Workers' compensation will pay for the physician, the X-rays, the cast, the traction equipment, and the home health nurse to care for him.
- Disability compensation will give Joe a percentage of his lost paycheck each month, so he will have the money to pay other bills, such as electricity, telephone, and rent, while he is recuperating.

Liability insurance is commonly part of a person's homeowners, or businessowners, insurance. This type of policy covers losses to a third party caused by the insured or something owned by the insured. In other words, the insurance company will pay for, or reimburse for, any harm or damage done to someone else (not a member of the household or the business).

CASE STUDY

Sarah goes over to Margaret's house for dinner. After a delicious meal, Sarah walks toward the door to leave and go home. As she turns to say goodnight to Margaret, Sarah trips and falls. Margaret calls the paramedics, and, at the hospital, the X-rays ordered by the attending physician confirm that Sarah has indeed broken her wrist. A cast is applied, and Sarah is sent home with a prescription for pain medication. The attending physician advises Sarah to see her primary care physician in one week for a follow-up.

Who will cover Sarah's medical expenses?

_____

_____

In this case, most often, it would be Margaret's liability insurance (included in her homeowners' insurance policy) that would pay for Sarah's damage (or medical expenses), not Sarah's health insurance policy. Margaret is the insured—it is her liability insurance policy on her house. Sarah is the third party—she does not live in the house; she is an outsider. If Margaret fell in her own house, she would *not* be a third party, and her injuries (medical expenses) would have to be covered by her health insurance plan, not the liability insurance.

CASE STUDY

A student slips down the stairs at school. Typically, the school's liability policy would cover the damage, or medical expenses. The school is the insured, and the student is the third party.

If a faculty member and a student are walking through the cafeteria of the school and both slip and fall, what types of policies will cover any injuries that might be caused by the fall?

_____

_____

The faculty member, being an employee of the school, will be covered by workers' compensation insurance, and the student, being a third party, will be covered by the school's liability insurance.

Key Term

Automobile insurance: Auto accident liability coverage will pay for medical bills, lost wages, and compensation for pain and suffering for any person injured by the insured in an auto accident.

Automobile insurance might become an issue for your office if you treat someone for an injury that was caused by the individual's involvement in an automobile accident. Full-coverage automobile policies usually include liability insurance that cover these expenses.

IMPORTANT NOTE

As you can see from this review, different types of insurance policies might be responsible for an individual's medical treatment. Therefore, in your job as medical insurance coder/biller, you must make certain that if an individual comes to the provider for treatment for an *injury* (rather than an *illness*), you must find out the *cause* of the injury. This will help determine which carrier will cover the charges.

METHODS OF PAYMENT TO YOUR OFFICE

There are several payment plans that insurance carriers (third-party payers) use to pay physicians and other health care providers for their services.

Fee-For-Service (FFS) Plans

Key Terms

Fee-for-service (FFS) plans: Payment agreements that outline, in a written fee schedule, exactly how much money the insurance carrier will pay the physician for each treatment and/or service provided.

Discounted FFS: An extra reduction in the rate charged to an insurer for services provided by the physician to the plan's members.

In **fee-for-service (FFS) plans**, the insurance company pays the health care provider for each individual service supplied to the patient, according to an agreed upon price list (also known as a fee schedule). When the physician's office agrees to participate in the plan, it is also agreeing to provide services and accept the amount of money indicated on that schedule for each of those services. This is like going to a restaurant with an à la carte menu. The menu lists a price for each item: the salad, the roast beef, the apple pie. The restaurant accepts the amount of money the guest pays for each item received. Different plans may pay different amounts of money for one particular service, just as different restaurants may charge different amounts for a similar dish.

Sometimes, when one insurance carrier pays a provider at a lower rate than other carriers, it is referred to as a **discounted FFS**. In a typical discounted FFS, the payments are reduced from the physician's regular rate. This is similar to the discount you might get at a store when showing your student ID card; you get a discount because you are a member of the school.

Example

Three people, each with a different insurance carrier, go to the same physician for a flu shot (injection). Insurance carrier #1 has agreed to pay the physician $20 for giving the injection. Insurance carrier #2 has agreed to pay the physician $22.50, and insurance carrier #3 has agreed to pay the physician $18 for the same injection. Your office should charge all patients the same amount. However, insurance carriers working with your office on a fee-for-service contract will pay only the amount stated on their fee schedule. That's all they will pay and no more. This is called the Allowed Amount.

Capitation Plans

With **capitation plans**, the insurance company pays the physician a fixed amount of money for every individual covered by that plan (often called members or subscribers) being seen by that physician. Physicians get this amount of money every month, as long as they are listed as the physician of record for that individual. Whether the insured person goes to see that physician once, three times, or not at all during a particular month, the physician's office will be paid the same amount. This plan is like the dinner special at your local restaurant. You pay one price, which includes soup, salad, all-you-can-eat entrée, and dessert. If you don't eat your soup, you do not pay any less; if you get seconds on the entrée, you do not pay any more.

Episodic Care

An **episodic care** agreement between insurer and physician means the provider is paid one flat fee for the expected course of treatment for a particular injury or illness. This is like the meal deal of health care. One package price includes all of the services and treatments necessary for the proper care of the patient's condition.

CASE STUDY

Ava Callahan fell off her bicycle and broke her arm. The X-ray shows that it is a simple, clean fracture and the physician applies a cast. The doctor schedules a follow-up appointment for her and expects that she will not need much other attention until the cast comes off in six weeks. At that time, an X-ray will confirm that the fracture has healed properly and the cast will be removed. This entire sequence of events, and treatment, is very predictable for a routine simple fracture. Therefore, the insurance company has agreed to pay the physician one flat fee for this event, rather than having the physician's office file a claim for each procedure and service individually: the first encounter; the first X-ray; the application of the cast; the follow-up encounter; the last encounter; the last X-ray; and removal of the cast.

What type of payment plan is in effect?

_____

_____

Ava Callahan's physician is being reimbursed under an episodic care agreement with the insurance carrier.

Diagnosis-Related Groups (DRG) are a type of episodic care payment plan used by Medicare to pay for treatments and services provided to hospital inpatients. DRGs are categorized by the principle (first-listed) diagnosis code, and take into consideration elements such as the patient's age, gender, and the presence of any complications or manifestations (additional diagnoses or conditions).

Individual Insurance Contributions

Patients with insurance policies often contribute to reimbursing providers for their health care services, in addition to paying monthly premiums. The following are the most common methods used for the individual's payments:

1. *Co-payment (also known as the co-pay).* The co-payment is usually a fixed amount of money that the individual will pay each time he or she goes to a health care provider. It may be $10, $15, $20, or more. Each policy is different. As a matter of fact, the co-pay on the same policy for the same patient may be different, depending on whether this is a visit to a family physician, a specialist, or the hospital.

2. *Co-insurance.* Co-insurance is different from the co-payment because it is based on a percentage of the total charge rather than a fixed amount. The percentage that the patient pays is most often calculated on the **usual, customary, and reasonable (UCR)** charge that has been determined for this type of visit or procedure. Frequently, the individual is required to pay 20% of the total amount charged by the physician or facility, but that might differ for various types of policies and carriers.

3. *Deductible.* This is the amount of money that patients must pay, out of their own pockets, before the insurance benefits begin. The deductible might be as little as $250 or as much as $1,000 or more. Patients have to pay the total amount until they have paid the whole deductible for that calendar year. After that, they will usually pay just the co-insurance amount.

Key Term

Usual, customary, and reasonable (UCR): The process of determining a fee for a service by evaluating: the <u>usual</u> fee charged by the provider; the <u>customary</u> fee charged by most physicians in the same community or geographical area; and what is considered <u>reasonable</u> by most health care professionals under the specific circumstances of the situation.

IMPORTANT NOTE

The various amounts for the co-pay, the co-insurance, and the deductible are good examples of why it is so essential that you call the insurance carrier for every patient to verify the patient's coverage, eligibility for certain procedures and treatments and to see if the deductible has been met for the year.

CHAPTER SUMMARY

A fundamental part of an insurance coding and medical billing specialist's job is to work with the insurance companies that will reimburse your health care facility for the services and procedures you provide to your patients. You need to: understand how your office will be paid (such as fee-for-service, capitation, or episodic care); be able to distinguish among the types of policies (such as HMOs, PPOs, and managed care policies, as well as Medicare, Medicaid, and TriCare plans); and quickly identify which is responsible for sending payment to you. This will help your billing efforts be more efficient and get paid more quickly.

Chapter Review

For the following multiple-choice questions, choose the best available answer.

1. Medical care is defined as

    a. Identification and treatment of illness and/or injury

    b. Services to prevent illness such as a routine check-up or wellness visit

    c. Laboratory services

    d. Only those services performed by a medical doctor

2. An organization that depends on the services of a gatekeeper is

    a. A preferred provider organization

    b. Medicare

    c. A health maintenance organization

    d. A not-for-profit hospital

3. A capitation plan pays the provider

    a. Per specific service

    b. Per member every month

    c. For treatments in a hospital only

    d. One flat fee per illness or condition

4. Medicare is a government plan that covers primarily

    a. Military personnel

    b. Poor and needy

    c. Those over the age of 65

    d. Government employees

5. Income lost as a result of a person's medical condition that makes him or her unable to work is covered by

    a. Liability insurance

    b. Health insurance

    c. Disability insurance

    d. Workers' compensation

6. CHAMPUS provides health care benefits for the dependents of

    a. State workers

    b. Those serving in the uniformed services

    c. Athletes

    d. Health care workers

7. Managed care plans promote the use of

    a. Experimental drugs

    b. Herbs and natural teas

    c. Acupuncture

    (d.) Preventive care

8. When the insured must pay a specific amount each time they see a health care provider, it is called a

    a. Deductible

    (b.) Co-payment

    c. Co-insurance

    d. Premium

9. When an individual pays a percentage of the total charge, it is called the

    a. Deductible

    b. Co-payment

    (c.) Co-insurance

    d. Premium

10. CMS stands for

    a. Centers for Medical Services

    b. Corporation of Medical Systems

    (c.) Centers for Medicare & Medicaid Services

    d. Cycle of Medical Selections

Match the situation with the type of insurance that would cover the expenses. Answers may be used more than once.

A. Health insurance   B. Workers' compensation   C. Medicaid

D. Disability insurance   E. Liability insurance   F. TriCare/CHAMPUS

G. Automobile insurance   H. Medicare

1. Mrs. Matthews, a teacher at Medical Coder Academy, slipped in her office, fell, and hurt her back. _____

2. Ralph broke his leg and must be in traction for nine months. What plan will help him pay his rent and electric bill? _____

3. Mary Lou was at the mall, shopping for a birthday present, when she slipped on a wet floor and broke her hip. _____

4. Keith was walking down the stairs in his house, fell over his son's toy, and twisted his ankle. _____

5. Marlene was driving to work when another car hit her from behind. The EMTs took her to the hospital with a sprained ankle and sore neck. _____

6. Harvey caught a cold when he went fishing last weekend. _____

7. Jared enrolled in the insurance coding program at the local college. While leaving after his first class, another student bumped into him, he banged his head on a shelf, and he got a scalp laceration. _____

8. At home after his 85th birthday party, Jack tripped on the rug, fell, and broke his hip. _____

9. Suzette's husband is in the Marines. She is pregnant with their first child. _____

10. James is out of work and has no prospects. He is broke and has a really bad sore throat. _____

Match the word or phrase to its best definition.

1. Co-payment ___C___

2. Fee-for-service ___D___

3. PPO ___B___

4. Medicaid ___E___

5. Auto insurance policy ___A___

A. May cover medical expenses caused by a car accident

B. Preferred provider organization

C. A fixed amount paid each visit by the individual

D. Payment, per service provided, from the insurance company

E. A government program for indigent and needy people

HIPAA's Privacy Rule Overview

2

OBJECTIVES

- Define the legal responsibilities of a health information specialist with regard to the regulations specified in the Health Insurance Portability and Accountability Act (HIPAA).
- Understand the importance of respecting patients' right to privacy.
- Apply and maintain good health care communications while protecting patients' privacy.
- Work within the law in the patients' best interests.
- Know the penalties for breaking the law.

It is understood that you are studying to work in a health care facility, not a law office. However, you have the responsibility for understanding and abiding by certain laws that directly apply to working in a health care office. The Health Insurance Portability and Accountability Act, more commonly known as **HIPAA** (pronounced hip-aah), is one such law. This law, enacted by the federal government, applies directly to you.

Like most federal laws, HIPAA covers many issues and concerns and creates rules about a lot of things, mostly relating to health care. The privacy rule is one part of the HIPAA law, and it is the section that you really have to know about and understand.

KEY TERMS

covered entities

disclosure

health care clearinghouses

health care provider

health plans

HIPAA

HIPAA's Privacy Rule

incidental use and disclosure

individually identifiable health information (IIHI)

limited data set

minimum necessary

privacy notice

protected health information (PHI)

treatment, payment, and/or operations

use

workforce

Key Terms

HIPAA (pronounced hip-aah): Health Insurance Portability and Accountability Act created to improve continuity of health insurance coverage and the administration of health care services.

HIPAA's Privacy Rule: Protects patients' information so it is available to those who need to see it, while protecting that information from those who should not.

HIPAA's Privacy Rule was written to protect an individual's privacy with regard to his or her personal health information, without letting that right to privacy get in the way of the flow of information that is necessary to provide appropriate care for that patient. Essentially, the lawmakers tried to make certain that *a patient's information is easily accessible to those who should have access to it* (such as the physician, insurance coder and biller, and radiologist) *yet is secured against unauthorized people* (such as potential employers, co-workers, and neighborhood gossips), so that they do not see things they have no business seeing.

WHO IS RESPONSIBLE FOR OBEYING THIS LAW

Although it was passed into law in 1996, HIPAA went into effect April 14, 2003. It concerns every physician's office, clinic, hospital, and health insurance carrier—every type of business that is directly involved in the delivery and/or payment of health care services—no matter how big. The largest of corporations owning hundreds of hospitals around the country and every office with one physician working alone are all included. HIPAA calls these businesses **covered entities**, and they all must comply with the terms of the law.

Covered entities are divided into three categories:

Key Terms

Covered entities: Organizations that access the personal health information of patients. They include health care providers, health plans, and health care clearinghouses.

Health care provider: Any professional who provides health care services.

Health plans: Companies whose main business focus is providing and/or paying for health care services.

- Health care providers
- Health plans
- Health care clearinghouses

You probably already know the definition of a **health care provider.** It is any person or organization that provides, and/or receives payment for health care services as the primary purpose of their business.

Example

Examples of health care providers as defined by HIPAA include physicians, dentists, hospitals, clinics, pharmacies, and laboratories.

Health plans are organizations that provide and/or pay for health care services as their primary business purpose. This, of course, includes health insurance carriers, HMOs, employee welfare benefit plans, government health plans (such as TriCare, Medicare, and Medicaid), and group health plans provided through employers and associations—all the types of plans and carriers that we reviewed in Chapter 1. It doesn't matter whether the plan is offered to an individual or a group; all companies offering this coverage are included.

Example

Examples of health care plans as defined by HIPAA include Medicare, Medicaid, TriCare, Blue Cross/Blue Shield, and Prudential.

In addition, technology has created another type of organization involved in this process. They are called **health care clearinghouses**. These companies help process electronic health insurance claim forms. Medical billing services, medical review services, and health information management system companies are included in this definition. We will learn more about clearinghouses later in this book, when we go over the creation and filing of electronic health claims.

Example

Examples of health care clearinghouses as defined by HIPAA include National Clearinghouse, NDC Electronic Claims, and WebMD Network Services.

The **workforce** of a covered entity is also included under HIPAA. A covered entity's workforce consists of every person who is involved with the company. Full-time staff, part-time staff, volunteer, intern, extern, physician, nurse, assistant—this has nothing to do with whether you are paid for work or not—you must comply with the terms of this law.

Example

Examples of a covered entity's workforce as defined by HIPAA include full-time staff members, part-time staff members, volunteers, interns, externs, and janitorial staff members.

Key Terms

Health care clearinghouses: Companies that process health claim forms, convert them into proper data format, and submit them to the correct insurance carrier.

Workforce: As defined in the HIPAA law, includes everyone involved with a covered entity, whether or not they are full-time, and whether or not they get paid.

WHAT THIS LAW COVERS

You are certainly familiar with the topic of doctor-patient confidentiality. It means that anything a patient tells his or her doctor must be kept private. The doctor is not allowed, under most circumstances, to reveal to anyone what was said. This includes family members, parents (in many cases), and friends. It is important that people feel comfortable being open and honest and tell their physician things that are very, very personal, possibly even embarrassing—private things that may have never been told to anyone else. In order for the physician to treat an individual properly, the physician must know everything.

IMPORTANT NOTE

HIPAA's Privacy Rule is mostly about protecting your patient's privacy.

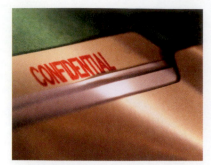

FIGURE 2-1

Confidentiality is an essential part of the health care relationship. It is also the law.

Key Terms

Individually identifiable health information (IIHI): Health care data that can be connected to a specific person.

Protected health information (PHI): Any identifiable patient health information, regardless of the form in which it is stored (for example, paper or computer file).

In order for you to do your job properly, you have access to confidential information (Figure 2-1). You need to know very personal and private things about every one of your patients in order to do your job. You know what is wrong with them (their diagnoses) now and in the past; you know why they came to see this health care provider and why they saw others before they came to your facility; and you know what the health care provider thinks (observations and impressions) about this patient, as well as what has been done, is being done, and will be done to treat this patient. You know these things because you have access to patients' health care records, including the physician's notes. HIPAA calls this personal health care information—past, present, and future conditions—**individually identifiable health information (IIHI)**. In other words, it is information that anyone could look at and know exactly which individual is being treated. Specific pieces of data, called **protected health information (PHI)**, is health information related to an individual that must be kept confidential. PHI is a grouping of facts that might cause someone to say, "Oh, my gosh, I know him! Oh, and he has that!"

CASE STUDY

A file is sitting on Mary Beth's desk, lying open. Mary Beth is not around; she had to go back to the storage room to find some supplies. The pieces of paper inside the file contain information about a specific patient, including records, charts, lab reports, and physician's notes that reveal many things about this person.

From the color of the folder, even from a distance, it is obvious that this is a patient of Dr. Monroe. The top piece of paper indicates that his patient has been diagnosed with a sexually transmitted disease. At this point, it is difficult to tell whose chart this is, because Dr. Monroe has hundreds of patients.

Right above the diagnosis, you can see that this patient is a male. Although this will eliminate some of Dr. Monroe's patients, there are still too many to know for certain.

On closer examination of the paperwork in the folder, you find out that the male patient with the sexually transmitted disease lives on Main Street in Our Town, Florida. The list of Dr. Monroe's patients that this file could be referring to is now getting very short.

It slips out that Dr. Monroe's male patient, of Main Street, Our Town, Florida, who has a sexually transmitted disease, was born on June 13, 1985. Doesn't John Smith live on Main Street in Our Town? Isn't his birthday June 13? It must be John who has that terrible disease!

Did Mary Beth fulfill her responsibility to protect John Smith's privacy? What could she have done differently to assure that this patient's PHI was protected?

John Smith's private health record is no longer private. His diagnosis of a sexually transmitted disease is health information. Once you added his gender, address, and birth date, it connected this diagnosis directly to one person. All of these details, and any other pieces of information, are protected and must be private under the law. This information is confidential and it is against the law for you to reveal any of it, with only a few exceptions:

1. You can tell other health care professionals who are directly involved in the course of doing your job.
2. You can tell anyone when you are given written permission from the patient to do so.
3. As outlined in the section "Permitted Uses and Disclosures" (Page 22) you can tell certain authorities.

The Use and Disclosure of PHI

HIPAA's Privacy Rule is very specific as to how you can handle the protected health information that you work with every day. The guidelines offer two terms to describe how you might deal with this data.

The term **use** (with regard to HIPAA) means that the information is being shared between people who work together in the same office or facility (Figure 2-2) and they need to exchange this PHI in order to better serve the patient.

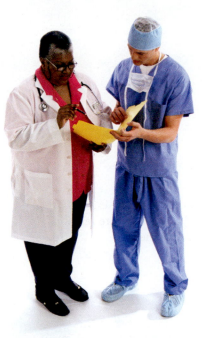

FIGURE 2-2
People who work together in the same facility use PHI to provide better patient care.

Example

You are getting ready to code the diagnosis for a patient and need additional information. You speak with the attending physician to discuss this patient's PHI so you can make certain you find the best, most appropriate diagnosis code. You are *using* that patient's PHI, because the information is being shared between you and the physician in the same office for the benefit of the patient.

HIPAA defines the term **disclosure** to mean that PHI is being revealed to someone outside of the health care office or facility. For example, you prepare a health insurance claim form to send to the patient's insurance company, so that it will pay your office for the procedures provided. On that claim form, you must put the patient's full name and address, birth date, diagnosis codes, and procedure codes. As you learned earlier in this chapter, each piece of data is not necessarily confidential. When you put all this information together in one place, it becomes PHI, because this health information (diagnosis code) is now connected to a specific person (identified by the name, address, and birth date) on one piece of paper. However, you must disclose this information to the insurance carrier in order to get paid. You are *disclosing* the information, because the insurance company personnel who will read this claim form do not work in your health care facility; they constitute an outside company.

Key Terms

Use: As defined by HIPAA, the sharing of information between people working in the same health care facility for the purpose of caring for a patient.

Disclosure: As defined by HIPAA, the sharing of information between health care professionals working in separate entities, or facilities, in the course of caring for a patient.

> **Example**
>
> Dr. Monroe indicates that his patient, John Smith, needs some lab work. Dr. Monroe will use Mr. Smith's PHI in his orders to indicate which tests should be performed. Then, you need to call the laboratory and *disclose* Mr. Smith's PHI—his name and diagnosis—along with what specific tests should be performed by the lab.

Remember that everyone in your office, along with everyone at the insurance carrier and the lab, are all members of a covered entity's workforce. You are all bound by the same terms of the HIPAA law and cannot reveal any patient's PHI, except under particular circumstances (such as use and disclosure), unless you have the patient's written permission.

Getting Written Approval

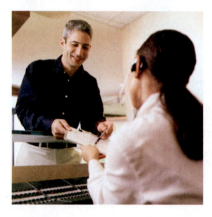

FIGURE 2-3

You must obtain a patient's written permission to release PHI.

In all situations, other than those mentioned in this chapter (such as use and disclosure, and other permitted circumstances that we will review later in this chapter), the health care provider must get a patient's written permission to disclose his or her PHI (Figure 2-3). Although there are many preprinted forms that your office or facility may purchase, HIPAA's Privacy Rule insists that all of these documents (Figure 2-4) contain specific information.

Releases must:

1. Be written in plain language (not legalese), so that the average person can understand what he or she is signing.
2. Be very specific as to exactly what information will be disclosed or used.
3. Specifically identify the person or organization who will be disclosing the information.
4. Specifically identify the person(s) who will be receiving the information.
5. Have a definite expiration date.
6. Clearly explain that the person signing this release may retract this authorization in writing at any time.

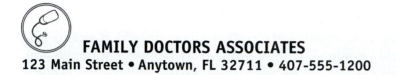

FAMILY DOCTORS ASSOCIATES
123 Main Street • Anytown, FL 32711 • 407-555-1200

AUTHORIZATION FOR RELEASE OF CONFIDENTIAL HEALTH INFORMATION

REGARDING:

_____

| PATIENT'S NAME | DATE OF BIRTH | SOCIAL SECURITY # | TELEPHONE NUMBER |

I AUTHORIZE _____

ADDRESS _____

CITY, STATE, ZIP _____

TO DISCLOSE _____
(EXACTLY WHAT INFORMATION HAS YOUR PERMISSION TO BE DISCLOSED)

_____

TO RECEIVING PARTY _____

ADDRESS _____

CITY, STATE, ZIP _____

NOTE TO RECEIVING PARTY: THIS INFORMATION IS DISCLOSED TO YOU FROM RECORDS WHOSE CONFIDENTIALITY IS PROTECTED BY LAW. ANY REDISCLOSURE IS STRICTLY PROHIBITED WITHOUT THE WRITTEN PERMISSION OF THE PATIENT/CLIENT/LEGAL REPRESENTATIVE IDENTIFIED BELOW.

THIS AUTHORIZATION FOR RELEASE OF CONFIDENTIAL HEALTH INFORMATION EXPIRES ON _____ AND MAY BE REVOKED AT ANY TIME WITH WRITTEN NOTIFICATION OF REVOCATION TO THE NAMED PARTY ABOVE.

_____   _____   _____

PATIENT/LEGAL REPRESENTATIVE'S SIGNATURE   RELATIONSHIP TO PATIENT   DATE

_____   _____   _____

WITNESS SIGNATURE   TITLE   DATE

FIGURE 2-4
Example of an authorization to release health information form.

Permitted Uses and Disclosures

HIPAA's Privacy Rule outlines six circumstances in which health care professionals are permitted, with or without written patient permission, to use their *best professional judgment* as to whether or not they should use and/or disclose a patient's PHI:

1. *To the individual.* Health care professionals can use their best professional judgment to decide whether or not a patient should be told certain things contained in their health care record. Questions may come up, especially when mental health issues and terminal conditions (when a patient is almost certain to die in the near future), are concerned and there is doubt if the patient can deal with the medical facts. In almost all cases, providing patients with their own PHI is allowed.

2. *Treatment, payment, and/or operations.* Health care professionals are free to use and/or disclose PHI when it comes to making decisions and coordinating and managing the *treatment* of a patient's condition. In addition, PHI can be disclosed for *payment* activities, such as billing and claims processing. *Operations* refers to the health care facilities management of case coordination and quality evaluations.

Key Term

Treatment, payment, and/or operations: As defined by HIPAA, three situations that permit covered entities to use or disclose PHI, when their best professional judgment deems it necessary.

Example

A physician needs to be able to discuss PHI details with a therapist, so that they can establish a proper course of treatment for the patient.

3. *Opportunity to agree or object.* This relates to a more informal situation, in which the patient is present, alert, and able to give or deny verbal permission with regard to a specific disclosure. Although it is much easier to simply ask someone and take his or her verbal approval than to get a piece of paper and make the patient sign first, it is in your best interest to get written approval whenever possible. People's memories may fail or they may change their minds later about what they told you. If there is nothing on paper, you cannot prove what was said. For your own protection, get it in writing whenever possible.

Example

The patient is about to hear the doctor explain his test results. The patient's wife is in the waiting room. The physician may ask the patient if it is okay to invite the wife in and permit her to hear this information. The patient then may say, "Yes, that is fine," or "No, I don't want her to know about this." The physician then must abide by what the patient requests.

4. *Incidental use and disclosure.* As long as reasonable safeguards are in place, this portion of the rule addresses the fact that information might accidentally be used or disclosed during the regular course of business (Figure 2-5). For example, imagine that a physician comes out of an examining room and approaches a nurse standing at the desk. This is a back area and patients are not generally in this hallway, so the physician speaks to the nurse in a normal tone of voice to instruct her on preparing the patient for a procedure. Suddenly, another patient comes around the corner, lost on her way back to the waiting room, and overhears the conversation. This is called incidental use and is understandable within a working environment; therefore, it is not considered a violation of the law. However, it is important to keep conversations such as this to include only the **minimum necessary** PHI to accomplish the goal. In other words, give the other person only the information they need to do what is necessary—no more than that. In the hallway outside the exam room, the physician would only need to say, "Marilyn, please prepare Mrs. Smith for her examination." She would not need to include other details about Mrs. Smith, such as "Marilyn, please prepare Mrs. Smith for her examination. You know she has a terrible rash on her thighs. I suspect that it's poison ivy. However, it could be a sexually transmitted disease. We'll have to find out how many sexual partners she has had in the past six months." Not only is it unnecessary, it is unprofessional.

5. *Public interest.* There are times when, in the public's best interest, you should disclose what you know about a patient. Very often, this is mandated by state laws, which then take priority over the federal HIPAA law. In other words, if the federal law says you are allowed to tell, and your state's law says you must tell, then you must. These situations include the reporting of suspected abuse (child abuse, elder abuse, or domestic violence) and the reporting of sexually transmitted and other contagious diseases. You are part of the health care team and must think about the community. The community must be warned if someone is walking around with a contagious (communicable) disease. Most states also require notification to the police when the patient has been shot or stabbed. It is your responsibility to find out what the laws are in your state and how to file a report correctly.

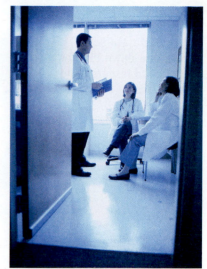

FIGURE 2-5
What's wrong with this picture? Take precautions to not accidently disclose PHI.

Key Terms

Incidental use and disclosure: The accidental release of PHI during the course of proper patient care.

Minimum necessary: Reveal only the smallest amount of information required to accomplish the task and no more.

Memory Tip

Incidental is close to the word *accidental*—someone accidentally overhears what you say.

IMPORTANT NOTE

Remember that when there is a state or federal mandate to report it means you have no choice; you must report to the proper authorities. This applies not only to the physician at your practice but also to you. If the physician does not report the suspected child abuse of one of your patients, it is your obligation to do so.

Key Term

Limited data set: Stripped-down PHI for approved research and statistics.

6. *Limited data set.* For research, public health statistics, or other health care operations, PHI can be revealed, but only after it has been depersonalized. In other words, if the data that connect this information to an individual is removed or blacked out, the information is no longer individually identifiable health information, so it no longer needs protection. The following is a portion of a record that can be shared without fear of violating anyone's privacy: *"_____ is 25 years old. Back in December, _____ was in a motor vehicle accident on the job. _____ is complaining about some neck pain. _____ has tingling into the right hand."* This is a quote from the medical record of a patient after the specified direct identifiers have been removed. This health information cannot be connected to any particular person; therefore, it is no longer protected, and it can be used for research and in other ways that may help the community (like this textbook, for example).

Example

You can release a health record that has no name, address, telephone number, e-mail address, Social Security number, or photographs attached to it. Even certain physicians' notes can be released after they have been stripped of personal data.

Privacy Notices

HIPAA instructs all of its covered entities to create policies and procedures with regard to the use and disclosure of PHI, including restrictions on access to PHI. In addition, the law states that once the covered entities' policies and procedures are developed, they must be put into practice and copies of the written policy must be given to every patient, along with posting a copy of the written **privacy notice** in a general area where it can be seen by all patients.

Privacy notices written in compliance with HIPAA's Privacy Rule must contain the following points:

Key Term

Privacy notice: A covered entity's written policies and procedures for protecting its patients' PHI.

1. A full description of how the covered entity may use and/or disclose each patient's PHI
2. A statement about the covered entity's responsibility to protect each patient's privacy
3. Complete information about the patients' rights, including contact information for the Department of Health and Human Services, should a patient wish to lodge a complaint that his or her privacy has been violated
4. An employee of the covered entity named as privacy officer; this person's name and contact information must be included in the written notice to handle patients' questions and complaints
5. Written acknowledgment from every patient stating that he or she received the written privacy notice must be obtained and placed in the patient's health record; this is usually one of the papers that one has to sign when going to a health care facility for the first time

One of the most important aspects of this portion of the Privacy Rule is that the law specifically says that the covered entity not only has to create these policies and procedures but also has to do what it says it will do in these policies. If it doesn't, that is considered a violation of federal law and punishable by monetary fines and/or imprisonment. Although some health care staff members feel that HIPAA and its Privacy Rule is a big pain in the neck, think about what this law actually means—respecting patients' privacy and dignity.

> **IMPORTANT NOTE**
>
> HIPAA assures every person coming to your health care facility that his or her personal, private information will be protected and treated with respect.

Don't you expect your health care professionals to keep what you tell them private when you go for help? It is not enough for the doctor alone to be bound to protect the patient's information as confidential, because the doctor is no longer the only person who has access. Your health care facility is no place for gossip or telling tales. You might find someone's hemorrhoids funny or someone else's rash gross. As a professional, you should not be concerned with entertaining your friends with your patients' private circumstances. How would you feel if it was your personal problem that your health care team members were giggling about with their friends? Or you might consider telling your brother that his girlfriend came in with a sexually transmitted disease. You must not. Everyone is entitled to privacy. As difficult as it may be, you must remain a professional.

> **IMPORTANT NOTE**
>
> The use of language in a health care facility is also a privacy consideration. Using medical terminology is not enough to disguise details about an individual—especially with medical dictionaries available on the Internet. In addition, languages other than English should not be used for any other reason than interpreting, in a private location, for a non-English speaking patient. Any other conversations in other languages may be considered a breach of confidentiality.

Violating HIPAA's Privacy Rule

Any individual who discovers that his or her privacy has been misused or disclosed without permission can file a complaint with the Department of Health and Human Services (DHHS) that his or her health care provider, his or her health plan, or a clearinghouse has not followed HIPAA's regulations. When writing this law, Congress included specifications for both civil and criminal penalties to be applied against any covered entity that fails to protect its patients' PHI. These penalties include fines that may be imposed for civil wrongdoings, as well as up to $250,000 and up to 10 years in prison for criminal breach.

A covered entity is responsible for any violations of HIPAA requirements by any of its employees, any of its business associates or any other members of its workforce, such as interns and volunteers. Generally, it is the senior officials of the covered entity who may be punished for the lack of compliance, however, middle managers and staff members are not exempt.

Civil Penalty

The civil penalty is $100 for each single violation of a HIPAA regulation, with a maximum of $25,000 for multiple violations of the same portion of the regulation during the same calendar year. Let's say you tell your best friend that Joe Smith, whom you both went to school with, came into your physician's office and tested positive for a sexually transmitted disease. You, of course, swear her to secrecy. Later that day, she bumps into Joe's fiancée and feels obligated to tell her about Joe's condition. Joe puts two and two together, after his fiancée breaks up with him, and he files a complaint that you disclosed his PHI without permission. You and/or your physician may be fined $100.

Criminal Penalties

The following are criminal penalties:

1. Up to $50,000 *and* up to one year in jail for the unauthorized or inappropriate disclosure of individually identifiable health information. After you are fined the $100 civil penalty for the inappropriate disclosure of Joe Smith's PHI, you and/or your physician may also be charged with criminal penalties for the same disclosure and have to pay up to $50,000; you can also be sentenced to up to one year in jail.

2. Up to $100,000 *and* up to five years in prison for the unauthorized or inappropriate disclosure of individually identifiable health information using deception. For example, you have a friend who has just gotten a great new job as a pharmaceutical representative. To help him, you give him a list of all your patients who have been diagnosed with diabetes, so he can advertise his company's new drug to them. You and he both know this is illegal, so you tell him that you got permission from each of the patients to release the information (and that is a lie). After a patient complains to the DHHS, the investigation turns up your relationship with your friend. You and your physician can both be fined up to $100,000 per occurrence (that's for each person on the list), as well as up to five years in prison.

3. Up to $250,000 *and* up to 10 years in prison for the unauthorized or inappropriate disclosure of individually identifiable health information using deception with intent to sell or use for business-related benefit, personal gain, or malicious purposes. Let's say a famous television star is a patient at the physician's office down the hall from yours. You get a call from a tabloid newspaper offering you a lot of money for any information on this celebrity's health, so you call the pathology lab and tell them you are filling in at the other physician's office and need test results for Mr. TV. Then you call the tabloid reporter and tell him what you found out. You used deception (you lied about working in the other physician's office) to get PHI, which you then sold for personal financial gain. You and possibly your physician can be fined for up to a quarter of a million dollars and be sentenced to up to 10 years in prison.

CHAPTER SUMMARY

The Health Insurance Portability and Accountability Act, commonly called HIPAA, is not a curse to the health care industry. It is a law that combines common sense with the reminder that health care professionals should always respect their patients and their patients' privacy, and treat them with dignity. We all expect this of anyone who has chosen an occupation that involves caring for others. However, some people do not take this obligation to care for others seriously, or they use the weak and sick for their own profit. This law is to protect us all from those who are not worthy of the title of health care professional.

Chapter Review

For the following multiple-choice questions, choose the best available answer.

1. According to HIPAA, covered entities include all of the following EXCEPT
    a. Health care providers
    b. Health plans
    c. Health care computer software manufacturers
    d. Health care clearinghouses

2. The HIPAA Privacy Rule is all about
    a. The training of medical assistants
    b. The use and disclosure of protected health information
    c. The security of health records
    d. Insurance billing and coding issues

3. An example of protected health information (PHI) is
    a. A patient's Social Security number
    b. A patient's next of kin
    c. A patient's next appointment date
    d. A patient's state of residence

4. HIPAA states that all covered entities must comply with the Privacy Rule as of
    a. October 16, 2003
    b. April 14, 2003
    c. September 15, 2003
    d. March 1, 2004

5. A patient calls your office and asks for the results of her recent blood tests. You
    a. Get her file and answer her questions honestly
    b. Tell her to hold on, so that she can speak with the doctor
    c. Explain that you cannot confirm the caller's identity, so you cannot give out that information
    d. Tell her she is breaking the law and hang up

6. Most state laws mandate that, when a health care professional suspects abuse of any kind, he or she must
    a. Call the appropriate authorities
    b. Talk to the patient about his or her suspicions
    c. Wait until he or she is absolutely certain
    d. Get a signed release, then call the police

7. All covered entities must create and implement written

   a. PHI information flow charts

   b. Customer service rules

   c. Privacy notices

   d. Coding guidelines

8. Protected health information (PHI) is

   a. Any health information that can be connected to a specific individual

   b. A listing of diagnosis codes

   c. Current procedural terminology

   d. A covered entity employee file

9. The term *use* when used in HIPAA's Privacy Rule refers to the exchange of information between health care personnel

   a. And health care personnel in other health care facilities

   b. And family members

   c. Within the same office

   d. And a pharmacist

10. The term *disclosure* when used in HIPAA's Privacy Rule refers to the exchange of information between health care personnel

    a. And health care personnel in other covered entities

    b. And family members

    c. Within the same office

    d. And the patient

11. HIPAA is a _____ law.

    a. Local

    b. County

    c. State

    d. Federal

12. Which of the following is NOT a covered entity under HIPAA?

    a. County hospital

    b. Blue Cross/Blue Shield

    c. Physician associates medical practice

    d. NDCMediSoft technical support

13. A woman enters a hospital emergency room. The attending physician suspects that her husband has been physically abusing her. The Privacy Rule says the physician is permitted, but not mandated, to disclose this information to the police. The state says the physician must report this to the police or lose his license. The physician should

   a. Call his attorney

   b. Get the patient to sign a release form before telling anyone

   c. Inform the police immediately

   d. Say nothing

14. A new pharmacy opens two blocks away from the office where you work. The manager of the store calls your medical practice and offers to pay for a copy of the names and addresses of your patients who are regularly prescribed medication. What should you do?

   a. Determine how much to charge the pharmacy for the list

   b. Explain that this would be against the law under HIPAA's Privacy Rule

   c. Provide the list for free to be a good neighbor

   d. Get the money for the list up front

15. A covered entity's workforce, with regard to who is included in the HIPAA rules and regulations, includes

   a. Only paid, full-time employees

   b. Only licensed personnel working in the office

   c. Volunteers, trainees, and employees, part-time and full-time

   d. Business associates' employees

16. There can be _____ penalties for any violation of HIPAA's rules.

   a. Civil

   b. Criminal

   c. Both civil and criminal

   d. No

17. Those who are permitted to file an official complaint with the DHHS are

   a. Health care providers

   b. Any individual

   c. Health plans

   d. Clearinghouses

18. Penalties for breaking any portion of HIPAA apply to

   a. Patients only

   b. Patients' families only

   c. All covered entities

   d. Health care office managers only

19. If you wrongly disclose PHI under false pretenses, you can be fined

    a. $100 for each occurrence

    b. Up to $50,000 and get up to one year in jail

    c. $10,000 and get up to two years in prison

    d. Up to $100,000 and get up to five years in prison

20. DHHS stands for

    a. Department of Home and Health Services

    b. Division of Health and Health Care Sciences

    c. Department of Health and Human Services

    d. District of Health and HIPAA Systems

Indicate if each of the following statements is true or false.

1. HIPAA's Privacy Rule's intent is to protect an individual's privacy while not interfering with the flow of information necessary to properly care for the patient's health.

    a. True

    b. False

2. Taking authorization for the release of protected health information over the phone from an individual is accepted, as long as you recognize the patient's voice.

    a. True

    b. False

3. Ensuring that patients' privacy is protected is only the responsibility of the doctor or health care provider who runs or owns the office or facility.

    a. True

    b. False

4. HIPAA's Privacy Rule has been carefully crafted to make medical records easier to see for those who should see them and much harder to see for those who shouldn't.

    a. True

    b. False

5. Protected health information includes the past, present, and future physical and mental health or condition of an individual.

    a. True

    b. False

3

Source Documents

KEY TERMS

accept assignment

birthday rule

eligibility confirmation

encounter form

group name or number

ID number (policy number)

patient

physician's (medical) notes

policyholder (insured)

primary insurance policy

referring physician/provider

responsible party (guarantor)

superbill

verification

OBJECTIVES

- Identify the types of documents involved in the patient care process.

- Define the terms used to describe patient condition and care.

- Understand the importance of each piece of data.

- Locate data on the correct documents.

You are probably already familiar with some of the documents used in health care facilities. For example, you must fill out a patient registration form the first time you see a provider, and, of course, you have to hand over your insurance card to be checked and copied when arriving for every appointment. Now you are on the other side of the desk, and you need these and other documents to find important information required to complete the health insurance claim form. Let's go over each source document, one at a time.

PATIENT REGISTRATION FORM

Let's look carefully at an example of a patient registration form (Figure 3-1). All health care providers have some variation of this form. They may look slightly different, but they contain about the same information. While at first glance you might worry, this form does not contain PHI, because

1. There is no personal health information on this form.
2. Typically, this form will only specify the **responsible party** (also known as the guarantor) and the **policyholder** (also known as the insured).

The top section of this form tells you about the responsible party. This is the person who is accepting financial responsibility for the charges from your office, and may be the **patient** but does not have to be.

Examples

Marlene lives in Georgia and her parents live in Iowa. Marlene goes to the hospital with a broken arm. She has health insurance, but her father, Harvey, has said he would pay anything the insurance company does not. Harvey will never be a patient of this physician because he lives in Iowa. However, he is guaranteeing payment for his daughter's treatment. Marlene is the patient and Harvey is the guarantor.

Joseph twists his knee playing basketball. As a vice president of the local telephone company, he has health insurance. He will pay anything not covered by his policy. Joseph is both the patient and the guarantor.

Also in the top section of this form, you will usually see information such as the Social Security number of the responsible party/guarantor. This, along with the address, phone number, work information, date of birth, and gender, is used to identify this person. If the responsible party/guarantor is also the policyholder (also known as the insured), there are certain boxes on the health insurance claim form that will require more information. In addition, this information would be important, should this account need to be sent to a collection agency.

The next section of the patient registration form provides space for the *dependents* of the responsible party and/or policyholder (see Chapter 1). This might include a spouse (husband or wife), a child, or a stepchild. It might include a significant other or a life/domestic partner (same-gender partner). You are not being nosey; you must know what the legal relationship is among all the people on the form. The insurance company needs to understand its responsibility with regard to paying for their health care charges. Generally, the person filling out the form lists dependent(s), because it is expected that, today or in the future, the dependent(s) will become a patient of this facility.

Key Terms

Responsible party (guarantor): The person who says he or she will pay any money due to the health care provider that is not paid by the insurance company.

Patient: The person seeking health care treatment or service.

Policyholder (insured): The person who gets the insurance policy, either directly or through work.

Memory Tip

A guarantor *guarantees* that the bill will be paid.

Memory Tip

The insured gets the *Insurance* policy.

PATIENT REGISTRATION FORM

RESPONSIBLE PARTY			DATE	
LAST NAME	FIRST NAME	MI	SOCIAL SECURITY #	DATE OF BIRTH
ADDRESS	CITY	STATE	ZIP CODE / SEX	MARITAL STATUS
HOME PHONE	WORK PHONE		REFERRED BY:	

EMPLOYER INFORMATION		WORK STATUS: FULL-TIME PART-TIME STUDENT	RETIRED
COMPANY NAME	ADDRESS	CITY, STATE, ZIP	DATE RETIR.

DEPENDENT INFORMATION

DEPENDENT'S NAME		DEPENDENT'S NAME		DEPENDENT'S NAME	
RELATIONSHIP	DATE OF BIRTH	RELATIONSHIP	DATE OF BIRTH	RELATIONSHIP	DATE OF BIRTH
SOC. SEC. #	SEX	SOC. SEC. #	SEX	SOC. SEC. #	SEX
EMPLOYER	WORK PHONE	EMPLOYER	WORK PHONE	EMPLOYER	WORK PHONE

INSURANCE INFORMATION—PRIMARY POLICY

COMPANY NAME	ADDRESS	CITY, STATE, ZIP
PHONE NUMBER	ID OR POLICY NUMBER	GROUP NUMBER OR NAME
INSURED'S NAME (IF DIFFERENT)	SOCIAL SECURITY #	RELATIONSHIP TO RESP. PARTY
INSURED'S ADDRESS (IF DIFFERENT)	INSURED'S CITY, STATE, ZIP	INSURED'S PHONE NUMBER

INSURANCE INFORMATION—SECONDARY POLICY

COMPANY NAME	ADDRESS	CITY, STATE, ZIP
PHONE NUMBER	ID OR POLICY NUMBER	GROUP NUMBER OR NAME
INSURED'S NAME (IF DIFFERENT)	SOCIAL SECURITY #	RELATIONSHIP TO RESP. PARTY
INSURED'S ADDRESS (IF DIFFERENT)	INSURED'S CITY, STATE, ZIP	INSURED'S PHONE NUMBER

OTHER INFORMATION

ALLERGIES	REASON FOR TODAY'S VISIT
PATIENT'S SIGNATURE	DATE

FOR OFFICE USE ONLY

CO-PAY $ _____   CO-INSURANCE $ _____   DEDUCTIBLE $ _____

CHECK ☐ # _____   CASH ☐   CHARGE ☐   PAID IN FULL ☐

ASSIGNED PROVIDER _____

FIGURE 3-1

Example of a patient registration form.

In the middle section of the form in Figure 3-1, you will find information regarding the patient's insurance coverage: first the **primary insurance policy**, then the secondary insurance policy. The terms *primary* and *secondary* refer to which company will be billed first (primary) and then second (secondary). What the primary insurance company does not cover and pay for will be billed to the secondary insurance policy. The order in which you bill these companies is very important. Most patients do not understand the impact of the billing sequence and may complete the two portions of this part of the form incorrectly. Therefore, you will have to confirm which policy should be billed first. If you send the bill to the wrong insurance company, it will delay payment to your office. You will find that many people have only one insurance policy, so the primary/secondary issue will not apply.

Determining the primary and secondary insurance policies is a different process for adults than it is for children.

Let's begin learning how to identify the correct order for adults with two policies. The insurance policy that names the patient as a policyholder, not as a dependent, is the primary policy for that person.

Key Term

Primary insurance policy: The contract that names the patient as the policyholder, or insured party.

Example

Alice has health insurance coverage from All County Insurance. Alice's husband, George, has her covered as a dependent on his Masters Insurance policy. In this situation, Alice's primary policy is All County Insurance—because this policy has her name on it. Her secondary policy is Masters Insurance—because this policy has her named as George's dependent. George has one policy, his primary, Masters Insurance.

CASE STUDY

Harold and Jane Mahoney have been married for 10 years. Harold has health insurance coverage with Blue Cross Blue Shield Insurance Companies. This is a group policy provided as a benefit of his employment at Category Printing. The company pays the insurance premiums in full for employees as well as their spouses, so Harold added Jane as a dependent on his policy. Jane's employer, Hillstone Computers LLC, also offers health insurance coverage for staff members, so Jane is insured through the company's group plan with Prudential Insurance. As the company also pays for spouses' coverage in full, at no cost to the employee, Jane has added Harold as a dependent to her policy.

Dr. Smothers has recommended that Jane have surgery.

When you call to verify Jane's eligibility with the insurance company that will pay for the upcoming procedures, in what order would you call for verification? When Harold becomes a patient with your health care facility, which plan is his primary insurance policy and which is his secondary plan?

_____

_____

The answer is that Jane's primary insurance policy is with Prudential. This is the policy on which she is the insured. Any fees that are not paid by Prudential would then be billed to Blue Cross Blue Shield, Jane's secondary insurance policy. This is her secondary insurance because Harold added her to his policy as a dependent. Harold's primary insurance policy is with Blue Cross Blue Shield and his secondary policy is Jane's with Prudential.

Now, let's look at children. The rules are different for determining the primary and secondary insurance policies for children. The first rule is:

> When both parents share custody, and both parents have insurance policies that identify the child as a dependent, then the parent whose birthday (month and day, *not* year) is closer to January 1 holds the primary policy.

Key Term

Birthday rule: Rule used to establish the primary insurance policy for a child by determining which parent has a birthday closer to January 1.

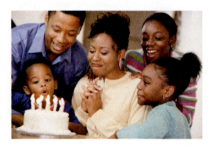

This is called the **birthday rule**. Therefore, you will need to know the parents' birthdates in order to make the decision.

Example

Bobby Smith comes to the office because he has a sore throat. His father has him listed as a dependent on his policy with Franklin Insurance. His mother has Bobby listed on her insurance policy with Nationwide, as well. Bobby's father's birthday is April 5, and his mother's birthday is January 7. Bobby's primary insurance policy is Nationwide, because his mother's birthday is closest to January 1.

Do not expect that the patient, or the patient's parents, know the rule. If the birthdates for both parents are not on the patient registration form, you will have to ask. It is important.

Whenever there is a rule, there is always an exception to the rule, and the birthday rule is no different. Exceptions to the birthday rule apply if the parents are divorced or legally separated. In this case, *the parent with custody of the child* will usually provide the primary insurance policy unless there is a court order stating something different. No matter what the rule, if the court has ordered one parent to provide health insurance for the minor child, then it doesn't matter who has custody. The court can overrule the birthday rule as well.

IMPORTANT NOTE

The following are exceptions to the birthday rule: 1. When the parents are divorced or legally separated, and both parents have insurance policies that identify the child as a dependent, then the parent who has custody of the child holds the primary policy. 2. When the court has ordered the noncustodial parent to provide health insurance, that policy is primary.

CASE STUDY

Stephanie and Phillip are married and have a five-year-old daughter, Maria. Phillip owns a plumbing company, which he started just three years ago. He is making pretty good money but has no employees. Stephanie works at a restaurant as an assistant manager. She gets health insurance through work and has Phillip and Maria covered as dependents on her policy. Phillip makes enough money from his business and has stated that he will pay all the bills. Maria must go to the doctor to get her shots so she can go to kindergarten.

Who is the patient? Who is the policyholder/insured? Who is the guarantor?

Maria   Stephanie   Phillip

The patient is Maria, because she is the one being treated by the health care provider. The policyholder/insured is Stephanie, because it is her insurance policy that will pay for Maria's shots. The guarantor is Phillip, because he is the one who has agreed to pay any charges that the insurance company does not pay.

Example

Latoya is single and a manager for Wal-Mart. Wal-Mart pays for her medical insurance. She goes to the doctor for her annual checkup. Can you identify the patient? The policyholder/insured? The guarantor? Latoya is all three: the patient, because she is the one being treated by the health care provider; the policyholder/insured, because it is her policy through her job; and the guarantor, because she will pay for any charges not paid by the insurance company.

CASE STUDY

Carolyn is divorced and has custody of her nine-year-old son, Jason. Carolyn, as a full-time employee of a local department store, gets insurance through her job and has Jason listed as a dependent on that policy. Carolyn's ex-husband, Robert, also has Jason listed as a dependent on his insurance policy. Carolyn has custody, so Carolyn's policy is Jason's primary insurance policy. Robert takes Jason to the physician because he has a sore throat and writes his insurance policy down as the primary insurance policy because he thinks it doesn't matter. He leaves the secondary insurance part blank because he doesn't have his ex-wife's policy information with him.

Is this correct? How would you know?

No   you would have to ask the father, if the mother had insurance, custody etc...

Even when working in a busy health care office, you must take the time to talk with your patients. When dealing with a child, it is important to ask questions of the adult bringing the child to the office. One question should be "Is this child covered by any other insurance policies?" This is a very polite way to get information on what might be a very sensitive subject (the divorce and the custody). In this case, Robert would answer yes, Jason is covered by another policy. Then you would ask for that information. If he does not have it, ask for the mother's phone number and offer to call her to get the information. Remember, if the parent gets annoyed ("What's the difference? He's covered by my insurance!"), you must be considerate, because they just do not know the rules. Try to be as sensitive as you can while getting the information you need to do your job correctly.

IMPORTANT NOTE

In the insurance section of the patient registration form, make certain to look on the line that says "Insured's Name (If Different from Responsible Party)." This is the line that will tell you if the policyholder/insured is different from the guarantor.

Key Terms

ID number (policy number): The number (or sometimes a combination of letters and numbers) that connects an individual to a specific insurance policy.

Group name or number: A number (or combination of letters and numbers) that connects one individual policy with a specific group of insureds.

In this same insurance section (Insurance Information—Primary Policy) of the standard patient registration form (see Figure 3-1), you will also find the ID number and the Group Name/Number for the policy. **ID number, policy number,** *contract number, subscriber number,* or *member number*—they are all the same thing. This is the number that identifies the individual's policy with the insurance company. Very often, this number is the policyholder's Social Security number, but not always. Never assume! Always check the patient registration form *and* the patient insurance ID card to make certain you get all the numbers correctly.

Many policies have a **group name or number,** even if it is an individual policy (that is, not one through a job). So be certain to look for it on both the patient registration form *and* on the *ID card* to make certain you have the correct number. (You may have difficulty reading the patient's handwriting on the form, so always double-check the number on the ID card. One wrong digit and your claim will be rejected!) Not all policies include a group number, so if there isn't one don't worry. But, if there is one, it must be included on the claim form.

The last part of the patient registration form contains a variety of information. The "Reason for Today's Visit" field indicates the individual's *chief complaint.* In other words, why did the person come to the provider's office today?

Also, there should be a place for the individual to write down any known allergies. Of course, this is critical information, because the physician needs to know—allergies can be deadly!

You will also find, if applicable, the name of a **referring physician,** also known as the **referring provider.** The name of the referring physician is very important information for several reasons. First, if the referral is required by the insurance policy (for example, from a primary care physician to a specialist under the terms of a typical HMO policy), you must make certain you have the referral form, signed by the referring physician, along with an authorization code and other information. Second, you must make certain that a note is made, so that your office sends a follow-up report to the referring physician.

Also included in the last part of the form is the place for the patient's signature and date. It is very important that the patient sign there and date the form. This signature covers the authorization for the health care provider to **accept assignment** of the benefits. What this means is that the insurance company will send the money directly to the physician's office, not to the policyholder. You must have the original patient's signature on file (and the policyholder's signature, if a different person). This signature usually also signifies that the patient is authorizing the health care provider to treat him or her (although sometimes the patient must sign a separate consent to treat form). You might think that the fact that the person came to the office to be treated would be enough; however, you must keep your paperwork in order. If, for some reason, the patient refuses to sign the patient registration form, be certain to tell your office manager or head (charge) nurse before the patient is treated by anyone in the office.

Box 3-1 lists some terms that you will need to be familiar with regarding the data that you will find on the patient registration form.

Key Terms

Referring physician (referring provider): The health care professional who recommended this individual see this specialist or another health care provider.

Accept assignment: The policyholder gives permission to the insurer to pay the benefits directly to the provider. When Medicare is the insurer, this also means that the provider agrees to accept the allowed amount from Medicare as payment in full.

BOX 3-1   Terms Common to Patient Registration Forms

Accept assignment—the term used to indicate that the insurance carrier is to pay the health care provider directly

Birthday rule—the rule used to determine the primary insurance policy for a minor child covered by policies from both parents

Dependent—an individual who is covered under someone else's insurance policy; very often this is a spouse or child, but not always

Group number or name—a number or name assigned to a specific group of insured people—most often, those working for the same company, used to identify the individual as a member of that group

Guarantor—the same as the responsible party

ID number—a number that identifies a particular insurance policy as belonging to a particular individual

Insured person—the same as the policyholder

Policyholder—the person who gets the insurance policy directly or through their employer

Policy number—the same as the ID number

Primary insurance policy—the insurance policy that gets billed for services first

Referring provider—a health care provider who recommends that a patient see another health care provider for more specific treatment

Responsible party—the person who guarantees payment of any charges not paid for by the insurance company

Secondary insurance policy—the insurance policy that will consider paying any charges not paid by the primary insurance policy for a particular health care event

INSURANCE CARD

Next, let's review an example of an insurance card (Figure 3-2). Every time someone goes to the doctor, they are asked for their insurance card. Now, you'll find out why. Remember, the only time a patient completes a patient registration form is when he or she is at a particular provider's office for the first time. Typically, the assistant who checks this new patient in for any appointments after the first one will simply ask this person if any information, such as address, phone number, or insurance coverage has changed. However, it is a good habit to always take a photocopy of the insurance card at each visit.

> **IMPORTANT NOTE**
>
> A health care facility's patient list is protected information under HIPAA, especially when the facility is one that specializes in a particular type of medicine, such as oncology or allergy (where mere attendance might imply a diagnosis). Therefore, please be careful when asking patients for personal information in a public location, such as the check-in desk in the waiting area, where others might easily overhear.

Each time you ask for a patient's insurance ID card, take it and copy both sides. The following is the information you will need to get from that card:

Key Terms

Verification: Calling the insurance carrier to confirm the patient has an active policy.

Eligibility: Confirming that the health issue to be addressed at this visit or the specific procedure will be covered by the patient's plan.

1. *Customer service phone number.* This phone number, usually a toll-free number, will tell you whom to call in order to verify coverage and confirm eligibility, known as **verification** and **eligibility confirmation.** You must do this every time the individual comes to the office for treatment. He or she may have lost coverage last week, or have today's health concern excluded as a preexisting condition. You wouldn't know that he or she does not have coverage for this visit unless you call. You also cannot accomplish this by simply asking the patient. Sometimes he or she does not realize that the insurance was lost when he or she quit a job; sometimes the person will try to fool you into thinking he or she has insurance because the person does not want to pay out-of-pocket. A call to the insurance company needs to be made *prior* to any services being given to the patient—*every* time.

2. *ID number or policy number.* You need to match the numbers and letters of the ID number or policy number to what the individual has written on the patient registration form. Sometimes it is difficult to read people's handwriting (a 5 and a 2 can look alike when written in a hurry, and so can a 4 and a 9). In addition, it can be easy to transpose numbers, such as writing 19 when you mean to write 91. This number may also be called different things. For example, on our sample card (see Figure 3-2), you will note that this number is called the contract number. No matter what it is called, it is still important, and it functions the same.

McGraw Insurance Companies	BlueMed
Tawney Johnson	
Contract No. XJW651-552973	
GROUP NO.	BM PLAN
9999PP3	909
Customer Service No. 800-555-6757	
Send claims to: PO Box 55, Cityville, FL 32901	

FRONT OF CARD

Type Contract	GROUP	
Type Coverage	GROUP	
	PPO	NON-PPO
Co-insurance	80%	60%
Deductible	----$2,000------	
Hospital per Adm Deductible	$0	$500
Family Physician Office Svs	$15co-pay	60%
All Other Physician Svs	80%	60%

Admission Certification Required Call 800-555-5971
24-month Preexisting Condition Limitation

BACK OF CARD

FIGURE 3-2
Example of a patient's insurance card.

3. *Group number.* Again, you will need to match what is shown on the card with what the individual has written on the patient registration form. This number is an important part of the ID number or policy number, and it must be shown on the claim form in order to have your claim with the insurance company processed efficiently.

4. *Co-pay or co-insurance.* On the back of the card, you will see the amount that the individual has to pay for different services. Look at Figure 3-2; you will see in the middle of the back of the card Co-insurance; Deductible; Hospital per Adm Deductible; Family Physician Office Svs; and All Other Physician Svs. You will see that there are two sets of numbers that tell you how much this insurance policy will pay for that type of service. The first column is for a PPO participating office and the second for a non-PPO participating office. This means you will have to know whether or not your office is a participating member of that plan, so that you will know how much to collect from the patient during this visit. A patient with insurance through an HMO may have different information on the back of the card. However, the basic information regarding co-pay or co-insurance and deductibles should be shown. You will also need to ask, during the verification phone call, to find out if the patient has met their deductible for the year.

5. *Admission certification.* If you need to admit this individual into the hospital, you might find a different phone number for admission certification. Just as in the office, when you must call to verify coverage before treating the individual, you may need to get approval to admit the individual into the hospital (unless it is an emergency) or get preauthorization to treat the patient. A *preadmission certificate* (PAC) is a request for a review by the insurance company, so that medical necessity can be established before the patient is treated as an inpatient in a hospital. *Preauthorization* gives a specialist or hospital the opportunity to get approval for payment from the insurance company for a health care service *before* the service is actually provided. You might need to do this if the procedure is elective or has unusual circumstances. Often, this is a different phone number than the regular customer service number for coverage verification.

Remember, just because the patient has an ID card does not mean that he or she has current insurance coverage. You must call to verify!

Box 3-2 highlights some important terms that you will need to know when working with the data from a patient's insurance card.

IMPORTANT NOTE
Once you have copied a patient's insurance card, write the date on the copy. This way, you have documented that the patient presented this card to you on that date, just in case there are any questions later.

BOX 3-2   Terms Common to an Insurance Card

Admission certification—prior approval from an insurance company to admit an individual to the hospital

Co-insurance—a percentage of the total charge to be paid by the insured

Co-pay—a fixed amount of money paid by the insured

Deductible—the total amount of money that an individual must pay, out of his or her own pocket, before the insurance benefits will begin to pay

Eligibility—the confirmation that an individual is eligible for the coverage of a service or procedure—for example, to make certain there is no preexisting condition exclusion in the individual's policy to prevent coverage for a particular type of procedure

Preadmission certificate (PAC)—confirmation by the insurance company that an upcoming inpatient treatment of an individual in a hospital has been determined to be a medical necessity

Preauthorization—when a provider gets approval (acceptance for payment) of a procedure or service by the insurance company before treatment is provided

Verification of coverage—confirmation from the insurance carrier: that an individual is covered by health insurance; regarding any limitations of the insurance plan; and regarding any other details pertinent to this particular provider-individual encounter

REFERRAL AUTHORIZATION FORM

When one physician recommends that an individual see another physician for a consultation or treatment, it is called a *referral*. Let's look carefully at a referral authorization form (Figure 3-3). Just as with the patient registration forms, different insurance companies have their own version of this form. Even though it may look a little different from the example in Figure 3-3, it should contain the same information. Also, some companies use electronic versions of this form. It doesn't matter what it looks like, as long as you get the information you need. Routinely, you should have the referral form, or its required information, before the individual arrives to meet with the provider. This will give you time to confirm that you have what you need to get proper authorization for payment for this encounter.

Primary Care Physician
Referral Authorization Form

Referral Authorization Number

TO BE COMPLETED BY PRIMARY CARE PHYSICIAN—PLEASE PRINT

Member ID No. _____   Member Name _____

Benefit Type: CM ☐ MC ☐ MD ☐ IN ☐

PCP Information:

PCP Name _____   Contact Name _____

Phone # _____   Fax # _____

Refer to Provider/Facility:

Name _____   Specialty _____

Address _____   Phone _____

_____   Provider Number _____

Clinical Information:

ICD code(s) must be completed

Primary Diagnosis _____   ICD-9 _____

Secondary Diagnosis _____   ICD-9 _____

Services Authorized   Specified Treatments/Procedures

___ Consultation w/Treatment   ___ Consultation   _____

___ Follow-Up visits   ___ Diagnostic Testing   _____

___ Follow-Up Visits w/Specified Treatments*

*Indicate specific procedure(s) to be performed AND/OR   _____

number of visits.   Number of Visits _____

Appointment Date   PCP Signature

                                                 Date _____

_____

Valid for ☐ 30 days   ☐ 60 days

Disclaimer: This referral does not guarantee member eligibility, service benefits, or payment.
For verification of member eligibility or contract benefits, please call Member Services at 800-555-9753.
This referral is not valid for any nonplan services.
Requests for nonplan services must be called in to Medical Services.

To the PCP: The issue of this form by the member's PCP authorizes the above listed services only. Any other services must be called in to Medical Services at 800-555-9297 or fax 800-555-1251. Please refer to your PCP Referral Authorization Form Process Quick Reference Sheet for specific instructions.

To the Patient: This form is your authorization to receive the above listed services. Contact your primary care physician for all other services. Please take your copy of this form with you to your appointment and give it to the staff. It is important they receive it to verify the request for services. Please verify your name, date of birth, and member ID number are correct.

To the Receiving Specialist/Facility: Please mail or fax consultation reports to the PCP within 10 days from date of service. This referral is authorized for the above services only. Please contact the PCP if additional services are required. Please ensure all patient identifying information conforms with your claim.

FIGURE 3-3

Example of a referral authorization form.

You will always need to get information regarding the provider making the referral; in certain insurance cases (such as HMOs), you will need to get prior authorization from the third-party payer to treat the individual. Particularly when a primary care physician is referring an individual to a specialist, the individual should bring with them, to the first appointment, a primary care physician referral authorization form. If the individual does not bring the form, you will need to call the referring physician to get the information over the phone. This form does *not* replace the need for the phone call to verify health insurance coverage. You will still have to do that. This is one version of a preauthorization.

Let's review key sections of the typical referral authorization form.

The upper right-hand corner of the form shows the *referral authorization number.* This is a critical piece of information, as it is the reference number indicating the insurance carrier's approval for the specialist to see the patient. You must have an authorization number in order to expect to get paid for the services.

The top section of the form contains information on the individual. On the sample form in Figure 3-3, you will note the individual (also known as patient) is referred to as the member. This is not unusual for HMO plans. Here, the member ID no. is the same as the ID or policy number for that individual with that insurance plan.

In addition, this section has the information about the referring physician, here called the *PCP (primary care physician).* This section gives you the name of the provider, the name of the contact person in the referring physician's office, and phone and fax numbers. You will need this information—at the very least—to send the physician reports on what the provider in your office has observed, provided, and/or recommended for this patient.

The last portion of the top section of the form, *Refer to Provider/ Facility,* should show your office's information or the data of the specialist to whom the patient is being referred.

The middle section includes the key *Clinical Information* that would form the basis for the referral—in other words, the diagnosis. You will note that the primary and secondary diagnoses must be indicated by words as well as the ICD-9-CM (diagnosis) code(s).

IMPORTANT NOTE

ICD stands for the International Classification of Diseases. ICD has one code to represent each diagnosis. You will learn more about these codes later in Chapter 5.

The lower middle section indicates the types of *Services Authorized.* As you can see, if *Specified Treatments/Procedures* or testing are required, the right-hand portion must also be completed. In addition, the insurance company will typically specify how many visits are approved for this one referral. You must make certain that, if the form says only one visit is approved, you call to get approval before permitting the individual to come back to see your provider a second time.

Below this, you will see the *Appointment* information, including the approved length of time this referral will remain valid. Often, the insurance carrier will approve a referral based on number of visits within a particular span of time, such as 30 or 60 days. Again, if your provider needs to continue treatment for this individual beyond either the number of visits or the span of time (beginning the date of the authorization), you will need to call the referring physician's office to get an extension on the referral authorization. It is one phone call that may make the difference between your office being paid for its services or not.

In the bottom section of the sample referral authorization form in Figure 3-3, you will find the instructions for the primary care physician (PCP), the patient, and the receiving specialist/facility. Notice that it says, "This referral is authorized for the above services only. Please contact the PCP if additional services are required." These instructional notes are standard on preprinted forms.

ENCOUNTER FORM AND SUPERBILL

Let's look carefully at a sample superbill (Figure 3-4). An **encounter form** is a piece of paper upon which the provider documents what happened during a visit between that provider and an individual. Basically, the encounter form identifies the individual, along with all appropriate diagnoses, a listing of all procedures performed or provided during the visit, and any remarks, such as the provider's request for a follow-up appointment with the patient. The provider completes this form during or immediately after the visit.

Many health care providers' offices use what is called a **superbill** (Figure 3-4). Superbills may look different than the sample in Figure 3-4. You will find that our sample lists the procedure codes (CPT) on the top and the diagnosis codes (ICD-9-CM) on the bottom. Some forms show them side by side; some show the ICD-9-CM codes first and then the CPT codes. Typically, remarks and orders for future appointments are placed in the lower right-hand corner of the form (Figure 3-4).

Key Terms

Encounter form: A form upon which a face-to-face visit between provider and patient is documented.

Superbill: An encounter form that is preprinted with the diagnosis (ICD-9-CM) codes, as well as the procedure (CPT) codes, most frequently used in that office. Also known as a routing slip or fee ticket.

IMPORTANT NOTE

CPT stands for *Current Procedural Terminology*. These codes indicate specific procedures and services that a health care professional could provide to a patient. We will learn more about CPT codes later on in Chapter 7.

After meeting with the patient, the provider simply checks off or circles the appropriate description and code and forwards it to the assistant in charge of completing the office's appointment process. Then, the form is sent to billing. Using a preprinted superbill saves time. Insurance coding and billing specialists still have work to do, but these certainly make the job a bit easier. You'll understand this better when we get to the coding section in Chapters 4 through 9.

FAMILY DOCTORS ASSOCIATES
123 Main Street
Anytown, FL 32711
(407) 555-1200

Date: _____   Attending Physician: _____

Patient Name: _____

CPT DESCRIPTION	CPT DESCRIPTION	CPT DESCRIPTION
OFFICE/HOSPITAL	**PATHOLOGY/LAB/RADIOLOGY**	**PROCEDURES/TESTS**
☐ 99201 OFFICE-NEW; FOCUSED	☐ 73100 X-RAY WRIST TWO VIEWS	☐ 12011 SIMPLE SUTURE, FACE
☐ 99202 OFFICE-NEW; EXPANDED	☐ 73590 X-RAY TIBIA/FIBULA, TWO	☐ 29125 SPLINT-SHORT ARM
☐ 99203 OFFICE-NEW; DETAILED	☐ 73600 X-RAY ANKLE TWO VIEWS	☐ 29355 WALKER CAST-LONG LEG
☐ 99204 OFFICE-NEW; COMPREHEN	☐ 76085 MAMMOGRAM-COMP DET	☐ 29540 STRAPPING-ANKLE
☐ 99205 OFFICE-NEW; COMPREHEN	☐ 76092 MAMMOGRAM SCREENING	☐ 45378 COLONOSCOPY-DIAGNOSTIC
☐ 99211 OFFICE-ESTB; MINIMAL	☐ 80050 BLOOD TEST-GEN HEALTH	☐ 45385 COLONOSCOPY-POLYP REM.
☐ 99212 OFFICE-ESTB; FOCUSED	☐ 80061 BLOOD TEST-LIPID PANEL	☐ 50390 ASPIRATION, RENAL CYST
☐ 99213 OFFICE-ESTB; EXPANDED	☐ 82947 BLOOD TEST-GLUCOSE	☐ 90703 TETANUS INJECTION
☐ 99214 OFFICE-ESTB; DETAILED	☐ 83718 BLOOD TEST-HDL	☐ 92081 VISUAL FIELD EXAM
☐ 99215 OFFICE-ESTB; COMPREHEN	☐ 85025 BLOOD TEST-CBC	☐ 93000 ECG, 12 LEADS, W/RPT
☐ 99281 EMER DEPT; FOCUSED	☐ 86403 STREP TEST, QUICK	☐ 93015 TREADMILL STRESS TEST
☐ 90844 COUNSELING – 50 MIN.	☐ 87430 ENZY IMMUNOASSAY-STREP	☐ 99173 VISUAL ACUITY SCREEN

ICD DESCRIPTION	ICD DESCRIPTION	ICD DESCRIPTION
☐ 034.0 STREP THROAT	☐ 522 LOW RED BLOOD COUNT	☐ V01.5 RABIES EXPOSURE
☐ 042 HUMAN IMMUNO VIRUS	☐ 538.8 STOMACH PAIN	☐ V16.0 FAM HISTORY-COLON
☐ 250.51 DIABETES W/VISION	☐ 643 HYPEREMESIS	☐ V16.3 FAM HISTORY- BREAST
☐ 250.80 DIABETES, TYPE II	☐ 707.14 ULCER OF HEEL/MID FOOT	☐ V20.2 WELL CHILD
☐ 307.51 BULIMIA NON-ORGANIC	☐ 788.30 ENURESIS	☐ V22.0 PREGNANCY-FIRST NORM
☐ 354.0 CARPEL TUNNEL SYNDROME	☐ 815.00 FRACTURE, HAND	☐ V22.1 PREGNANCY-NORMAL
☐ 362.01 RETINOPATHY (DIABETIC)	☐ 823.2 FRACTURE, TIBIA	☐ E816.2 MOTORCYCLE ACCT
☐ 401.9 HYPERTENSION, UNSPEC	☐ 831.00 DISLOCATION, SHOULDER	☐ E826.1 FALL FROM BICYCLE
☐ 482.30 PNEUMONIA	☐ 845.00 SPRAINED ANKLE	☐ E849.0 PLACE OF OCCUR-HOME
☐ 490 BRONCHITIS, UNSPECIFIED	☐ 880.03 OPEN WOUND UPPER ARM	☐ E881.0 FALL FROM LADDER
☐ 493.92 ASTHMA, UNSPECIFIED	☐ 912.0 ABRASION, SHOULDER	☐ E906.0 DOG BITE

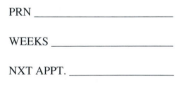

FOLLOW-UP

PRN _____

WEEKS _____

NXT APPT. _____

TIME _____

FIGURE 3-4   Example of a superbill.

PHYSICIAN'S NOTES

Just like the notes you take in class, **physician's notes** document all of the important facts of the discussion, as well as the examination, any procedure(s) provided and/or ordered, any recommendations or prescriptions made by the provider during this visit, and the diagnosis. The physician's notes may include the individual's history (especially if this is the first meeting between this individual and this provider). The notes also include the specific concern that brought the individual to see the provider this day, any allergies, and any symptoms or circumstances related to the illness, injury, or condition. Some providers still handwrite their notes, but most of the time the notes are dictated by the doctor and typed up by a medical transcriptionist.

The insurance specialist needs to be able to read and understand physician's notes for several reasons:

1. There may be information contained in the notes that is not on the superbill, such as the cause of an injury, days unable to work, or dates of hospitalization. This is required on the health insurance claim form. Also, this additional information may help you more easily find the best, most appropriate code(s).

2. The superbill may be incomplete and you may require further information to complete the claim form properly. The superbill cannot begin to list every code in the entire procedure code (CPT) or diagnosis code (ICD-9-CM) books, so the superbill shows only those codes used most frequently in that office. However, after reading the notes, you may find that another code would be more accurate and actually pay your office more money.

3. The CPT codes indicated on the superbill may not be medically necessary with relation to the ICD-9-CM code on the same bill, requiring you to do further investigation. Perhaps the physician accidentally circled the wrong code or made a check so big it went through two different codes.

Key Term

Physician's notes: The written or dictated notations of an encounter between a provider and an individual. Also known as medical notes or provider's notes.

CASE STUDY

Harriet Samuels makes an appointment to see her regular physician, Dr. Seymours. When the medical office assistant asks her why she needs to see the doctor, Harriet states that she has hurt her knee. After the encounter, the physician marks the superbill with the diagnosis (ICD-9-CM) code 844, sprain of knee or leg, along with procedure (CPT) codes 99212, office visit, and 73560, knee X-ray. This paperwork then gets processed and passed along to the insurance coder/biller (you) for this office. However, this documentation is not complete. All of the details that you need to code this visit properly are not there. Information that is not usually included on preprinted superbills is required data, in most states, in order to get your claim paid promptly.

Do you know what is missing?

_____

_____

An experienced coder would notice right away that more information is needed. Once reviewing the physician's notes, you would see that the injury to the knee was (1) a sprain of the lateral collateral ligament of the knee (requiring the fourth digit, changing the ICD-9-CM code to 844.0), and (2) an E code is needed. An E code is a diagnosis code that explains how and/or where the injury occurred. The notes will explain that the injury to the knee was caused by the patient's involvement in an automobile accident. Now you know what E code to add, as well as to which insurance company the claim should be sent. Remember what you learned in Chapter 1? Now you would know that you should probably send this claim to Harriet's automobile insurance carrier, rather than her health insurance carrier. Without this information, the claim would have been sent to the health insurance carrier, who would have rejected the claim, awaiting more information regarding the cause of the injury to determine which plan should pay these charges. At the very least, your office's payment is now delayed.

You will learn more about E codes, when we get to diagnostic coding (ICD-9-CM), later on, in Chapter 5.

Using Physician's Notes to Support Medical Necessity

John has all the symptoms of the flu, so he makes an appointment to see his physician. The physician's diagnosis is 487.8, stomach influenza. The physician circles that code on the superbill, along with 99211, office visit, established patient, problem focused and advises John to drink lots of fluids and to get some rest. While in the examining room, John says, "As long as I'm here, doctor, my wrist has been really painful for a while," so the doctor sends John down the hall for a wrist X-ray and circles CPT code 73100, wrist X-ray.

When you get this superbill for processing, you need to look at both the ICD-9-CM codes' descriptions and the CPT codes' descriptions and make certain they belong together. In this example, clearly the diagnosis of the stomach flu does not give a good reason to send the patient for a wrist X-ray. You need to note this before filing the health claim form, because if you don't, the insurance company will certainly deny the claim. What you need to do is go to the physician's notes. There you will see that the doctor ordered the wrist X-ray to confirm a diagnosis of a hairline fracture of the wrist. Now you know what ICD-9-CM code to add to the claim to justify the wrist X-ray. This is called looking for medical necessity. The ICD-9-CM code (the diagnosis) must show that there was a medical reason to perform the procedure or treatment (the CPT code). The diagnosis of hairline fracture of the wrist is a good reason to get a wrist X-ray—the stomach flu is not! Therefore, the procedure is medically necessary—in other words, a medical necessity.

If you do not find anything in the physician's notes to direct you to a diagnosis that supports the procedure or treatment performed, you may need to speak to the doctor directly. However, you need to read the notes carefully and be certain the information is not there before you approach the provider.

Learning How to Understand Physician's Notes

Many providers dictate their notes into a tape recorder and have a medical transcriptionist type them into the computer. Others handwrite their notes on pages inserted into the patient's file. Whichever method is used in the office or hospital where you work, the information must be accurately recorded into the patient's health record, and possibly on the health insurance claim form.

Members of the health care industry use many abbreviations, particularly in physician's notes. In order for you to be able to read and interpret the notes properly, you need to be able to understand what is written. Many of these abbreviations come from commonly used medical terms. This is one of the reasons that you need to study and understand medical terminology as well as anatomy and physiology. As you probably already know, many medical terms come from the Latin language.

You need to pay close attention to whether the abbreviation is in capital letters or lowercase. A capital letter may mean something totally different than a lowercase letter.

Examples

K (capital letter) means potassium or kidney, but k (lowercase letter) means kilo.

D&C (with the ampersand) means dilation and curettage, whereas dc (with no punctuation) means discharge.

If periods are shown, they are important and must not be left out, because there might be another abbreviation with the same letters and no periods, meaning something else.

Read the entire paragraph and look at the context of what is written. This will help you understand the meaning of the abbreviation. Box 3-3 contains a short list of some of the most frequently used medical abbreviations and what they mean. Anyone responsible for insurance coding and/or the creation of health insurance claim forms needs to understand these abbreviations to do their job correctly. You should note that each physician might use his or her own versions of these abbreviations. Therefore, it is wise to check with the facility where you work, so you can learn what abbreviations are approved for use there. These and additional abbreviations are shown in Appendix A at the back of this textbook. In addition, the health care industry, as a whole, is working on creating a universal abbreviation list to enable consistency among providers. Watch for it over the next few years.

Consider the following example:

- *Physician's notes: NP* presented to this physician's office is a 7 yo male with a *FH* of diabetes. *Ht 4'2" Wt 93 lbs. UA pos* for diabetes. *Pt* presents with open wound on *rt ft.*
- *Translation into English:* A *new patient* presented to this physician's office is a seven-year-old boy with a *family history* of diabetes. *Height* 4 feet 2 inches, *weight* 93 *pounds.* The *urinalysis* was *positive* for diabetes. The *patient* came to see the doctor with an open wound on his *right foot.*
- *The coder needs to know:*
  - The *new patient* presented to this *physician's office* = type of CPT Evaluation and Management code for the office visit.
  - The *urinalysis* = CPT code for the urinalysis.
  - . . . an *open wound* on his *right foot* = ICD-9-CM code for the reason the patient came to see the doctor today.
  - The urinalysis was positive for *diabetes* = ICD-9-CM code for the diagnosis of diabetes.

Hopefully you can now see how important it is that the insurance coding and billing specialist be able to read physician's notes. It's a good idea to keep a medical dictionary handy, so you can completely understand all of the details shown.

BOX 3-3   Frequently Used Medical Abbreviations

Abbreviation	Meaning	Abbreviation	Meaning
abd	abdomen	lbs	pounds
b.i.d.	two times a day	LLL	left lower lobe
BI or BX	biopsy	LLQ	left lower quadrant
BP or B/P	blood pressure	LMP	last menstrual period
Ca or CA	cancer or carcinoma	LT or lt	left
CBC	complete blood count	LUQ	left upper quadrant
CC	chief complaint	mg.	milligrams
ch	check-up	neg	negative
CO or C/O or c/o	complains of	NP	new patient
comp	comprehensive	PA	posterior anterior
compl	complete	PE or Ph ex or phys.	physical examination
Con or Cons	consultation	PID	pelvic inflammatory disease
Cont. or cont.	continue	PND	postnasal drip
COPD	chronic obstructive pulmonary disease	PO or postop	postoperative
		pos.	positive
CPX or CPE	complete physical examination	Post.	posterior
CVA	cardiovascular accident	PRN or p.r.n.	as necessary
CXR	chest X-ray	Pt or pt	patient
D&C	dilation and curettage	PT	physical therapy
DC	discharge	RBC	red blood cell
dc	discontinue	re	about, for
Dx or Dg	diagnosis	RLQ	right lower quadrant
ECG or EKG	electrocardiogram	RO or R/O	rule out
EEG	electroencephalogram	RT	respiratory therapy
EENT	eye, ear, nose, and throat	rt.	right
FBS	fasting blood sugar	RUQ	right upper quadrant
FH	family history	Rx or RX	prescription
Fx	fracture	STD	sexually transmitted disease
G	gravida (number of pregnancies)	T	temperature
g or gm	gram	TB or Tb or tbc	tuberculosis
GI	gastrointestinal	TIA	transient ischemic attack
HBP	high blood pressure	TPR	temperature/pulse/respiration
hct	hematocrit	UA or U/A	urinalysis
HCVD	hypertensive cardiovascular disease	UCR	usual, customary, and reasonable
HEENT	head, eyes, ears, nose, throat	UGI	upper gastrointestinal
Hgb or Hb	hemoglobin	UTI	urinary tract infection
Ht	height	WBC	white blood cell
hx, Hx	history	WNL	within normal limits
K	potassium or kidney	Wt or wt	weight
k	kilo	yo	years old

Styles of Physician's Notes

SOAP Notes

SOAP notes are written in an outline format using four sections: *Subjective*, *Objective*, *Assessment*, and *Plan*. SOAP is an acronym for the four section titles.

Subjective (impressions and patient observations) is the first section and will include the patient's reason for the visit today: the chief complaint in his or her own words; status regarding current medications and/or treatments; history (family history; problem-focused history [of the current condition] and/or social history e.g., personal habits affecting health such as smoking, drinking); and an itemization of the reported symptoms.

Objective (facts), section two, will contain the results of any physical examination performed, e.g., including vital signs, height/weight, physician's observations; and the results of any diagnostic testing related to the concern at hand or the patient's general health status.

Assessment is the diagnosis, and/or the physician's conclusions. If there is no definitive diagnosis, the coder must reread the objective portion of the notes to look for positive test results (such as a statement reading "X-ray showed lateral fracture of the tibia") for coding a diagnosis. If there is no confirmed diagnosis as a result of the testing, then the patient's symptoms must be coded. (More about this in Chapter 4.)

Plan, the last part of these notes, documents the physician's orders for the patient. These may include diagnostic tests to be done in the future, procedures to be performed ("Colonoscopy scheduled for one week"), recommendations for lifestyle changes ("Patient is advised to quit drinking alcoholic beverages as soon as possible"), and follow-up care ("Recheck CBC in two weeks").

Many physicians like SOAP notes because they are orderly and thorough. With this format, they are reminded to address each portion as they are dictating, or writing, to document all aspects of the encounter with the patient.

In Figure 3-5, you will find an example of SOAP notes taken from a family practitioner. See if you can distinguish each of the four SOAP terms by the content of each paragraph or section.

<u>PROGRESS NOTE</u>

PT NAME: ROBBINS, ARLENE   **DATE:** 03/03/06
DOB: 05/27/88
MRN: 05003579

S: This pt is an 18-year-old white female, g 0, LMP 2/18, not sexually active, not on any birth control who presents today with two main complaints. The first complaint is she feels a lump in her right groin. The second complaint is a vaginal discharge, no odor or itching, just feels irritated.

O: Pelvic exam revealed the external genitalia to be within normal limits. The vagina was without lesions. Scant discharge seen. Wet mount neg for Trichomonas, clue cells or hyphae. Increased bacteria in the background noted. Inspection of the rt groin revealed no abnormality. The pt was asked to point out the area of abnormality and this felt to be dilated areas within one of the vessels in the groin. These were less than the size of a pea and did not feel like lymphadenopathy. Similar areas were felt on the lt side as well. The patient was reassured.

A: Possible nonspecific vaginitis

P:

    1. Cleocin vaginal cream qhs times seven nights.
    2. Follow up in one month for reinspection of the rt groin.
    3. Otherwise follow up with us prn. She verbalized understanding.
    4. All questions were answered. She will follow up with us prn or for her yearly Pap smear.

_____

Harold Doctor, M.D.

D: 03/03/06
T: 03/08/06 nk

FIGURE 3-5
Example of SOAP notes.

> **IMPORTANT NOTE**
>
> In Figure 3-5, you will notice the abbreviation MRN (Medical Record Number). At the bottom, under the physician's signature, you will see the date the notes were dictated (identified by the D), the date the notes were transcribed (identified by the T), and the initials of the medical transcriptionist (identified by the initials nk).

Narrative Notes

Some physicians prefer to dictate their notes using the narrative format, as shown in Figure 3-6. This means that they tell the story of the encounter with the patient, including all the details. This is typed and presented in paragraph format.

Generally, it seems that family physicians, who may plan more time between appointments and have a wider scope of interest with regard to their patients' health (the whole body), tend to prefer SOAP notes, whereas specialists, who see their patients in sequenced appointments with more regularity and for a more singular focus (one particular part of the body and often one concern), tend to prefer narrative notes. It may be because specialists typically will not have vital signs taken and documented with each visit, unless they are applicable to the problem, as well as the fact that each consecutive visit with a specialist is a follow-up to the original concern.

However, this is usually the physician's personal preference. For the coder and biller in the office, the only difference is that SOAP notes' outline format can make it easier and faster to find the diagnosis, whereas the narrative format requires a more thorough reading of the entire encounter.

> **IMPORTANT NOTE**
>
> In narrative notes, the initials of the transcriptionist are shown, in lower-case, at the end of each paragraph. OV stands for office visit.

<u>PROGRESS NOTE</u>

PT NAME: DAWSON, KATIE
DOB: 07/13/85
MRN: 06002795

DATE: 09/08/06

OV This patient is coming along well since her colonoscopy. She is having minimal problems. Examination reveals mild colitis. She was told I would not put her on any type of treatment at this time. The patient doesn't want to take steroids; she is not having enough problems to warrant steroids. We will see her again in three months. ks

DATE: 12/18/06

OV This patient is getting along exceptionally well. She was scoped up to 40 cm and has colitis up this far. However, the worst of it is in the last 10 centimeters. The patient will be given another course of Flagyl to see if we can get this to resolve. We will check her in three weeks. ks

DATE: 01/09/07

OV This patient is in today and she still has her colitis. It is getting worse. We will start her on some Rowasa. We will give her one a night for three weeks. We will see her after that and see how she is getting along. She will probably have to take it for six weeks before we will see a difference. ks

_____
                            Suzanne Example, M.D.

FIGURE 3-6
Example of narrative notes.

Procedure Notes

Procedure notes, and operative reports, as shown in Figure 3-7, contain different types of information than standard office visit documentation. This is why these notes take on a different format.

For extensive procedures that need operative support, such as those usually done in same-day surgical centers, the attending physicians may use an IPIP (Indications, Procedures, Impressions, Plans) outline format for their reports. In these cases, there is not typically time spent discussing things with the patient or other evaluation and management services. Often, the patient goes in, the procedure is performed, and the patient goes home. Follow-up will be done when the patient sees the physician in the office for his or her next appointment.

The sections on these notes include the following:

_I_ndications—a statement of the diagnosis that is the reason for the procedure

_P_rocedures—a step-by-step accounting of what was done during the encounter

_I_mpressions—the physician's impression of the results or findings of the procedure

_P_lans—the steps or actions for the patient's continued treatment

Hospital operative reports (Figure 3-8) are similar but typically include a preoperative diagnosis and a postoperative diagnosis, along with a report of what was done during the procedure and what the findings were.

PROCEDURE NOTE

PT NAME: DAWSON, KATIE
DOB: 07/13/85
MRN: 06002795

DATE: 07/29/06
PROCEDURE PERFORMED: Colonoscopy
PHYSICIAN: Suzanne Example, M.D.

INDICATIONS: History of colitis

PROCEDURE: The patient was given no premedication at her request and the Olympus PCF-130 colonoscope was used. The mucosa of the rectum was essentially normal apart from some mild nonspecific edema. Photographs and biopsies were obtained. The remainder of the rectum was normal. The sigmoid was normal as was the descending colon, splenic flexure, transverse colon, hepatic flexure, right colon, and cecum. No evidence of polyps, tumors, masses, or inflammation. The scope was then withdrawn, these findings confirmed. The procedure was terminated and the patient tolerated it well.

IMPRESSION: Normal colonic mucosa through the cecum.

PLAN: Await results of rectal biopsies.

_____
                                  Suzanne Example, M.D.

FIGURE 3-7
Example of procedure notes.

FAMILY DOCTORS ASSOCIATES
123 MAIN STREET • ANYTOWN, FL 32711 • 407-555-1200

PATIENT: DOE-SMITH, JANE
ACCOUNT/EHR #:   DOESMJA010

DATE OF OPERATION: 11/9/2004
PREOPERATIVE DIAGNOSIS: Hallux limites, right foot
POSTOPERATIVE DIAGNOSIS: Same
OPERATION: Shortening, osteotomy, first metatarsal, right foot, with screw
                                        fixation and cheilectomy, first metatarsal head, right foot.

SURGEON: Mark C. Welby, D.P.M.
ASSISTANT: n/a
ANESTHESIA: IV sedation with local anesthesia

DESCRIPTION OF OPERATIVE PROCEDURE: Following the customary sterile preparation and draping the right limb was elevated approximately 5 minutes in order to facilitate circulatory drainage at which time the pneumatic cuff, which had previously been placed on her right ankle, was inflated to a pressure of 250 mmHg. The right limb was then placed in the operative position. The operative site was injected with 2% Xylocaine mixed with 0.5% Marcaine. Upon having achieved anesthesia, a curvilinear incision was created on the plantar medial aspect of the first metatarsophalangeal joint of the right foot. The incision was deepened with sharp dissection, traversing veins were cauterized. Capsule was identified on the medial and dorsomedial aspect. Capsule was longitudinally incised on the dorsomedial aspect and meticulously dissected on to expose the head of the first metatarsal into the operative site. At this point, it was noted that the cartilage of the first metatarsal head was healthy, however there was distinct irritation to the dorsal portion of the metatarsal head with an apparent flattening of the metatarsal head secondary to the hallux limites. Using a rongeur, the hypertrophic exuberant portion of the first metatarsal head was resected, and the remaining surface was rasped smooth in order to recreate a ball joint. Using an oscillating saw, an osteotomy was performed from medial to lateral in a V-shaped fashion with the apex centrally located and the dorsal arm longer than the plantar arm. A segment of bone was removed from the dorsal arm in order to shorten and plantar flex the metatarsal head. Upon having done so, two 2.0 mm screws were obliquely driven into the osteotomy site, following range of motion was noted that the osteotomy remained stable. At this point, the hallux had approximately 90 degrees of motion to the metatarsal shaft. The area was copiously irrigated with sterile saline. The capsular tissue was repaired using 4-0 Vicryl, subcutaneous tissue was repaired using 5-0 Vicryl. Operative site was injected with dexamethasone, Betadine-soaked adaptic was applied to the incision site, sterile gauze and Kling. The pneumatic cuff was deflated. Normal color, circulation was noted to return to all digits immediately. The patient tolerated the surgery well. Vital signs remained stable throughout the entire procedure. The patient returned to the recovery room in good condition.

_____

Mark C. Welby, D.P.M.

MCW/mg   D: 11/9/04 09:50:16   T: 11/12/04 12:55:01

FIGURE 3-8
Example of operative notes.

CHAPTER SUMMARY

Documentation is possibly the most important concept in the entire process of health insurance coding and billing. When the term "documentation" is used, it includes all of the forms we reviewed in this chapter:

- patient registration form
- insurance card
- referral authorization form
- encounter form and superbill
- physician's notes
    - SOAP notes
    - narrative notes
    - procedure notes
    - operative notes

You must have the paperwork (or digital files) supplied to you by the health care provider before you can do anything. In addition, you must know what pieces of data you need to do your job correctly and on which document the data can be found. This is critical to your success.

You will need to learn how to read and interpret the documents used in the office in which you work. Ask about an office-approved list of abbreviations that are acceptable for use in your facility. This will help you get used to the way the physician in your office writes his or her notes.

Chapter Review

Who Am I?

1. The person who promises to pay the medical bills, whatever the insurance company does not pay, is the _____.

2. The person who brings the health insurance policy to the family is the _____.

3. The person who comes to the provider, seeking advice and treatment, is the _____.

4. The person whose name is on the health insurance policy is the _____.

5. The provider who recommends that a patient see a specialist is the _____ provider.

6. The provider who is primarily in charge of this patient's care in this office is the _____ provider.

7. The person, often a spouse or child, who is covered under someone else's insurance policy is the _____.

8. The provider who is in charge of monitoring an individual's well-being and makes all the referrals is the _____ _____ _____.

9. The person who creates the medical notes is the _____.

10. The person who reads the medical notes in order to convert diagnoses and procedures into codes for the health insurance claim form is the _____.

Translate the notes into everyday English.

1. This NP is 63 yo African American male with prior Dx. HBP. Wt. 185 lbs, BP 130/70, T 99.5°.

   _____

   _____

2. Pt is 15 yo female. CC: sore throat, and PND. Rx. Antihistamine PRN and aspirin b.i.d. re ch 60 days.

   _____

   _____

3. Pt. is 60 yo female. CC: stiffness and tiredness. Wt. 134 lbs. BP 116/72, T 98.6°. Dx. Exhaustion Rx. Prednisone 5 mg. b.i.d., ck CBC and UA in 4 wks.

_____

_____

4. 21 yo female Pt. CC: pain in RLQ of abd, 2 days, T 102°, BP 110/72, Wt. 120. PE shows rebound tenderness with radiation to the RUQ and RLQ. Lab tests shows WBC 19.1; RBC 4.61. UA within normal limits.

_____

_____

5. NP is 75 yo male with hx of COPD. CC cough. BP 125/85, T 98.6°, Wt. 178 lbs. EKG normal. CBC and UA normal limits. Rx. RT prn.

_____

_____

Where will you find it? Match the piece of information to its source.

1. Patient's name _____A_____

2. Guarantor's name _____A_____

3. Policyholder's name _____B_____

4. Patient's date of birth _____A_____

5. Policy ID number _____B_____

6. Diagnosis _____C_____

7. Procedures performed _____C_____

8. Next appointment or follow-up _____C_____

9. Referral authorization number _____D_____

10. Patient's allergies _____A_____

11. Patient's signature _____A_____

12. Referring physician's name _____D_____

13. Insurance company phone number _____B_____

14. Co-payment amount _____B_____

15. Policyholder's employer information _____A_____

A. Patient registration form

B. Insurance ID card

C. Encounter form/superbill

D. PCP referral form

E. Physician's notes

4 Introduction to Coding—Guidelines Overview

OBJECTIVES

- Explain the purpose of health care coding.
- Follow correctly the appropriate steps to coding.
- Use official guidelines provided to apply the best, most accurate code.
- Detect ethical danger zones that might exist in the workplace.
- Know the AHIMA *Code of Ethics* and *Standards of Ethical Coding.*
- Know the AAPC *Code of Ethical Standards.*

The purpose of coding is to make every effort to ensure clear and concise communication among all parties involved. In most cases, these parties are the health care providers and the insurance companies (third-party payers). Insurance coding is simply translating health care terms and definitions into a predetermined set of numbers and letters (alphanumeric codes).

This and the following chapters will take you through two books that you will use in the process of translating **diagnoses** and **procedures** into codes: ICD-9-CM and CPT, to properly identify the reason for this encounter, and which services were provided.

The *International Classification of Diseases (ICD)* is a directory of every diagnosis that could be assigned by a health care provider for a patient. You may also see reference to **ICD-9-CM**, which stands for *International Classification of Diseases—9th revision—Clinical Modification.*

Current Procedural Terminology—4th edition (**CPT**) is similar to the ICD-9-CM book, except that, instead of listing codes for diagnoses, the CPT book catalogs codes for procedures, treatments, and services provided to patients.

Each set of numbers and letters means something so specific that a code number just one digit off could mean something totally unrelated. That difference could cause the claim to be rejected, resulting in your office not getting paid for the work it did. This is why it is critical to be careful and accurate when coding and always *double-check* your codes.

Key Terms

ICD-9-CM: *International Classification of Diseases—9th revision—Clinical Modification, Volumes I and II,* the book of diagnosis codes.

CPT: *Current Procedural Terminology*—4th edition, the book of service and procedure codes.

Example

ICD-9-CM code 915 is a superficial injury of finger;
ICD-9-CM code 951 is an injury to cranial nerve.
    Big difference!

EIGHT STEPS TO ACCURATE CODING

There is an eight-step process to code a health care encounter for billing in the approved manner. As you gain experience, it will take less time. However, remember that time is not the number one consideration—no matter what anyone says—*accuracy* is the most important factor. The steps are as follows:

1. Read through the superbill and the physician's notes for this encounter completely, from beginning to end. Make a copy of the pages relating to this visit, so that you can write on these copies without marking the originals.
2. Reread through the physician's notes and highlight key words regarding diagnoses and procedures directly relating to this encounter. Pulling out the key words is also called **abstracting** physician's notes.
3. Make a list of any questions you have regarding unclear or missing information necessary to code this encounter. **Query**, or ask, the health care provider who treated the patient. Never assume. Code only what you know from actual documentation. If it is not documented, it doesn't exist or it didn't happen.
4. Code the diagnosis(es) as stated by the physician and/or the appropriate symptoms describing *why* the patient came to see the health care provider for this encounter. Use the best, most appropriate code available based on the documentation.
5. Code the procedure(s) as stated in the notes describing *what* the provider did for the patient. Use the best, most appropriate code(s) available based on the documentation.

Key Terms

Abstracting: The process of finding the key words in the physician's notes used in the coding process.

Query: To ask.

Memory Tip

Patient = WHO came to see the provider for health care
Diagnosis = WHY the individual came to see the provider for this visit
Procedure = WHAT the provider did for the individual

6. Link every procedure code to at least one diagnosis code shown on the same claim form to document medical necessity. Use this step to double-check the codes you have assigned.

7. Confirm that the codes you've chosen are correct. Code backwards (in other words, look up the numbers you have chosen and make certain the description in the code book matches the physician's notes. This is one method of confirming that your codes are correct). Use a medical dictionary, if necessary.

> **IMPORTANT NOTE**
>
> Medical necessity, or medically necessary, is the determination that the provider was acting according to standard practices in providing a procedure or service for an individual with a specific diagnosis.

8. Enter the information carefully and precisely into the computer and create the claim form. (You'll find more details on creating claim forms later in Chapters 10 and 11.)

Following these steps will help you code precisely, resulting in a greater number of your claims getting paid quickly, rather than having them rejected and dealing with the same cases again and again.

CODING FROM SUPERBILLS INSTEAD OF PHYSICIAN'S NOTES

Each individual has his or her own way of tackling a task. Health information management administrators are the staff members responsible for choosing the system that their health care facilities use to handle the routine of coding diagnoses and procedures to create health insurance claim forms—in other words, how their facilities process billing. Some outsource this very important job to an independent company. Large facilities, such as hospitals and large physician groups, typically establish a separate department, which may or may not be located in another office. Smaller practices and physicians' offices may opt to have one or two people in their office handle this process.

Health care facilities differ in more ways than simply the logistics of where coding occurs. Some have their coders use only superbills to create the first health claim form and refer to the physician's notes only if that claim is rejected. This may happen because the staff believes that it is the quickest way to process claim forms. When an office is dealing with 60 or 100 patients a day, this seems to make sense: "Get those claim forms coded and sent as soon as possible and we will deal with the rejected ones later! We don't have time for people to sit around, reading physician's notes."

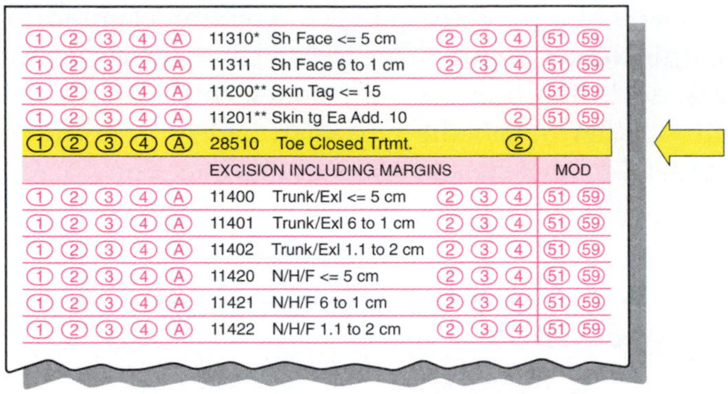

① ② ③ ④ Ⓐ	11310*	Sh Face <= 5 cm	② ③ ④	51 59
① ② ③ ④ Ⓐ	11311	Sh Face 6 to 1 cm	② ③ ④	51 59
① ② ③ ④ Ⓐ	11200**	Skin Tag <= 15		51 59
① ② ③ ④ Ⓐ	11201**	Skin tg Ea Add. 10	②	51 59
① ② ③ ④ Ⓐ	28510	Toe Closed Trtmt.	②	
		EXCISION INCLUDING MARGINS		MOD
① ② ③ ④ Ⓐ	11400	Trunk/Exl <= 5 cm	② ③ ④	51 59
① ② ③ ④ Ⓐ	11401	Trunk/Exl 6 to 1 cm	② ③ ④	51 59
① ② ③ ④ Ⓐ	11402	Trunk/Exl 1.1 to 2 cm	② ③ ④	51 59
① ② ③ ④ Ⓐ	11420	N/H/F <= 5 cm	② ③ ④	51 59
① ② ③ ④ Ⓐ	11421	N/H/F 6 to 1 cm	② ③ ④	51 59
① ② ③ ④ Ⓐ	11422	N/H/F 1.1 to 2 cm	② ③ ④	51 59

FIGURE 4-1
Superbill with CPT procedure code.

On the surface, it appears that coding from superbills saves time and, therefore, money (fewer hours for coders = lower payroll expenses). The reality is that coding only from superbills is not efficient with regard to either time or money. The policy of coding from superbills can result in a higher number of rejected or underpaid claims. When this happens, the facility loses money in several ways:

1. Extra time is needed for the coder to go back over the claim if it is rejected or denied.
2. If a claim is rejected, money will be lost because it will take longer for your health care office to get paid by the third-party payer.
3. There may be a better code that is more accurate that is not included on the superbill. This means the office is not getting paid as much money as it is entitled to for its legitimate work.

See Figure 4-1 for a portion of a superbill used at a local family physician's office. The CPT procedure code shown is

28510 Toe Closed Treatment.

However, when you look up this code in the CPT book, you see that the full description is

28510—Closed treatment of fracture, phalanx, or phalanges, other than great toe; without manipulation, each.

It is the only code related to a toe fracture offered on this office's preprinted form. Let's double-check this in the CPT book. You will note a few facts:

- 28510 can be used only for any of the other four toes (the great toe is not included).
- If this were a closed treatment of the great toe, without manipulation, the correct code would be 28490.
- If a manipulation was performed during the procedure, the correct code changes to 28515. Due to the fact that 28515 is the code including manipulation (more work on the physician's part), it would pay at a higher rate.

If this physician's office had the policy of creating claim forms only from superbills, this office would have received a lesser payment than it actually deserved. The only way the coder could know which toe was treated and whether or not the physician had to perform manipulation would be to read the physician's notes of this encounter.

CASE STUDY

Sasha White came to the health care office where you work to see Dr. Healer. She had been in a car accident and was concerned about the neck pain she was experiencing. Figure 4-2, on the next page, is the superbill completed by Dr. Healer during this encounter with Ms. White. Do you think the information you have is enough for you to do a proper job coding and then billing this case? To which type of insurance carrier should you send the claim: health insurance; automobile insurance; liability insurance; workers' compensation? Do you think the diagnosis of a shoulder abrasion supports the three X-rays, especially the chest and spine X-rays?

Now, look at Dr. Healer's notes for his encounter with Ms. White (Figure 4-3). From what you already learned in Chapter 1, you can see that this will probably be a workers' compensation claim and not a health insurance claim or an automobile insurance claim, because she was driving while on the job.

As you will learn in Chapter 5, you will need to add a diagnosis code for the neck pain (nothing close to that is included on the superbill). The neck pain code will support the taking of the C spine and chest X-rays, in addition to the upcoming MRI. While you are at it, if you look up diagnosis code 912.0 the description is "abrasion or friction burn without mention of infection." Not exactly what is described in the notes. On the next page of the ICD-9-CM book a much more accurate code can be found—923.09 "contusion of upper limb, multiple sites" (multiple sites = upper arm and shoulder). This matches the notes perfectly. You will also need to add ICD-9-CM code E812 "Motor vehicle collision," to identify that the injury happened in a car accident.

Good job! You coded accurately and certainly made it easier for the third-party payer to approve the claim. And, hopefully, you found this case study to be a good example of the advantages of taking the time to review the physician's notes rather than simply relying on the superbill.

Family Doctors Associates
123 Main Street • Anytown, FL 32711
(407) 555-1200

Date: *September 16, 2005*   Attending Physician: *J. Healer, MD*

Patient Name: *Sasha White*

CPT DESCRIPTION	CPT DESCRIPTION	CPT DESCRIPTION
OFFICE/HOSPITAL	**PATHOLOGY/LAB/RADIOLOGY**	**PROCEDURES/TESTS**
☐ 99201 OFFICE-NEW; FOCUSED	☒ 710200 X-RAY CHEST TWO VIEWS	☐ 12011 SIMPLE SUTURE, FACE
☒ 99202 OFFICE-NEW; EXPANDED	☒ 72040 X-RAY SPINE-C, TWO VIEWS	☐ 29125 SPLINT-SHORT ARM
☐ 99203 OFFICE-NEW; DETAILED	☒ 73030 X-RAY SHOULDER COMP	☐ 29355 WALKER CAST-LONG LEG
☐ 99204 OFFICE-NEW; COMPREHEN	☐ 76085 MAMMOGRAM-COMP DET	☐ 29540 STRAPPING-ANKLE
☐ 99205 OFFICE-NEW; COMPREHEN	☐ 76092 MAMMOGRAM SCREENING	☐ 45378 COLONOSCOPY-DIAGNOSTIC
☐ 99211 OFFICE-ESTB; MINIMAL	☐ 80050 BLOOD TEST-GEN HEALTH	☐ 45385 COLONOSCOPY-POLYP REM.
☐ 99212 OFFICE-ESTB; FOCUSED	☐ 80061 BLOOD TEST-LIPID PANEL	☐ 50390 ASPIRATION, RENAL CYST
☐ 99213 OFFICE-ESTB; EXPANDED	☐ 82947 BLOOD TEST-GLUCOSE	☐ 90703 TETANUS INJECTION
☐ 99214 OFFICE-ESTB; DETAILED	☐ 83718 BLOOD TEST-HDL	☐ 92081 VISUAL FIELD EXAM
☐ 99215 OFFICE-ESTB; COMPREHEN	☐ 85025 BLOOD TEST-CBC	☐ 93000 ECG, 12 LEADS, W/RPT
☐ 99281 EMER DEPT; FOCUSED	☐ 86403 STREP TEST, QUICK	☐ 93015 TREADMILL STRESS TEST
☐ 90844 COUNSELING – 50 MIN.	☐ 87430 ENZY IMMUNOASSAY-STREP	☐ 99173 VISUAL ACUITY SCREEN

ICD DESCRIPTION	ICD DESCRIPTION	ICD DESCRIPTION
☐ 034.0 STREP THROAT	☐ 522 LOW RED BLOOD COUNT	☐ V01.5 RABIES EXPOSURE
☐ 042 HUMAN IMMUNO VIRUS	☐ 538.8 STOMACH PAIN	☐ V16.0 FAMILY HISTORY-COLON
☐ 250.51 DIABETES W/VISION	☐ 643 HYPEREMESIS	☐ V16.3 FAMILY HISTORY- BREAST
☐ 250.80 DIABETES, TYPE II	☐ 707.14 ULCER OF HEEL/MID FOOT	☐ V20.2 WELL CHILD
☐ 307.51 BULIMIA NON-ORGANIC	☐ 788.30 ENURESIS	☐ V22.0 PREGNANCY-FIRST NORM
☐ 354.0 CARPEL TUNNEL SYNDROME	☐ 815.00 FRACTURE, HAND	☐ V22.1 PREGNANCY-NORMAL
☐ 362.01 RETINOPATHY (DIABETIC)	☐ 823.20 FRACTURE, TIBIA	☐ E816.2 MOTORCYCLE ACCT
☐ 401.9 HYPERTENSION, UNSPEC	☐ 831.00 DISLOCATION, SHOULDER	☐ E826.1 FALL FROM BICYCLE
☐ 482.30 PNEUMONIA	☐ 845.00 SPRAINED ANKLE	☐ E849.0 PLACE OF OCCUR-HOME
☐ 490 BRONCHITIS, UNSPECIFIED	☐ 880.03 OPEN WOUND UPPER ARM	☐ E881.0 FALL FROM LADDER
☐ 493.92 ASTHMA, UNSPECIFIED	☒ 912.0 ABRASION, SHOULDER	☐ E906.0 DOG BITE

FOLLOW-UP

PRN _____

WEEKS _____

NXT APPT. _____

TIME _____

FIGURE 4-2
Sasha White's superbill.

FAMILY DOCTORS ASSOCIATES
123 MAIN STREET • ANYTOWN, FL 32711 • 407-555-1200

PATIENT: WHITE, SASHA
ACCOUNT/EHR#:   WHITSA001

DATE: 09/16/05

ATTENDING PHYSICIAN: James Healer, MD

S: This new Pt is a 25-year-old female who was involved in a 2 car MVA while driving on the job. She is complaining about some neck pain. She has tingling into her hand and her feet. She states that her arm hurts when she tries to pull it overhead. She apparently was told by a friend that she should see a spine doctor, but somehow she came to see me first. PMH is remarkable for kidney trouble. Past bronchoscopy, laparoscopy, and kidney stone surgery, otherwise noncontributory as per the medical history form completed by the patient and reviewed at this visit.

O: Ht 5'5" Wt. 179 lbs. R 16. Pt presented in a sling. She was told to use it by the same friend. She states if she does not use it her arm does not feel any different, so I had her remove it. On exam, the left shoulder demonstrates full passive motion. She has normal strength testing. She has no deformity. She has some tenderness over the trapezial area. The reflexes are brisk and symmetric. X-rays of her chest 2 views and C spine AP/LAT are relatively benign, as are complete X-rays of the shoulder.

A: Contusion of upper arm and shoulder

P: 1. MRI to rule/out torn ligament
      2. Rx Naprosyn.
      3. Referral to PT
      4. Referral to spine doctor.

_____

James Healer, MD

JHW/mg D: 9/16/05 09:50:16 T: 9/18/05 12:55:01

FIGURE 4-3
Physician's notes for Sasha White's encounter.

ICD-9-CM OFFICIAL GUIDELINES FOR CODING AND REPORTING

In Appendix B of this text, as well as in the front of your ICD-9-CM book, you will find the Official Guidelines for Coding and Reporting as issued by the Centers for Medicare & Medicaid Services (CMS) and the National Center for Health Statistics (NCHS), two departments within the U.S. federal government's Department of Health and Human Services (DHHS). You should read all of these pages carefully, so that you can become familiar with these rules. They will guide you toward the best, most accurate code and make it easier for you to make coding decisions.

The guidelines are divided into four sections:

I. ICD-9-CM Conventions, General Coding Guidelines, and Chapter-Specific Guidelines
II. Selection of Principal Diagnosis(es)
III. Reporting Additional Diagnoses
IV. Diagnostic Coding and Reporting Guidelines for Outpatient Services (outpatient services include procedures performed at physicians' offices)

All of these guidelines are the same for, and are applicable to, coding for both inpatient (patients admitted into the hospital) and outpatient (including outpatient departments, same-day surgical centers, and physicians' offices) with a few exceptions. These exceptions are important.

- Section II: Selection of Principal Diagnosis(es) for Inpatient, Short-Term, Acute Care Hospital Records—H. Uncertain Diagnosis. The guidelines state that, with regard to a diagnosis documented as "probable," "suspected," "likely," "questionable," "possible," or "still to be ruled out," you should "code the condition as if it existed or was established."

However, see the following section:

- Section IV: Diagnostic Coding and Reporting Guidelines for Outpatient Services—Paragraph I. The guidelines state, "Do not code diagnoses documented as "probable," "suspected," "questionable," "rule out," or "working diagnosis." Rather, code the condition(s) to the highest degree of certainty for that encounter/visit, such as symptoms, signs, abnormal test results, or other reasons for the visit."

These two rules are not conflicting. They are letting you know that, in this case, the rules are different when assigning diagnostic codes for a hospital inpatient than they are for a patient seen in a physician's office. You will have to learn only one set of rules. Which set will depend on what type of health care facility in which you are working.

Example

Our case study on page 66 of Dr. Healer's encounter with Sasha White is an excellent example of the differences in these rules. We did not code the torn ligament noted in the last portion of the notes (1. MRI to rule/out torn ligament) because this encounter was in the doctor's office. If Ms. White had been an inpatient in a hospital, the torn ligament would have been coded.

You should also note that there are specific guidelines and rules related to some of the individual sections of the ICD-9-CM book, as well. In Section I—Conventions, General Coding Guidelines and Chapter-Specific Guidelines, Part C, you will find detailed rules affecting your decisions when coding certain diseases, conditions, illnesses, and injuries. The headings, or sections, of the guidelines are very specific. They are

C1. A. Human Immunodeficiency Virus (HIV) Infections
C1. B. Septicemia, SIRS, and Septic Shock
C2. Neoplasms
C3. A. Diabetes mellitus
C7. A. Hypertension
C7. B. Cerebrovascular Accident (CVA)
C7. C. Postoperative cerebrovascular accident
C7. D. Late effects of cerebrovascular disease
C8. A. COPD and asthma
C8. B. COPD and bronchitis
C11. Complications of Pregnancy, Childbirth, and the Puerperium
C15. Newborn (Perinatal) Guidelines
C16. Sign, Symptoms, and Ill-defined conditions
C17. Injury and Poisoning
C18. Classification of Factors Influencing Health Status and Contact with Health Services (also known as V codes)
C19. Supplemental Classification of External Causes of Injury and Poisoning (also known as E codes)

Example

In Section C17, you would learn that a fracture not indicated in the physician's notes as open or closed should be coded as closed.

In addition to the guidelines, some coders find the American Hospital Association's *Coding Clinic for ICD-9-CM* very beneficial to accurate diagnostic coding.

CPT PROCEDURE CODING GUIDELINES

The official guidelines you will use to ensure that you are coding procedures correctly are presented in a different manner than those for the diagnosis coding in ICD-9-CM.

In your CPT book, you will notice gray-toned pages in front of each of the six sections of the book: Evaluation and Management; Anesthesia; Surgery; Radiology; Pathology and Laboratory; and Medicine. These gray pages identify important items that the coder must understand when assigning codes from each section.

Some of the guidelines provided to you in the gray pages are

- Evaluation and Management Services Guidelines, including the definitions of commonly used terms
- Surgery Guidelines, including a listing of services that are bundled into the surgical package definition
- Medicine Guidelines, including instructions on how to code multiple procedures and the proper use of add-on codes

Example

In the medicine section, home health procedure codes (99500–99600) are to be used for the services provided by non-physician health care professionals. When services are provided by a physician in the patient's home, the service should be coded as a home visit using E/M codes (99341–99350) in addition to regular CPT codes for procedures provided.

Take a minute to look through the CPT book and the gray pages before each of the sections of the book. You might also find the monthly newsletter, *CPT Assistant*, from the American Medical Association, to be helpful for up-to-date coding information.

RULES FOR ETHICAL AND LEGAL CODING

As a coder, you have a very important responsibility—to yourself, your patients, and your facility. The work you do results in the creation of health claim forms, which are legal documents. What you do can help your facility stay healthy (businesswise) or contribute to the business being fined and shut down by the Office of the Inspector General and your state's attorney general. It is important that you clearly understand the ethical and legal aspects of your new position. The following are some issues, with regard to the ethics and legalities of coding, with which you should become very familiar.

1. It is very important that the codes indicated on the health claim form represent the services actually performed and be supported by the notes and other documentation in the patient's health record. Don't use a code on a claim form without having the **supporting documentation** in the file.
2. Some health care providers **code for coverage**. This means that codes (both diagnostic and procedural codes) are not chosen for the best, most accurate code available but, rather, with regard to what procedures the insurance company will pay for, or "cover." This is dishonest and is considered fraud. If you find yourself in an office or a facility that insists you code for coverage rather than code to accurately reflect the documentation and the services actually performed, you should discuss this with your instructor or someone else you trust. Some providers will rationalize this process by saying they are doing it so the patient can get the treatment he or she really needs to be paid for by the insurance company. Altruism aside, it is still illegal.

Key Terms

Supporting documentation: The paperwork in the patient's file that corroborates the codes presented on the claim form for a particular encounter.

Coding for coverage: To change a code to fit what the insurance company will pay for, rather than accurately reflect the procedure that was performed.

Key Terms

Upcoding: Using a code on a claim form that indicates a higher level of service than that which was actually performed.

Double billing: Submitting two claims for one encounter.

Unbundling: Coding individual parts of a specific procedure instead of using one combination, or bundle, code that includes all of the components.

Correct Coding Initiative (CCI): A computerized system used by Medicare to prevent overpayment for procedures.

Mutually exclusive codes: Codes that are identified in the coding book as not permitted to be used on the same claim form with other specified codes.

3. If you find yourself in an office or a facility that insists that you include codes for procedures that you know, or believe, were never performed, talk to someone you trust about what you suspect. This might be a case of fraud. This includes **upcoding**—using a code that claims that a higher level of service was given than that which was actually performed. Upcoding is considered falsifying records. Even if all you do is simply fill out the claim form, it is still an unethical and illegal act.

Example

Using a code for a colonoscopy when a sigmoidoscopy was actually done is an example of upcoding. A colonoscopy is a much more complex procedure that requires patient preparation as well as anesthesia or a sedative. Therefore, it costs more to perform than a sigmoidoscopy, which can be done in the office with not much preparation and no sedation.

4. If you resubmit a claim that has been lost, make certain to identify it as a "tracer" or "second submission." If you don't, you might be found guilty of **double billing**—billing the insurance company twice for a service provided only once. This also constitutes fraud and can result in your getting into legal trouble.

5. It is not permissible to code and bill for individual (also known as component) services when a comprehensive or combination (bundle) code is available. This is referred to as **unbundling** and it is illegal. For Medicare billing, be certain to refer to the Medicare National **Correct Coding Initiative (CCI)**, which lists standardized bundled codes. The CCI is used to find coding conflicts, such as unbundling, the use of **mutually exclusive codes**, and other unacceptable reporting of CPT codes. Claims upon which these errors are discovered, are pulled for review and may be subject to possible suspension or rejection.

6. You must code all conditions or complications that are relevant to the current encounter. Failure to do this can be considered unethical.

Examples

The physician's notes indicate that the patient received an MMR vaccine. Reporting 90704 Mumps virus vaccine, 90705 Measles virus vaccine, and 90706 Rubella virus vaccine separately instead of using the combination code of 90707 Measles, Mumps, and Rubella virus vaccine would be unbundling and unethical.

In the CPT codebook, you'll find the instruction "Do not report 43752 in conjunction with critical care codes 99291-99292." In this case, the book is telling you it is unethical to place both 43752 and 99291 on the same claim form and your claim would most likely be rejected.

7. Separating the codes relating to one encounter and placing them on several claim forms over the course of several days is not legal or ethical. This not only indicates a lack of organization in the office but also can cause suspicion of duplicating service claims. Even if you are reporting procedures that were done for diagnoses that actually exist, remember that the claim form is a legal document. All data on that claim form, including dates of service, must be accurate. Do not submit the claim form until you are certain it is complete, with all the correct diagnosis and procedure codes listed. If, after you submit a claim, an additional service provided comes to light (such as a lab report with an extra charge that didn't come across your desk until after you filed the claim), then you must file an amended claim. While not illegal because you are identifying that this claim contains an adjustment, most third-party payers dislike amended claims. You can expect an amended claim to be scrutinized.

All of the previously mentioned activities are considered fraud and are against the law. HIPAA included the creation of the Health Care Fraud and Abuse Control Program. This program, under the direction of the attorney general and the secretary of the Department of Health and Human Services, acts in accordance with the Office of the Inspector General (OIG) and coordinates with federal, state, and local law enforcement agencies to catch those who attempt to defraud or abuse the health care system, including Medicare and Medicaid. In 2002, approximately $1.4 billion was returned to the Medicare Trust Fund and another $59 million in restitution was returned to Medicaid. In that year alone, 480 defendants were convicted for health care fraud–related crimes, and 3,448 individuals and organizations were forbidden from working with any federally sponsored programs (such as Medicare and Medicaid).

IMPORTANT NOTE

Always remember to read the complete descriptions in the provider's notes in addition to referencing the encounter form/superbill and then carefully find the best available code for medical necessity, according to the documentation. The American Health Information Management Association (AHIMA) offers a free e-newsletter called *CodeWrite Community News*. This monthly resource is free and has great articles on ICD-9-CM, ICD-10-CM, and CPT coding issues.

American Health Information Management Association (AHIMA) Code of Ethics

The American Health Information Management Association (AHIMA) is the preeminent professional organization for health information workers, including insurance coding specialists. The AHIMA House of Delegates designated the elements in Box 4-1 as being critical to the highest level of honorable behavior for its members.

BOX 4-1   AHIMA Code of Ethics

The following ethical principles are based on the core values of the American Health Information Management Association and apply to all health information management professionals.

Health information management professionals

1. Advocate, uphold, and defend the individual's right to privacy and the doctrine of confidentiality in the use and disclosure of information
2. Put service and the health and welfare of persons before self-interest and conduct themselves in the practice of the profession so as to bring honor to themselves, their peers, and the health information management profession
3. Preserve, protect, and secure personal health information in any form or medium and hold in the highest regard the contents of the records and other information of a confidential nature, taking into account the applicable statutes and regulations
4. Refuse to participate in or conceal unethical practices or procedures
5. Advance health information management knowledge and practice through continuing education, research, publications, and presentations
6. Recruit and mentor students, peers, and colleagues to develop and strengthen a professional workforce
7. Represent the profession accurately to the public
8. Perform honorably health information management association responsibilities, either appointed or elected, and preserve the confidentiality of any privileged information made known in any official capacity
9. State truthfully and accurately their credentials, professional education, and experiences
10. Facilitate interdisciplinary collaboration in situations supporting health information practice
11. Respect the inherent dignity and worth of every person

"This Code of Ethics sets forth ethical principles for the health information management profession. Members of this profession are responsible for maintaining and promoting ethical practices. This Code of Ethics, adopted by the American Health Information Management Association, shall be binding on health information management professionals who are members of the Association and all individuals who hold an AHIMA credential."

In this era of payment based on diagnostic and procedural coding, the professional ethics of health information coding professionals continues to be challenged. See Box 4-2 for standards of ethical coding, developed by AHIMA's Coding Policy and Strategy Committee and approved by AHIMA's board of directors, offered to guide coding professionals in this process.

BOX 4-2   AHIMA Standards of Ethical Coding

1. Coding professionals are expected to support the importance of accurate, complete, and consistent coding practices for the production of quality health care data.

2. Coding professionals in all health care settings should adhere to the ICD-9-CM (*International Classification of Diseases—9th revision—Clinical Modification*) coding conventions, official coding guidelines approved by the Cooperating Parties*, the CPT (*Current Procedural Terminology*) rules established by the American Medical Association, and any other official coding rules and guidelines established for use with mandated standard code sets. Selection and sequencing of diagnoses and procedures must meet the definitions of required data sets for applicable health care settings.

3. Coding professionals should use their skills, their knowledge of currently mandated coding and classification systems, and official resources to select the appropriate diagnostic and procedural codes.

4. Coding professionals should only assign and report codes that are clearly and consistently supported by physician documentation in the health record.

5. Coding professionals should consult physicians for clarification and additional documentation prior to code assignment when there is conflicting or ambiguous data in the health record.

6. Coding professionals should not change codes or the narratives of codes on the billing abstract so that meanings are misrepresented. Diagnoses or procedures should not be inappropriately included or excluded because payment or insurance policy coverage requirements will be affected. When individual payer policies conflict with official coding rules and guidelines, these policies should be obtained in writing whenever possible. Reasonable efforts should be made to educate the payer on proper coding practices in order to influence a change in the payer's policy.

---

*The Cooperating Parties are the American Health Information Management Association, American Hospital Association, Health Care Financing Administration, and National Center for Health Statistics. All rights reserved. Reprint and quote only with proper reference to AHIMA's authorship.

BOX 4-2   (Continued)

7. Coding professionals, as members of the health care team, should assist and educate physicians and other clinicians by advocating proper documentation practices, further specificity, and re-sequencing or inclusion of diagnoses or procedures when needed to more accurately reflect the acuity, severity, and occurrence of events.

8. Coding professionals should participate in the development of institutional coding policies and should ensure that coding policies complement, not conflict with, official coding rules and guidelines.

9. Coding professionals should maintain and continually enhance their coding skills, as they have a professional responsibility to stay abreast of changes in codes, coding guidelines, and regulations.

10. Coding professionals should strive for optimal payment to which the facility is legally entitled, remembering that it is unethical and illegal to maximize payment by means that contradict regulatory guidelines.

American Academy of Professional Coders (AAPC) Code of Ethical Standards

The American Academy of Professional Coders (AAPC) is another influential organization in the health information management industry. Their members, and their certifications, are well respected throughout the United States and the world. Their code of ethical standards (Box 4-3) also illuminates the importance of an insurance coding and billing specialist exhibiting the most ethical and moral conduct.

"This Code of Ethical Standards for members of the American Academy of Professional Coders strives to promote and maintain the highest standard of professional service and conduct among its members. Adherence to these standards assures public confidence in the integrity and service of professional coders who are members of the American Academy of Professional Coders. Failure to adhere to these standards may result in the loss of credentials and membership with the American Academy of Professional Coders."

(Copyright © 2004 American Academy of Professional Coders. All Rights Reserved.)

BOX 4-3   AAPC Code of Ethical Standards

Members of the American Academy of Professional Coders shall be dedicated to providing the highest standard of professional coding and billing services to employers, clients and patients. Behavior of the American Academy of Professional Coders members must be exemplary.

American Academy of Professional Coders members shall maintain the highest standard of personal and professional conduct. Members shall respect the rights of patients, clients, employers and all other colleagues.

Members shall use only legal and ethical means in all professional dealings, and shall refuse to cooperate with or condone by silence, the actions of those who engage in fraudulent, deceptive or illegal acts.

Members shall respect the laws and regulations of the land, and uphold the mission statement of the American Academy of Professional Coders.

Members shall pursue excellence through continuing education in all areas applicable to their profession.

Members shall strive to maintain and enhance the dignity, status, competence and standards of coding for professional services.

Members shall not exploit professional relationships with patients, employees, clients or employers for personal gain.

Above all else, we will commit to recognizing the intrinsic worth of each member.

CHAPTER SUMMARY

Once you assign a diagnosis code or procedure code to a patient's claim form, the form becomes a legal document and a permanent part of the patient's health care record. A mistake might result in some major problems for you, your health care facility, and even your patients. It is your responsibility, as a professional in the health information management industry, to assure that you always behave in an ethical and legal manner and protect yourself, your patients, and your facility.

Chapter Review

1. The seven steps to accurate coding are

    1. _____

    2. _____

    3. _____

    4. _____

    5. _____

    6. _____

    7. _____

2. The most important factor in coding is

    a. Speed of coding process

    b. Accuracy of codes

    c. Quantity of codes

    d. Level of codes

3. When you find unclear or missing information in the physician's notes, you should

    a. Ask a co-worker

    b. Figure out the information yourself; you should know what the doctor is thinking

    c. Query the physician

    d. Place the file at the bottom of the pile

4. Diagnostic codes identify

    a. What the provider did for the patient

    b. Who the policyholder is

    c. At which facility the patient was seen by the provider

    d. Why the patient saw the provider

5. Procedure codes identify

    a. What the provider did for the patient

    b. Who the policyholder is

    c. At which facility the patient was seen by the provider

    d. Why the patient saw the provider

6. Coding from superbills instead of physician's notes can cause the facility to

    a. Lose time

    b. Lose money by undercoding

    c. Lose money by delaying payments received

    d. All of the above

7. ICD-9-CM official guidelines

    a. Are generalized and do not provide details about any one section of the book

    b. Identify specific rules for coding

    c. Apply only to hospital coders

    d. Apply only to coders working in physicians' offices

8. ICD-9-CM official guidelines

    a. Must be memorized by professional coders

    b. Can be found in the front of every CPT book

    c. Can be found in the front of every ICD-9-CM book

    d. Can be found in the front of every ICD-9-CM section

9. CPT guidelines

    a. Must be memorized by professional coders

    b. Can be found in the front of every CPT section

    c. Can be found in the front of every CPT book

    d. Change every two months

10. An example of a CPT guideline is

    a. The proper way to read a superbill

    b. The way to determine the principle diagnosis

    c. The alphabetical listing of procedures and services

    d. The proper use of add-on codes

11. Changing a code to one you know the insurance company will pay for is called

    a. Coding for coverage

    b. Coding for packaging

    c. Unbundling

    d. Double billing

12. Unbundling is an illegal practice in which coders

    a. Bill for services never provided

    b. Bill for services with no documentation

    c. Bill using several individual codes instead of one combination code

    d. Bill using a code for a higher level of service than what was actually provided

13. Upcoding is an illegal practice in which coders

    a. Bill for services never provided

    b. Bill for services with no documentation

    c. Bill using several individual codes instead of one combination code

    d. Bill using a code for a higher level of service than what was actually provided

14. Medicare's Correct Coding Initiative (CCI) looks for

    a. Unbundling

    b. The improper use of mutually exclusive codes

    c. Unacceptable reporting of CPT codes

    d. All of the above

15. Coding improperly on a claim form can cause that claim to be

    a. Rejected

    b. Reviewed

    c. Suspended

    d. All of the above

Coding Diagnoses: ICD-9-CM

5

OBJECTIVES

- Explain the foundation of diagnosis codes using ICD-9-CM.

- Identify the best way to determine the key words located in physician's notes as they relate to the diagnoses for a specific encounter.

- Describe the rules regarding the determination of choosing the best, most appropriate code.

- Use the determined diagnosis codes for establishing medical necessity.

- Use the diagnosis codes for creating a valid claim form.

As mentioned in Chapter 4, the National Center for Health Statistics (NCHS) put together a committee to create the *International Classification of Diseases—9th revision—Clinical Modification* (ICD-9-CM)* in February 1977. The members of the committee represented a wide variety of organizations, including the American Hospital Association, the American College of Physicians, and the American Psychiatric Association. This revision was designed to serve as an indexing system to classify data relating to diseases. It was determined that a more precise listing of codes was needed to establish a more complete picture of patient care.

*Enhance the learning process by pairing this chapter with a current copy of the International Classification of Diseases—9th revision—Clinical Modification Volumes 1 and 2.

KEY TERMS

Alphabetic Index to Diseases
adverse reaction
anatomical site
causal condition
condition
eponyms
E (External cause) code
greatest specificity
highest degree of certainty
manifestation
neoplasm
Tabular List of Diseases
underlying condition
V code

The contents of ICD-9-CM translate almost everything that could affect the human body into three-, four-, and five-digit numbers. The ICD-9-CM code(s) placed onto a health care claim form specifically describe the reasons the individual has come to see the health care provider on a given day. The health claim form does not describe the individual's entire medical history, or any other condition, injury, or illness. As a coder, the only thing you are interested in is the specific explanation (diagnosis as determined by the health care provider) as to why an individual has consulted with a health care professional on a given day, along with any other conditions that might be related to this visit. The patient's chief complaint is usually a key element in properly coding this explanation.

The health care provider does not get paid according to which diagnosis codes are shown on the claim form, and the insurance company does not pay for anything with regard to the diagnosis directly. The payment is for service—the procedures performed. However, the insurance carriers must know what the concern or problem is with the individual in order to justify providing the indicated health care service at the time. For example, a health care provider gives a patient an injection. Don't you agree that there should be a good medical reason for giving that injection? This is called medical necessity.

Requiring medical necessity to be established helps make certain the health care provider is not just performing tests and giving injections for no good medical reason. The ICD-9-CM diagnosis codes explain *why* the individual came to see the physician and support the physician's rationale for providing the appropriate services (the *what* as explained by the CPT codes).

Medical necessity is one of the main reasons it is so important to code the diagnosis correctly. One small number off, and you could accidentally cause the claim to be rejected, because the diagnosis indicated by the wrong code would not rationalize or justify the procedure that was actually done.

Memory Tip

ICD-9-CM codes = *why* the patient saw the provider

Example

Sarita is 33 weeks pregnant and having trouble with her legs. Dr. Timmons diagnoses her with varicose veins and prescribes physical therapy. The coder was in a hurry and reported 571.0 for the diagnosis code. The claim was denied. Here's why:

571.0 Alcoholic fatty liver

The correct code is 671.0 Varicose veins of legs

One number—big difference!

GETTING READY TO CODE

First, let's discuss the parts of the ICD-9-CM book, so you can understand where to look to find the best, most appropriate code. There are three sections in the book, referred to as volumes.

Volume 1, the **Tabular List of Diseases**, is the section of the book that lists all of the ICD-9-CM codes, in numerical order from 001 to 999.9, then the V codes V01–V85.4, and then E codes E800–E999.1. (More details about V and E codes, in the pages to come.)

Volume 2 is the **Alphabetic Index to Diseases**, the alphabetical portion of the book that lists all of the diagnoses in alphabetical order. Diagnoses are listed by

- **Condition**
- **Anatomical site**
- **Eponyms**
- Other descriptors (such as history)

In the back of Volume 2 is Section 2, which contains the

- Table of Drugs & Chemicals
- Index to External Causes, the alphabetical listing for the causes of injury and poisoning

---

IMPORTANT NOTE

Volume 1—Tabular List of Diseases is located after Volume 2—Alphabetic Index to Diseases in your ICD-9-CM book.

Volume 3, **the Procedure Classification**, is typically used only by hospitals to code inpatient services. These are the ICD-9-CM procedure codes that some hospitals use instead of CPT procedure codes. The first part is the alphabetic listing, followed by the numerical listing. We will discuss this section further in Chapter 8.

IMPORTANT NOTE

ICD-9-CM Volume 3 lists procedure codes, in alphabetical order, then numerical order, which hospitals use instead of CPT procedure codes.

Many physicians' offices are specialized, so you will most likely be working with a limited number of sections within the ICD-9-CM book. This will make the entire process of coding from the huge ICD-9-CM book less intimidating. However, because you do not know what type of health care facility you will be working in, and you may go to work in a hospital or clinic that typically sees a wide range of illnesses and injuries, this text will cover the entire spectrum.

Key Terms

Tabular List of Diseases: The portion of the ICD-9-CM book listed in numerical order.

Alphabetic Index to Diseases: The portion of the ICD-9-CM book listed in alphabetical order from *A* to *Z*.

Condition: The situation, such as infection, fracture, or wound.

Anatomical site: The place in the body, such as the knee or heart.

Eponyms: A condition named after a person, such as Epstein-Barr syndrome or Cushing's disease.

Example

If you are working for a gastroenterologist you would rarely use codes for Mental disorders 290–319.

Particularly for inexperienced coders, it is easiest to look in Volume 2, the alphabetic listing, first to find the diagnosis, as indicated by the key words in the physician's notes. Once you find the diagnosis in the alphabetic listing, use the code number shown to look in Volume 1, the tabular (numeric) listing. This is very important because the tabular listing may have additional information that makes another code more accurate.

You use the alphabetical listings to get to the correct page or area in the tabular (numerical) volume. From there, you need to look around in the tabular (numerical) listings, so you can make certain that you find the best code, to the highest level of specificity, according to the physician's notes for an individual encounter. You must look up to the beginning of the category, where the three-digit code is shown, and as far down as you need to in order to be certain you have the best code. Read all of the notations carefully: the "includes" notations; "excludes" notations; as well as any instructions to "code additional" aspects; or to "code first" an underlying condition.

When you begin, you will find that looking for a diagnosis in the alphabetic listing is not as easy as it sounds. Remember that accuracy is the most important issue. It is not a race. You need to be careful and meticulous. Sometimes you find the code right away; other times, it is like looking for a contact lens on a carpet—you have to look very carefully. The first thing to do is break apart the diagnosis, as noted by the physician. If you recall from Chapter 4, this is called abstracting the physician's notes.

Let's look at a sample diagnosis: *family history of colon cancer.* There are four key words: *family, history, colon,* and *cancer.* Let's take them one at a time.

CANCER: If we look up *cancer* in the alphabetical listing, we find that the ICD-9-CM book refers us to *neoplasm, by site, malignant.* You know from medical terminology class that *malignant neoplasm* is the proper term for what is commonly called cancer. However, you must note that this individual does not *have* a malignant neoplasm, just a family history. If you follow this lead and go to the neoplasm listings, you will see that none of the headings match family history. The column headings malignant, benign, uncertain behavior, and unspecified are the only ones shown. Nothing indicates a family history. You now know that this part of the diagnosis will not lead to the correct ICD-9-CM code for this patient.

Let's go to the next word in the diagnosis.

COLON: When you look up the word *colon* in the alphabetic listing, the book directs you to *see condition.* This does not mean to go to the listing for the word condition; it means that you should go back to the physician's notes and look for the condition of this patient's colon. What is wrong with his colon? Well, there isn't anything in the notes indicating there is something wrong with his colon. So this is not going to get you any closer to the correct code. Don't get frustrated. Look at this as a treasure hunt. The correct answer is in the book; you just have to find it. Let's go to the next word in the diagnosis—*family.*

Key Term

Neoplasm: Abnormal tissue; malignant neoplasm is another term for cancer; carcinoma is any of a variety of types of malignant neoplasms.

FAMILY: Next to the word *family* you see the book directs you to *see also condition*. Underneath, you see codes indicated for . . .

> **Family, familial**—*see also* condition
>   disruption V61.0
>   Li-Fraumeni (syndrome) V84.01
>   planning advice V25.09
>   problem V61.9
>   specified circumstance NEC V61.8
> retinoblastoma (syndrome) 190.5
>
> None of these descriptions match what we are looking for.

Because the diagnoses specifically mentioned under the word *family* don't match the physician's notes, you need to move on to the last key word in the diagnosis.

HISTORY: Looks like we struck gold! There are over a page and a half of diagnosis codes listed under the word *history (personal) of*. So, what kind of history does this individual have? A *family* history. Look down the column under the word *history* until you get to *family*.

You will notice that beneath the word *family*, there is an indented column, in alphabetical order, of codes for conditions that individuals might have a family history of. Look down the listing to see if the word *colon* appears. It does not. That's because you can't have a family history of having a colon. Just about everyone has one. What does this individual actually have? He has a *family history* of a *malignant neoplasm* (cancer) of the colon. Let's continue down the list.

> History
>   Family
>   Malignant neoplasm (of) NEC V16.9.

This translates to a Family History of a Malignant Neoplasm <u>N</u>ot <u>E</u>lsewhere <u>C</u>lassified (NEC). But, that's not your situation. Keep going down the new indented list under *malignant neoplasm:*

> Colon V16.0. We found it!

IMPORTANT NOTE

When looking through these long lists with lots of indentations, you must be conscientious and go down the columns carefully. Use a ruler or your finger to keep things in line.

Each word or phrase indented below another word or phrase includes the one above. Look above to Family indented once under the heading History. You read this as Family History. Then, Malignant neoplasm is indented once under Family, which is indented once under History. So, we read this as Family History of Malignant Neoplasm. This can get a little confusing, so use a ruler or your finger to keep track of what is indented at which level. If you let your eyes jump ahead, you might accidentally look at the next column under History, which says malignant neoplasm (of) V10.9. If you look at the indentations of the columns, you will see that this means History of Malignant Neoplasm (indicating that the patient him- or herself had been previously diagnosed) and not *Family* History of a Malignant Neoplasm (indicating that someone in the family, not this individual, was diagnosed)—a big difference. Of course, you would be able to catch this mistake as soon as you went to the tabular (numeric) listing to check the V10 code, as it specifically states V10 *Personal history of malignant neoplasm* in comparison with V16 *Family history of malignant neoplasm.*

Now, we can turn to the numeric listings (Volume 1—Tabular) to make certain V16.0 is the best, most specific code available. It matches the physician's notes perfectly, so we know we have the correct code.

IMPORTANT NOTE

Never code from the alphabetical listings (Volume 2—Alphabetic Index to Diseases). *Always check* the tabular listing before deciding on the best code.

THREE CATEGORIES OF ICD-9-CM DIAGNOSTIC CODES

ICD-9-CM Codes

The majority of the ICD-9-CM book contains ICD-9-CM codes, which are three-, four-, and five-digit numbers that directly connect to specific, confirmed diagnoses of illness (disease) or injury. These codes specifically define why the individual met with the health care professional.

V Codes

Sometimes individuals go to see a health care provider without any particular illness or injury. It may be for services to ensure they continue to be healthy, such as a flu shot or an annual physical. Perhaps an individual has a personal history of a particular disease and wishes to get tests to assure that the disease has not returned, or he or she has a family history that might cause the person to be watchful. Because the individual does not have any illness or disease, you cannot use a standard ICD-9-CM code. However, you must have a diagnosis code to justify performing a test on, or giving an injection to, the individual. A standard ICD-9-CM code would indicate a confirmed diagnosis. You must, instead, use a **V code.**

Key Term

V code: Code used to describe an encounter between a provider and an individual without a specific current health care illness or injury.

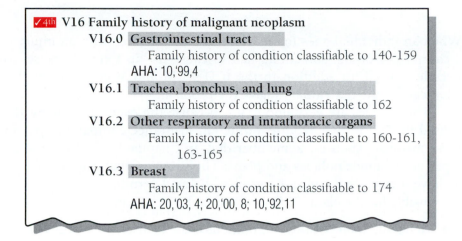

FIGURE 5-1
V Code for family history of malignant neoplasm.

Example

Harriet, a 22-year-old female, goes to her physician's office for a mammogram because she has a family history of malignant neoplasm of the female breast (breast cancer). The appropriate code would *not* be:

174 Malignant neoplasm of female breast

Using this code would indicate that Harriet has been confirmed to have a diagnosis of breast cancer, but she does not. The physician's notes do state that she has a family history of malignant neoplasm of the breast. Therefore, the correct code (Figure 5-1) is

V16.3 Family history of malignant neoplasm, breast

Take a few minutes to look through the V code section in the tabular listing of the ICD-9-CM book. Get a feeling for the category headlines and sections. The descriptions for all V codes are included in Volume 2, the Alphabetic Index to Diseases, so the ICD-9-CM book will guide you as to when to use them.

Example

V codes cover screenings, such as a mammogram or a colonoscopy; preventive medicines, such as vaccinations; fertility testing and treatments; prenatal checkups; and well-baby exams.

Memory Tip
V in **V** code stands for pre**V**entive.

CASE STUDY

Drew just found out that his son's best friend has come down with a case of rubella. His son was over at his house, playing, just two days ago. So, Drew takes his son to his pediatrician to get checked. Dr. Morgan writes in his notes that the reason for the visit was Exposure to Rubella. What is the best ICD-9-CM code to use on the claim form?

The correct code is: V01.4 Exposure to Rubella.

E Codes

Key Term

E (External cause) code: A code that explains *how* an injury or poisoning happened, and/or *where* it happened.

When an individual goes to see a health care provider with an injury or a case of poisoning, something had to cause it—an External cause. An **E code** is used, in addition to the ICD-9-CM and V codes, to explain what caused the individual to have the problem.

These codes are very important, because the event or element that caused the injury may require a different insurance company to pay for these medical expenses. Remember that, in Chapter 1, we discussed the types of insurance policies and plans. The situation that caused a person to have a fractured arm, for instance, helps determine which policy is responsible for the claim. If the individual hit her head

- *At work,* then Workers' Compensation insurance would pay the medical bills, not the health care plan
- While *shopping at a store,* the store's liability insurance might pay for the medical bills
- *In an automobile accident,* then her automobile insurance would probably be billed
- After slipping in her bathtub *in her own home,* then her health care policy would be billed

Therefore, you, as an insurance coder, must explain what happened, so the billing personnel and the insurance company will know who is responsible for these medical bills. The way you tell them is by adding an E code after the diagnosis code.

To make it easier to find the correct E code, Section 2 of Volume 2 has a separate Index to External Causes. This is the alphabetic listing of all the possible situations that might cause an injury or a poisoning to a human. Then, you can confirm that code in the E code section of the tabular listing.

IMPORTANT NOTE

In some circumstances, you need to include two E codes to tell the whole story—the how and the where.

In some cases, one E code will include both the cause and the location, such as (Figure 5-2)

E816 Motor vehicle traffic accident due to loss of control, without collision on the highway

This E code includes both the how (motor vehicle accident) and the where (on the highway).

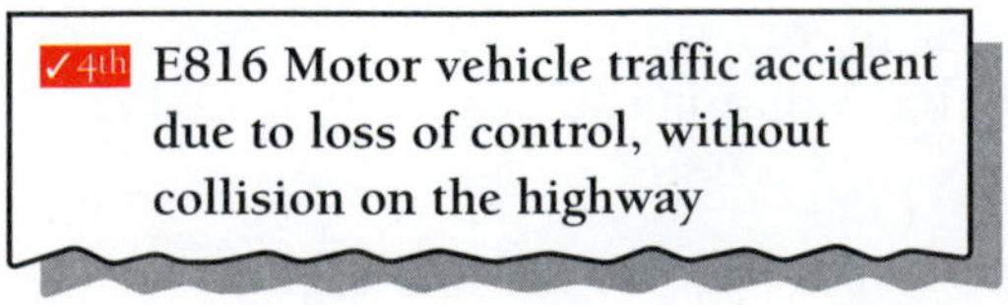
✓4th **E816 Motor vehicle traffic accident due to loss of control, without collision on the highway**

FIGURE 5-2
Example of one E code including both How and Where.

Remember, the main purpose of the E code is to help guide you in your determination as to which insurance policy should be responsible for paying the claim. Therefore, be certain you know the whole story, so your codes can tell the whole story. Although E codes are not required in all states, including them on your health care claim form will speed the process and get your claim paid faster, and that's what this is all about!

IMPORTANT NOTE

An E code can never be a principal, or first-listed, code. In other words, it cannot be first on a claim form.

Occasionally, the ICD-9-CM book reminds you to include an E code. However, you should learn when an E code is needed, because they are not included in the main alphabetic listing. Remember, they have their own alphabetic list in Volume 2, Section 2. This means that you have to look them up separately from the other diagnosis codes.

Examples

If a person comes to the physician's office with a brain concussion, something external had to hit her in the head, or bang against her head, to cause that concussion. One doesn't just wake up one day with a concussion. One can't catch a concussion from someone else, and one can't inherit a concussion from one's parents. An E code explains what caused the injury.

Keith sprains his ankle, falling from a ladder while changing a lightbulb in the foyer of his home. You need the codes:

845.00 Sprained ankle unspecified site.

E881.0 Fall from ladder

E849.0 Place of occurrence, home

Now, you and the insurance carrier will know that Keith's medical bills will be the responsibility of his own health insurance plan.

Memory Tip

The **E** code explains the **E**xternal cause of an individual's injury or poisoning.

CASE STUDY

Eric was walking barefoot through his living room when he jammed his toe against the leg of the coffee table. He was in so much pain, he went to his doctor. The X-ray confirmed a fracture of the great toe (closed). What are the best, most appropriate ICD-9-CM code(s)?

The correct codes are: 826.0 Fracture of one or more phalanges of foot (closed)

E917.3 striking against furniture without subsequent fall

E849.0 Place of occurrence, home

THREE, FOUR, OR FIVE NUMBERS—HOW DO YOU KNOW?

Key Term

Greatest specificity: The most detail available.

The primary purpose of coding is to be able to describe, with the **greatest specificity**, what is going on with regard to an individual. You need to explain, in as much detail as possible, exactly why the provider saw the patient. Five-digit codes have more detail, or specificity, than four-digit codes, which have more detail, or specificity, than three-digit codes.

> **IMPORTANT NOTE**
>
> The letter in V codes counts as a digit, but the E in E codes does not.

Three Digits

Each condition, illness, or injury is divided into a separate category identified by a three-digit number. Sometimes the three-digit number is all that is needed, as in the case of ICD-9-CM code (Figure 5-3)

> 325 Phlebitis and thrombophlebitis of intracranial venous sinuses

This three-digit code is complete and requires no further information or detail.

FIGURE 5-3

Example of a complete three-digit code.

> 325 Phlebitis and thrombophlebitis of intracranial   **cc**
>   venous sinuses
>
> | Embolism | } of cavernous, lateral, or |
> | Endophlebitis | other intracranial |
> | Phlebitis, septic or suppurative | or unspecified |
> | Thrombophlebitis | intracranial |
> | Thrombosis | venous sinus |

Example

Alexander, a 56-year-old male, is seen at the physician's office and diagnosed with unspecified bronchitis. When you look for bronchitis in the alphabetic listing, you see the code 490. Because there are no other specifications to the bronchitis, you will go with the Bronchitis (simple) 490. When you turn to the numerical listing for 490, you see *Bronchitis, not specified as acute or chronic.* As you look down the column, you find this definition is best and most specifically matches the physician's notes. Therefore, the three-digit code 490 is correct.

> **IMPORTANT NOTE**
>
> ICD-9-CM books are printed by several different publishers. Each publisher uses their own colors and symbols for notations throughout the book. For example, in the following pages, we will review red boxes that direct you to add a digit to the code. Some publishers use black boxes, others a circle through a line Ø. Don't let this throw you—they will all direct you to the best code.

Four Digits

In some cases, a fourth digit is required to indicate a more specific description. In these cases, you will see a small red box with a check mark and "4th" next to the three-digit code ✓4th or a red dot ● that directs you to the legend across the bottom of the page that a fourth digit is needed. Let's use our example from before, the individual with the diagnosis of a family history of a malignant neoplasm of the colon. You found code V16.0 in the alphabetic listing and now must go to Volume 1, the numeric listing, to make certain this is the best, most specific code available.

✓4th V16 Family history of malignant neoplasm

You will notice the small red box with the check mark and the "4th" next to the V16. This reminds you that you must keep reading to find the correct four-digit code. If you continue reading down the column, you will see codes

V16.0 Gastrointestinal tract

V16.1 Trachea, bronchus and lung

V16.2 Other respiratory and intrathoracic organs

V16.3 Breast

The details you will need in order to determine which code is correct should be found in the physician's notes. In this example, the notes state that the family history was of a malignant neoplasm of the colon. You should remember from your anatomy course that the colon is part of the gastrointestinal tract. Therefore, V16.0 is the correct four-digit code for this diagnosis.

To make certain that this is the correct code, take a look at the notation under the V16.0 gastrointestinal tract listing: Family history of condition classifiable to 140–159. Let's use this note to double-check your work and go to code 140 Neoplasm. As you look through all the following codes, you get to code 153 Malignant neoplasm of colon. Code 153 is within the range shown, 140–159. Now you can be certain that the code V16.0 is the correct diagnosis code for an individual with a family history of colon cancer.

CASE STUDY

Abby, a 19-year-old female, was having a really bad time emotionally. Her counselor referred her to a psychiatrist, Dr. Crandle. After a thorough series of tests, Dr. Crandle diagnosed Abby with chronic paranoid psychosis, a delusional disorder.

What is the best, most accurate ICD-9-CM code?

Abby's diagnosis would be indicated with the code _____

297.1 Delusional disorder.

Five Digits

When an additional level of detail is available, a fifth digit is needed for the ICD-9-CM code. Similar to the fourth-digit red box, the need for the fifth digit is indicated by a similar red box, with a check mark and a "5th" next to the four-digit code ✓5th. A good example of this is the ICD-9-CM code

✓4th 368 Visual disturbances

Next to the 368 code is a red box with a check mark and "4th" next to it. This tells you that a fourth digit is required, so you keep reading down the column. The next code shown is

✓5th 368.0 Amblyopia ex anopsia

You can see that next to the 368.0 is a red box with a check mark and "5th." This tells you that you need to give even more detail with a fifth digit. When you keep reading down the column, you see codes

368.00 Amblyopia, unspecified

368.01 Strabismic amblyopia

368.02 Deprivation amblyopia

368.03 Refractive amblyopia

The red boxes that indicate a fourth or fifth digit are not suggestions: these boxes are telling you that the extra digit *is required*. They are helping guide you to the best, most appropriate code. If the extra digit is required and you do not include it, your claim will be denied.

IMPORTANT NOTE

A ✓4th box or a ✓5th box is *not* a suggestion for an additional digit. It means you *must* keep looking for a more specific code—a code with that additional digit.

Consider Barbara, a 15-year-old female, seen by her physician and diagnosed with non-organic bulimia. In the alphabetic listings, you see *Bulimia non-organic origin 307.51*. You go to the numerical listing for

✓4th 307 Special symptoms or syndromes, not elsewhere classified

and see that a fourth digit is required. As you move down the column, you find

✓5th 307.5 Other and unspecified disorders of eating

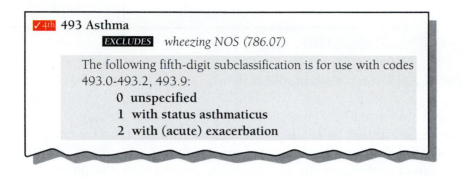

FIGURE 5-4
Boxes contain information that can apply to several diagnosis codes.

This requires a fifth digit, as indicated by the red box. You move farther down the column and see

307.51 Bulimia nervosa, overeating of non-organic origin

This matches the physician's notes, so you now know this is the correct five-digit code:

307.51 Bulimia, non-organic origin

On some pages in the ICD-9-CM book, you will find the fourth or fifth digit not by reading farther down in the column but, rather, by reading up—toward the top of the column, page, or sometimes to the page beforehand—to a pink box. This saves space when the addition of this digit means the same additional information for many different codes. A good example is ICD-9-CM code

✓4th 493 Asthma

showing the red box requiring a fourth digit. As you read down the column, you see a pink box (Figure 5-4).

Reading farther down the column, you see the definitions for the four-digit codes in this category.

✓5th 493.0 Extrinsic asthma

✓5th 493.1 Intrinsic asthma

✓5th 493.2 Chronic obstructive asthma

✓5th 493.8 Other forms of asthma

✓5th 493.9 Asthma, unspecified

All of these four-digit descriptions show red boxes with check marks and "5th" next to them. Here, you must first read down from the three-digit code to find your fourth digit. Then go back up, reading toward the top of the page, to find your fifth-digit code in the box.

Now, let's look at a case that will help us practice what we have learned so far.

CASE STUDY

Bobby Appleton is a 6-year-old male who is being seen in the office by his regular primary care physician for an open wound on his upper arm. Bobby's mother, Janet, tells the doctor that a strange dog from the neighborhood bit the boy, causing the wound. They do not know where the dog lives. It seems wild, or certainly has not been cared for in quite a while, and the people in the area believe the dog to be a stray. The doctor concludes from this scenario that the child should be treated as if he has been exposed to rabies.

Which key words will you use to find the ICD-9-CM codes? What are the best, most appropriate codes?

_____

_____

Begin by pulling out the elements of the diagnosis: open wound on upper arm. The key words are *open, wound, upper arm*. In the alphabetic listing, you see no description for *upper arm*, and *arm* directs us to *see condition*. That would be the wound. Wound, open is actually one listing. You read down the column to Arm, and indented under the word *arm* you find Upper 880.03. That sounds pretty good, so let's go to the numerical listing to confirm (Figure 5-5).

The code

✓4th 880 Open wound of shoulder and upper arm

indicates the need for a fourth digit. You have to look down past the pink box to find the four-digit choices. Because the physician's notes make no mention of complications, you will add the fourth digit of zero.

✓5th 880.0 Open wound of shoulder and upper arm without mention of complication

FIGURE 5-5
Numeric listing for wound, open, upper arm.

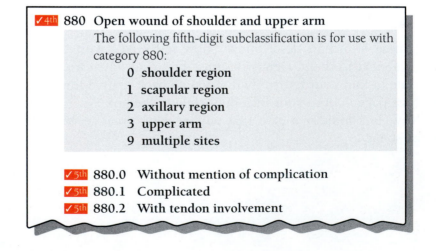

✓4th 880 **Open wound of shoulder and upper arm**
          The following fifth-digit subclassification is for use with category 880:

          0 shoulder region
          1 scapular region
          2 axillary region
          3 upper arm
          9 multiple sites

✓5th 880.0 **Without mention of complication**
✓5th 880.1 **Complicated**
✓5th 880.2 **With tendon involvement**

So far, this code description is in agreement with the notes. However, you will see that this code requires a fifth digit. You have to look back up the column, to the box, to find your choices. You know from the physician's notes that the boy's wound is on his upper arm. This leads you to the fifth digit of 3. This gives you the final, correct code of

880.03 Open wound of upper arm without mention of complication

You know that a wound is an injury, not an illness. Therefore, you must explain what external factor caused the wound. This means that you need to add an E code.

1. Go back to the physician's notes and see that the child's wound was the result of being bitten by a dog.
2. Go to the alphabetic listing and look up dog bite. Wow, it's actually right there, under D for Dog bite—see Wound, open, by site. This notation is the book directing us back to the wound itself, not an E code. Hmmm. If you look under B for Bite(s), then animal, the book gives you the same instruction. The reason this does not lead to an E code is because you mistakenly used the Alphabetic Index to Diseases (the regular alphabetic listing), not the E code alphabetic listings (Index to External Causes).
3. Remember, when an E code is needed, you must use the second alphabetic listing—the Index to External Causes in Volume 2, Section 2, right after the Table of Drugs & Chemicals. When you turn to the Index to External Causes and look under D for dog, it's right there.

Dog bite E906.0—of course, you should turn to the E code section in Volume 1 to double-check that this is the best available code, and it is!

IMPORTANT NOTE

When an E code is needed, you must use the separate alphabetic listing—the Index to External Causes in Volume 2, Section 2—immediately after the Table of Drugs & Chemicals.

Are you done? Not yet. You will remember that the physician's notes also mention that the dog is a stray and that the child has been exposed to rabies. When you go to the word *exposure* in the alphabetic listing and go down the column, you see

Exposure

   To

      Rabies V01.5

When you go to the V code section of the numerical listings, you can see that this is the correct code. The claim form for this encounter will show the three diagnoses codes: 880.03, E906.0, and V01.5. Now you are done. Good job!

Example

Dr. Hesse's notes state that Mrs. Alexander is diagnosed with unspecified asthma with acute exacerbation. What is the best ICD-9-CM code?

You first find the code for asthma, 493, and continue reading down the column to get the fourth digit, which is 493.9 for asthma, unspecified. Because a fifth digit is also required (as you can tell by the red box with the check mark and "5th" next to the 493.9 code), you move back up the page to the box and add the fifth digit for acute exacerbation. This gives you the final and correct code of

493.92 Asthma, unspecified, with acute exacerbation

WHAT TO CODE OR NOT CODE

The diagnosis codes that must be used on the health insurance claim form are the codes that explain or describe the answer to the question "Why did this individual come to see this health care provider today?" That is it. The health claim form does not relate the individual's medical history. Only the symptoms, conditions, problems, or complaints that directly correlate with why the individual is in this office on this day are to be coded and included on this health insurance claim form.

CASE STUDY

John Longenstein, a 48-year-old male, goes to see his physician because of a sore on his foot. He states that the sore has been present for three weeks and is not healing. John has a history of bronchial asthma. After examination, the physician notes that the patient has an ulcer on his right midfoot due to his type II diabetes.

First, *why did this individual come to see this health care provider today?* The reason is the ulcer on his foot. This is your first diagnosis code listed on the health insurance claim form. This is the principal—the number one—reason that the patient came to the physician's office today.

Second, you must include a code for the diabetes, because the diabetes is the **underlying condition** that has influenced this man's health and resulted in the ulcer.

Third, the patient has a history of bronchial asthma. The asthma would not be coded here because it has nothing to do with why the patient came to see the physician today. If the physician had addressed the asthma in any way (such as renewing a prescription), then you would code it. In this case, it is not coded.

Key Term

Underlying condition: One disease that affects or encourages another condition. Also referred to as a causal condition.

> ## IMPORTANT NOTE
>
> In some cases there are issues that are typically related to another diagnosis. In the ICD-9-CM book, this may be indicated by a small gray box, next to the code description with two letter Cs. `CC` stands for **c**omplication/**c**omorbidity. A small blue box with an MC in it `MC` means that this diagnosis code is a **m**ajor **c**omplication of another diagnosis. When the diagnosis code is for a condition that is either a complication or comorbidity element of an HIV-positive status, a small black box with "HIV" may also be present `HIV`. In all of these cases, these boxes indicate that an additional diagnosis code *may* be required.

Let's code this case by first going to look up Ulcer, foot in the alphabetic listing, Volume 2. The code 707.15 is indicated. Now, let's go to the tabular listing to double-check.

707.15 Ulcer of other part of foot `CC`

But wait, look right above that at

707.14 Ulcer of heel and midfoot `CC`

That matches the physician's notes exactly. This is another reminder why you should never code from the alphabetic listings. Also, did you notice the `CC` box? That's there to remind you to code the diabetes.

Look up the column, toward the descriptions for the four-digit version of this code:

707.1 Ulcer of lower limbs, except decubitus

and take a look at the notation below:

Code, if applicable, any causal condition first:
Diabetes mellitus (250.80–250.83)

This patient does have diabetes and, as noted by the physician, it is a causal, or underlying, condition. Let's go back to the alphabetic listings to (Figure 5-6)

Diabetes
Ulcer (skin) 250.8 ✓5ᵗʰ *[707.9]*

Keep looking. We always want to check our options.

Lower extremity 250.8 ✓5ᵗʰ *[707.10]*
Foot 250.8 ✓5ᵗʰ *[707.15]*

Ta da! Now not only do you have the code for the diabetes but you also have been able to verify the correct code for the ulcer. But you are not done yet. Remember that red box. You must go to the tabular listing and check for the fifth digit, and you find

250.80 Diabetes with other specified manifestations, type II, not stated as uncontrolled

FIGURE 5-6
Alphabetic listing showing
required secondary code.

ulcer (skin) 250.8 ☑ *[707.9]*
   lower extremity 250.8 ☑ *[707.10]*
      ankle 250.8 ☑ *[707.13]*
      calf 250.8 ☑ *[707.12]*
      foot 250.8 ☑ *[707.15]*
      heel 250.8 ☑ *[707.14]*
      knee 250.8 ☑ *[707.19]*
      specified site NEC 250.8 ☑ *[707.19]*
      thigh 250.8 ☑ *[707.11]*
      toes 250.8 ☑ *[707.15]*
   specified site NEC 250.8 ☑ *[707.8]*
   xanthoma 250.8 ☑ *[272.2]*

Are you done now? Yes, because the asthma does not get coded. It has nothing to do with this visit to the provider, so the claim form will show two diagnosis codes:

707.14

250.80

However, did you notice something? There is a notation underneath the 250.8 code listing. It says

Use additional code to identify **manifestation,** *as:*
Any associated ulceration (707.10–707.9)

Remember the notation underneath the 707.1 code listing. See what it says (Figure 5-7).

Code, if applicable, any causal condition first:
atherosclerosis of the extremities with ulceration (440.23)
diabetes mellitus (250.80–250.83)

Key Term

Manifestation: A condition caused by or developed from the existence of another condition, similar to a side effect.

FIGURE 5-7
Example of a Code First notation.

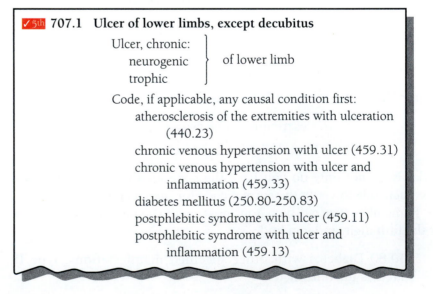

☑5th **707.1   Ulcer of lower limbs, except decubitus**

   Ulcer, chronic:
      neurogenic ⎫
            ⎬ of lower limb
      trophic ⎭

   Code, if applicable, any causal condition first:
      atherosclerosis of the extremities with ulceration
         (440.23)
      chronic venous hypertension with ulcer (459.31)
      chronic venous hypertension with ulcer and
         inflammation (459.33)
      diabetes mellitus (250.80-250.83)
      postphlebitic syndrome with ulcer (459.11)
      postphlebitic syndrome with ulcer and
         inflammation (459.13)

And even the alphabetic listing told us not only do we need two codes but it tells us in which order they need to be shown.

Foot 250.8 ✓5ᵗʰ [707.15]

That seems to directly apply to this case, doesn't it? Therefore, you must change the order of your codes and put the diabetes not the ulcer, first. Isn't it great the way the book tells you exactly how to do this properly? So, the claim form will show two diagnosis codes:

250.80

707.14

CASE STUDY

Ashley Matthews, a 33-year-old female, goes to see her regular physician, Dr. Montoya, in his office with complaints of coughing and feeling very weak. After the appropriate tests, Dr. Montoya diagnoses her with pneumonia due to streptococcus, unspecified. Ashley was found to be HIV positive two years ago.

How many diagnosis codes should be used? What are the best, most accurate codes?

_____

_____

There would be two ICD-9-CM codes shown on the health insurance claim form:

042 Human immunodeficiency virus [HIV] disease

482.30 Pneumonia due to streptococcus, unspecified

You must show both codes, because the 482.30 Pneumonia is a complication of the patient's 042 HIV condition. Also be aware of the notation that the ICD-9-CM book shows under the 042 code. This guides you to the fact that the 042 code must be assigned first, then the manifestation, the pneumonia.

IMPORTANT NOTE

Be certain to double-check the physician's notes before choosing any "other" or "unspecified" description of a code. Make sure that either the physician wrote the word *unspecified* or there really is no indication of any more detail. When possible, ask the physician for more information to increase your opportunity to avoid an unspecified code.

FIGURE 5-8
Example of Other Specified and
Unspecified code descriptions.

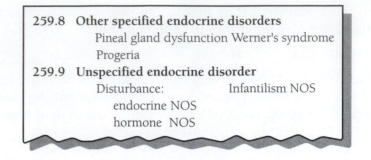

259.8   **Other specified endocrine disorders**
          Pineal gland dysfunction Werner's syndrome
          Progeria
259.9   **Unspecified endocrine disorder**
          Disturbance: Infantilism NOS
            endocrine NOS
            hormone NOS

You will see *unspecified* and other types of vague code descriptions in a few different ways, such as (Figure 5-8):

259.8 *Other specified* endocrine disorders

This means that the physician did specify the dysfunction but the ICD-9-CM book did not include the same detail in any of the other codes in the category. (In other words, none of the codes available 259.0–259.4 matched what the physician wrote.) This is a similar notation to NEC, Not Elsewhere Classified.

259.4 Dwarfism, *Not elsewhere classified*

Not Elsewhere Classified (NEC) means that the physician *did* specify the specific aspect of the condition but the ICD-9-CM book did not include the same detail in any of the other codes in the category.

259.9 *Unspecified* endocrine disorder

Unspecified means that the physician was not specific in his or her notes. *Never* assume or make up any detail of the description; if you have no more specific information available to you, you have to choose this code.

261 Nutritional marasmus, severe malnutrition NOS

Not Otherwise Specified (NOS) can mean the same thing as Unspecified indicating that the documentation did not mention additional detail.

There may be times when the ICD-9-CM book directs you with an *includes* or *excludes* notation (Figure 5-9). In these cases, below the description of the code, the notation will either: further describe other variations of the condition that is included in this code; or describe variations that are not included in this code, which means they are excluded.

FIGURE 5-9
Example of an Excludes notation.

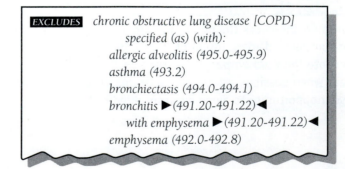

EXCLUDES   *chronic obstructive lung disease [COPD]*
                specified (as) (with):
            allergic alveolitis (495.0-495.9)
            asthma (493.2)
            bronchiectasis (494.0-494.1)
            bronchitis ▶*(491.20-491.22)*◀
                with emphysema ▶*(491.20-491.22)*◀
            emphysema (492.0-492.8)

CASE STUDY

Anita Carnahan is a 23-year-old female who is 18 weeks pregnant. She goes to see her OB-GYN physician, Dr. Harrison, because she has been vomiting quite a lot over the past few days. After a complete examination, Dr. Harrison diagnoses her with hyperemesis.

What are the best, most appropriate ICD-9-CM codes?

____

____

The alphabetical listing directs you to code

643 Excessive vomiting in pregnancy

When you continue to read, you will see the notation below that description

INCLUDES hyperemesis arising during pregnancy

The white box outlined in black shows the word *Includes* INCLUDES. This indicates that there are more descriptive words that are encompassed by this code. This tells you that you are in the correct category. Good work! (Figure 5-10.) These notations, along with all the others, are additional examples of how the ICD-9-CM book will guide you to the correct code, if you pay attention.

ICD-9-CM codes are to be used to indicate the **highest degree of certainty.** This means that those diagnoses that are not definite, those that are described as *probable, suspected, to be ruled out,* or *working,* are *not coded.* In these cases, you code only the symptoms, as directed by the *Official Guidelines Section IV: Diagnostic Coding and Reporting Guidelines for Outpatient Services* (e.g., physician's office, ambulatory surgery center, clinic).

Key Term

Highest degree of certainty: What we know for a fact.

✓4th **643 Excessive vomiting in pregnancy**

INCLUDES hyperemesis
vomiting:
persistent
vicious
} arising during pregnancy
hyperemesis gravidarum

FIGURE 5-10
Example of an Includes notation.

IMPORTANT NOTE

The coding guideline that states the coder should *not* code those conditions described as probable, suspected, rule out, or working is *only* for outpatient coding. This rule changes for those coding for inpatient treatments.

When variations of a diagnosis, or similar diagnoses, are not a part of a code or group of codes, the ICD-9-CM book may list those other conditions with an ▮EXCLUDES▮ notation. This black box with white letters will direct you to other, possibly better, codes depending upon what the physician has written.

Examples

A 9-year-old male is seen by the physician and diagnosed with enuresis. The physician does not know at this point in time what is causing the problem. The coder finds

307.6 Enuresis

You can't get much better than that, can you? Well, actually, if you continue reading, you will see the description Enuresis (primary) (secondary) of non-organic origin. The physician did not write in her notes that the origin (or cause) of the enuresis is non-organic, so this code may not be correct after all. If you keep reading, you will see the black box with the word *Excludes* ▮EXCLUDES▮ below the description. You then see

▮EXCLUDES▮ enuresis of unspecified cause (788.3). Aha!!

When you turn to 788.3, you see

✓5th 788.3 Urinary incontinence

    788.30 Urinary incontinence, unspecified

      Enuresis NOS

This matches the information in the physician's notes.

A patient was seen in the physician's office with a complaint of nausea and vomiting every morning; the physician will run a test to rule out pregnancy. Because the pregnancy is to be ruled out, and has not been confirmed, you would code only the vomiting and nausea. When a specific diagnosis has not yet been confirmed, you need to code the signs and/or symptoms, because the patient's symptoms are the only things you know for a fact.

787.01 Nausea with vomiting

Memory Tip

If you don't *know,* don't *code!*

NOTATIONS AND EXPLANATIONS

Punctuation is also used in ICD-9-CM to add information and to help you further in your quest for the best, most appropriate code.

[ ] These brackets show you alternate terms or phrases to provide additional detail or explanation to the description.

[ ] Italicized, or slanted, brackets surround additional code(s) (secondary codes) that *must* be included with the initial code. This notation will only show up in the alphabetic listing of ICD-9-CM.

( ) Parentheses show you additional descriptions, terms, or phrases that are also included in the description of a particular code.

: A colon (two dots, one on top of the other) emphasizes that the following descriptors are also included in the notation. This notation shows up only in the tabular (numerical) listing of ICD-9-CM.

} A brace indicates that a list of words or terms is affected by the word or phrase to the right of the brace.

MULTIPLE AND ADDITIONAL CODES

Sometimes a patient has several conditions or concerns at the same time. When the physician indicates more than one diagnosis, it is easier for you to know what additional codes are to be included on that health insurance claim form.

In this case, the physician's notes indicate the patient suffers from a fractured hand (closed) and a dislocated shoulder ligament (closed):

815.00 Fracture, of metacarpal bone(s), closed, site unspecified

831.00 Dislocation, shoulder, closed, unspecified

Therefore, you will have one code for the dislocation and an additional code for the fracture. Whenever, there are two diagnoses concurrently (at the same time) but one is not the result of, or caused by, the other, you put the codes onto the health insurance claim form in order of severity, with the more severe condition first. In our example, a fracture is more severe than a dislocation, so this claim form will place the fracture code as first-listed. (If you noticed that the above case would also require an E code to identify what caused the patient's dislocation and fracture, give yourself a cheer—good job!)

When a provider indicates a differential diagnosis using the word *versus* or *or* between two diagnostic statements, you need to code both as if they were confirmed.

FIGURE 5-11
Sometimes the ICD-9-CM book points you in a specific direction.

> **692.72 Acute dermatitis due to solar radiation**
> Berlogue dermatitis
> Photoallergic response
> Phototoxic response
> Polymorphus light eruption
> Acute solar skin damage NOS
> **EXCLUDES** *sunburn (692.71, 692.76-692.77)*
> Use additional E code to identify drug, if drug induced

There are times, however, when you will need to look for and code an underlying disease or condition that caused the reason the patient came to see the health care provider today. We reviewed this earlier in this chapter when we learned about major complications, coexisting conditions, and comorbidities. In addition to the small boxes indicating the possibility that another diagnosis is involved, the ICD-9-CM book will sometimes come right out and tell you when an additional code is necessary. Let's look at some codes that do exactly this.

330 Cerebral degenerations usually manifest in childhood. Use additional code to identify associated mental retardation.

This note is shown below the description of the code and not only directs you to add a code but also sends you in a specific direction (Figure 5-11).

333.3 Tics of organic origin. Use additional E code to identify drug, if drug induced.

Again, the ICD-9-CM book gives you fair warning that you might need an additional code.

590.81 Pyelitis or pyelonephritis in diseases classified elsewhere. Code first underlying disease as: tuberculosis (016.0).

This note is telling you that you need to code the disease or condition that existed first or perhaps caused the other diagnosis. When this is indicated, you put the diagnosis code 016.0 on the claim form first, followed by 590.81. Just as you saw with the patient suffering from a diabetic ulcer on his foot, the ICD-9-CM book is not only guiding you but also actually giving you the other code.

These notes are only included in the tabular section (Volume 1) of the ICD-9-CM book and not in the alphabetic listing (Volume 2). This is another good reason that you should *never code from Volume 2—the alphabetic listing*. However, these notations are not shown in all cases where a second code is required, so you will still have to read the physician's notes carefully.

The alphabetic listing (Volume 2) has a different way of letting you know that a second code is required (Figure 5-12). In these cases, next to the listing and code for a particular diagnosis, you may see a second code enclosed in brackets and italicized:

Epstein-Barr infection (viral) 075

chronic 780.79 *[139.8]*

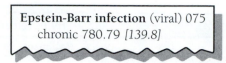

Epstein-Barr infection (viral) 075
chronic 780.79 [139.8]

FIGURE 5-12
Secondary diagnosis code shown in brackets.

The code shown first, 780.79, is actually described as Other malaise and fatigue. You may notice that there is no "Use additional code" or "Code first underlying disease" notation. The second code, shown in the italicized brackets, is

139.8 Late effects of other and unspecified infectious and parasitic diseases

This is an example of how the alphabetic listing (Volume 2) can help you code correctly as well. Again, you must then check both codes in the numeric listing to be certain both codes match the patient's condition, according to the physician's notes for this visit.

Example

Marjorie Katz was seen by her regular physician in his office with a complaint of chest pain and shortness of breath. Dr. Healer admitted her into the hospital with a differential diagnosis of congestive heart failure versus pleural effusion with respiratory distress. Here, you would code the

1. Congestive heart failure (428.0)
2. Pleural effusion (511.9)
3. Respiratory distress (786.09)

TABLES IN THE ALPHABETIC LISTINGS

There are three conditions in Volume 2, which include extended information using a multicolumn table within the listing. These tables are

- Hypertension (commonly referred to as high blood pressure)
- Neoplasms (commonly referred to as tumors, whether cancer or not)
- Drugs & Chemicals

Hypertension Table

When you turn to hypertension in the alphabetic listing (Figure 5-13), you see a three-column table to the right of the indented column of descriptions. The three columns are titled

- Malignant
- Benign
- Unspecified

You will first look down the column of descriptions to find the definition that matches the physician's notes. Then, once you have found the correct description, you will look across the line to the right to find the correct code.

	Hypertension, hypertensive		
	Malignant	**Benign**	**Unspecified**
Hypertension, hypertensive (arterial) (arteriolar) (crisis) (degeneration) (disease) (essential) (fluctuating) (idiopathic) (intermittent) (labile) (low renin) (orthostatic) (paroxysmal) (primary) (systemic) (uncontrolled) (vascular) ...	401.0	401.1	401.9
with			
heart involvement ▶(conditions classifiable to 429.0-429.3, 429.8, 429.9 due to hypertension)◀ (see also Hypertension, heart)	402.00	402.10	402.90
with kidney involvement—see Hypertension, cardiorenal			
renal involvement (only conditions classifiable to 585, 586, 587) (excludes conditions classifiable to 584)			
(see also hypertension, kidney)	403.00	403.10	403.90
renal sclerosis or failure	403.00	403.10	403.90
with heart involvement—see Hypertension, cardiorenal failure (and sclerosis)			
(see also Hypertension, kidney)	403.01	403.11	403.91
sclerosis without failure (see also Hypertension, kidney)	403.00	403.10	403.90
accelerated—(see also Hypertension by type, malignant)	401.0	—	—
antepartum—see Hypertension, complicating pregnancy, childbirth, or the puerperium			
cardiorenal (disease)	404.00	404.10	404.90
with			
heart failure	404.01	404.11	404.91
and renal failure	404.03	404.13	404.93
renal failure	404.02	404.12	404.92
and heart failure	404.03	404.13	404.93
cardiovascular disease (arteriosclerotic) (sclerotic)	402.00	402.10	402.90
with			
heart failure	402.01	402.11	402.91
renal involvement (conditions classifiable to 403) (see also Hypertension, cardiorenal)	404.00	404.10	404.90
cardiovascular renal (disease) (sclerosis) (see also Hypertension, cardiorenal)	404.00	404.10	404.90
cerebrovascular disease NEC	437.2	437.2	437.2
complicating pregnancy, childbirth, or the puerperium	642.2 ✓	642.0 ✓	642.9 ✓
with			
albuminuria (and edema) (mild)	—	—	642.4 ✓
severe	—	—	642.5 ✓
edema (mild)	—	—	642.4 ✓
severe	—	—	642.5 ✓
heart disease	642.2 ✓	642.2 ✓	642.2 ✓
and renal disease	642.2 ✓	642.2 ✓	642.2 ✓
renal disease	642.2 ✓	642.2 ✓	642.2 ✓
and heart disease	642.2 ✓	642.2 ✓	642.2 ✓
chronic	642.2 ✓	642.0 ✓	642.0 ✓
with pre-eclampsia of eclampsia	642.7 ✓	642.7 ✓	642.7 ✓
fetus or newborn	760.0	760.0	760.0
essential	—	642.0 ✓	642.0 ✓
with pre-eclampsia of eclampsia	—	642.7 ✓	642.7 ✓
fetus or newborn	760.0	760.0	760.0
fetus or newborn	760.0	760.0	760.0
gestational	—	—	642.3 ✓
pre-existing	642.2 ✓	642.0 ✓	642.0 ✓
with pre-eclampsia or eclampsia	642.7 ✓	642.7 ✓	642.7 ✓
fetus or newborn	760.0	760.0	760.0
secondary to renal disease	642.1 ✓	642.1 ✓	642.1 ✓
with pre-eclampsia or eclampsia	642.7 ✓	642.7 ✓	642.7 ✓
fetus or newborn	760.0	760.0	760.0
transient	—	—	642.3 ✓
due to			
aldosteronism, primary	405.09	405.19	405.99
brain tumor	405.09	405.19	405.99
bulbar poliomyelitis	405.09	405.19	405.99
calculus			
kidney	405.09	405.19	405.99
ureter	405.09	405.19	405.99
coarctation, aorta	405.09	405.19	405.99
Cushing's disease	405.09	405.19	405.99
glomerulosclerosis (see also Hypertension, kidney)	403.00	403.10	403.90
periarteritis nodosa	405.09	405.19	405.99
pheochromocytoma	405.09	405.19	405.99
polycystic kidney(s)	405.09	405.19	405.99
polycythemia	405.09	405.19	405.99
porphyria	405.09	405.19	405.99
pyelonephritis	405.09	405.19	405.99
renal (artery)			
aneurysm	405.01	405.11	405.91
anomaly	405.01	405.11	405.91
embolism	405.01	405.11	405.91
fibromuscular hyperplasia	405.01	405.11	405.91
occlusion	405.01	405.11	405.91
stenosis	405.01	405.11	405.91
thrombosis	405.01	405.11	405.91

FIGURE 5-13

The Hypertension Table, in part.

IMPORTANT NOTE

You still need to go to the numeric listing to double-check the code to be certain it is correct and has the correct number of digits (see Figure 5-13).

- *Malignant.* This is a rather unusual diagnosis, which signifies extremely high blood pressure accompanied by swelling of the optic nerve behind the eye (known as papilledema). Most typically, this condition is associated with other organ damage, such as heart failure, kidney failure, and hypertensive encephalopathy. This diagnosis occurs in only about 5% of all patients who have hypertension.
- *Benign.* This is a standard case of high blood pressure and is typically brought under control with medication and diet. This type of hypertension is fairly stable over many years.
- *Unspecified.* Choose codes in this column when the physician's notes do not include any specific information regarding the nature of the hypertension. However, this code should always be a last resort only after you have read all of the physician's notes thoroughly and/or spoken to the physician.

IMPORTANT NOTE

Even though 95% of all hypertension cases are benign, you cannot assume. Code benign or malignant only when the physician specifically uses these words in the notes. If the physician does not use either of those words, you must code the hypertension as unspecified.

CASE STUDY

A 65-year-old female is seen by the physician and diagnosed with hypertension. The physician's notes state that this is a result of her prior diagnosis of Cushing's disease.

How would you code this diagnosis?

_____

_____

First, go to the alphabetic listing and look under Hypertension. Look down the column and see *"due to"* (which is the same as "result of" stated in the physician's notes). Review the indented listing under *"due to"* until you get to *"Cushing's disease."* Now that you have found the basic description, according to the physician's notes, you need to look across the table to find the correct code. Look back at the physician's notes and you will see that this diagnosis was not specified as malignant or benign. Therefore, you are going to go all the way across and use

405.99 Hypertension, due to Cushing's disease, unspecified

Then, add 255.0 Cushing's syndrome

Remember, you are not to assume anything when you are coding. It can be very easy to look at these physician's notes and think, "Well, the physician didn't specify, and malignant hypertension is so unusual. I don't want to bother the doctor, so I will just code it as benign. I'm sure that's right." No. *Never assume.* Never put words in the mouth—or pen—of the physician. You can go only by what is documented in the patient's record. Ask the physician. If you cannot, then code only what you know.

Neoplasm Table

Turn to Neoplasm in the alphabetic listing and you will see a table as well (Figure 5-14). Neoplasms are listed by anatomical site in alphabetical order down the description column. This means that the first column is in order by the part of the body where the tumor is located. This table has six columns across: Primary, Secondary, Ca in Situ, Benign, Uncertain Behavior, and Unspecified. Let's review what each of these titles mean.

- *Primary.* This indicates the anatomical site (the place in the body) where the neoplasm originated—the first place a tumor was seen and identified as malignant. If the physician's notes do not specify primary or secondary, then the site mentioned is primary.
- *Secondary.* This identifies an anatomical site to which the malignant neoplasm has spread or metastasized. One very strange thing about cancerous cells is that they travel through the body and do not necessarily spread to adjoining body parts. Cancer can be identified primarily in the breast and metastasize to the liver, not actually interacting with anything in between. Notes will state that this site is "secondary to [primary site]," "metastasized from [primary site]," or "[primary site] metastasized to [secondary site]."
- *Ca in Situ.* This indicates that the tumor has undergone malignant changes but is still limited to the site where it originated and has not spread. Ca is short for carcinoma, and you can remember *situ* like the word *situated.* Think of this as cancerous cells that are staying in place.
- *Benign.* This means there is no indication of invasion of adjacent cells. Generally, *benign* means not cancerous.
- *Uncertain Behavior.* This classification indicates that the pathologist is not able to specifically determine whether this is benign or malignant, because indicators of both are present.
- *Unspecified.* Choose a code from this column when the physician's notes do not include any specific information regarding the nature of the tumor.

IMPORTANT NOTE

It can be easier, and more accurate, to look up the histologic type of malignancy, such as melanoma, before going to the neoplasm table.

Neoplasm, bone   Index to Diseases

Neoplasm, neoplastic — continued	Malignant Primary	Malignant Secondary	Malignant Ca in situ	Benign	Uncertain Behavior	Unspecified
bone — continued						
atlas	170.2	198.5	—	213.2	238.0	239.2
axis	170.2	198.5	—	213.2	238.0	239.2
back NEC	170.2	198.5	—	213.2	238.0	239.2
calcaneus	170.8	198.5	—	213.8	238.0	239.2
calvarium	170.0	198.5	—	213.0	238.0	239.2
carpus (any)	170.5	198.5	—	213.5	238.0	239.2
cartilage NEC	170.9	198.5	—	213.9	238.0	239.2
clavicle	170.3	198.5	—	213.3	238.0	239.2
clivus	170.0	198.5	—	213.0	238.0	239.2
coccygeal vertebra	170.6	198.5	—	213.6	238.0	239.2
coccyx	170.6	198.5	—	213.6	238.0	239.2
costal cartilage	170.3	198.5	—	213.3	238.0	239.2
costovertebral joint	170.3	198.5	—	213.3	238.0	239.2
cranial	170.0	198.5	—	213.0	238.0	239.2
cuboid	170.8	198.5	—	213.8	238.0	239.2
cuneiform	170.9	198.5	—	213.9	238.0	239.2
ankle	170.8	198.5	—	213.8	238.0	239.2
wrist	170.5	198.5	—	213.5	238.0	239.2
digital	170.9	198.5	—	213.9	238.0	239.2
finger	170.5	198.5	—	213.5	238.0	239.2
toe	170.8	198.5	—	213.8	238.0	239.2
elbow	170.4	198.5	—	213.4	238.0	239.2
ethmoid (labyrinth)	170.0	198.5	—	213.0	238.0	239.2
face	170.0	198.5	—	213.0	238.0	239.2
lower jaw	170.1	198.5	—	213.1	238.0	239.2
femur (any part)	170.7	198.5	—	213.7	238.0	239.2
fibula (any part)	170.7	198.5	—	213.7	233.0	239.2
finger (any)	170.5	198.5	—	213.5	238.0	239.2
foot	170.8	198.5	—	213.8	238.0	239.2
forearm	170.4	198.5	—	213.4	238.0	239.2
frontal	170.0	198.5	—	213.0	238.0	239.2
hand	170.5	198.5	—	213.5	238.0	239.2
heel	170.8	198.5	—	213.8	238.0	239.2
hip	170.6	198.5	—	213.6	238.0	239.2
humerus (any part)	170.4	198.5	—	213.4	238.0	239.2
hyoid	170.0	198.5	—	213.0	238.0	239.2
ilium	170.6	198.5	—	213.6	238.0	239.2
innominate	170.6	198.5	—	213.6	238.0	239.2
intervertebral cartilage or disc	170.2	198.5	—	213.2	238.0	239.2
ischium	170.6	198.5	—	213.6	238.0	239.2
jaw (lower)	170.1	198.5	—	213.1	238.0	239.2
upper	170.0	198.5	—	213.0	238.0	239.2
knee	170.7	198.5	—	213.7	238.0	239.2
leg NEC	170.7	198.5	—	213.7	238.0	239.2
limb NEC	170.9	198.5	—	213.9	238.0	239.2
lower (long bones)	170.7	198.5	—	213.7	238.0	239.2
short bones	170.8	198.5	—	213.8	238.0	239.2
upper (long bones)	170.4	198.5	—	213.4	238.0	239.2
short bones	170.5	198.5	—	213.5	238.0	239.2
long	170.9	198.5	—	213.9	238.0	239.2
lower limbs NEC	170.7	198.5	—	213.7	238.0	239.2
upper limbs NEC	170.4	198.5	—	213.4	238.0	239.2
malar	170.0	198.5	—	213.0	238.0	239.2
mandible	170.1	198.5	—	213.1	238.0	239.2
marrow NEC	202.9 ✓	198.5	—	—	—	238.7
mastoid	170.0	198.5	—	213.0	238.0	239.2
maxilla, maxillary (superior)	170.0	198.5	—	213.0	238.0	239.2
inferior	170.1	198.5	—	213.1	238.0	239.2
metacarpus (any)	170.5	198.5	—	213.5	238.0	239.2
metatarsus (any)	170.8	198.5	—	213.8	238.0	239.2
navicular (ankle)	170.8	198.5	—	213.8	238.0	239.2
hand	170.5	198.5	—	213.5	238.0	239.2
nose, nasal	170.0	198.5	—	213.0	238.0	239.2
occipital	170.0	198.5	—	213.0	238.0	239.2
orbit	170.0	198.5	—	213.0	238.0	239.2
parietal	170.0	198.5	—	213.0	238.0	239.2
patella	170.8	198.5	—	213.8	238.0	239.2
pelvic	170.6	198.5	—	213.6	238.0	239.2
phalanges	170.9	198.5	—	213.9	238.0	239.2
foot	170.8	198.5	—	213.8	238.0	239.2
hand	170.5	198.5	—	213.5	238.0	239.2
pubic	170.6	198.5	—	213.6	238.0	239.2
radius (any part)	170.4	198.5	—	213.4	238.0	239.2
rib	170.3	198.5	—	213.3	238.0	239.2
sacral vertebra	170.6	198.5	—	213.6	238.0	239.2

Neoplasm, neoplastic — continued	Malignant Primary	Malignant Secondary	Malignant Ca in situ	Benign	Uncertain Behavior	Unspecified
bone — continued						
sacrum	170.6	198.5	—	213.6	238.0	239.2
scaphoid (of hand)	170.5	198.5	—	213.5	238.0	239.2
of ankle	170.8	198.5	—	213.8	238.0	239.2
scapula (any part)	170.4	198.5	—	213.4	238.0	239.2
sella turcica	170.0	198.5	—	213.0	238.0	239.2
short	170.9	198.5	—	213.9	238.0	239.2
lower limb	170.8	198.5	—	213.8	238.0	239.2
upper limb	170.5	198.5	—	213.5	238.0	239.2
shoulder	170.4	198.5	—	213.4	238.0	239.2
skeleton, skeletal NEC	170.9	198.5	—	213.9	238.0	239.2
skull	170.0	198.5	—	213.0	238.0	239.2
sphenoid	170.0	198.5	—	213.0	238.0	239.2
spine, spinal (column)	170.2	198.5	—	213.2	238.0	239.2
coccyx	170.6	198.5	—	213.6	238.0	239.2
sacrum	170.6	198.5	—	213.6	238.0	239.2
sternum	170.3	198.5	—	213.3	238.0	239.2
tarsus (any)	170.8	198.5	—	213.8	238.0	239.2
temporal	170.0	198.5	—	213.0	238.0	239.2
thumb	170.5	198.5	—	213.5	238.0	239.2
tibia (any part)	170.7	198.5	—	213.7	238.0	239.2
toe (any)	170.8	198.5	—	213.8	238.0	239.2
trapezium	170.5	198.5	—	213.5	238.0	239.2
trapezoid	170.5	198.5	—	213.5	238.0	239.2
turbinate	170.0	198.5	—	213.0	238.0	239.2
ulna (any part)	170.4	198.5	—	213.4	238.0	239.2
unciform	170.5	198.5	—	213.5	238.0	239.2
vertebra (column)	170.2	198.5	—	213.2	238.0	239.2
coccyx	170.6	198.5	—	213.6	238.0	239.2
sacrum	170.6	198.5	—	213.6	238.0	239.2
vomer	170.0	198.5	—	213.0	238.0	239.2
wrist	170.5	198.5	—	213.5	238.0	239.2
xiphoid process	170.3	198.5	—	213.3	238.0	239.2
zygomatic	170.0	198.5	—	213.0	238.0	239.2
book-leaf (mouth)	145.8	198.89	230.0	210.4	235.1	239.0
bowel—see Neoplasm, intestine						
brachial plexus	171.2	198.89	—	215.2	238.1	239.2
brain NEC	191.9	198.3	—	225.0	237.5	239.6
basal ganglia	191.0	198.3	—	225.0	237.5	239.6
cerebellopontine angle	191.6	198.3	—	225.0	237.5	239.6
cerebellum NOS	191.6	198.3	—	225.0	237.5	239.6
cerebrum	191.0	198.3	—	225.0	237.5	239.6
choroid plexus	191.5	198.3	—	225.0	237.5	239.6
contiguous sites	191.8	—	—	—	—	—
corpus callosum	191.8	198.3	—	225.0	237.5	239.6
corpus striatum	191.0	198.3	—	225.0	237.5	239.6
cortex (cerebral)	191.0	198.3	—	225.0	237.5	239.6
frontal lobe	191.1	198.3	—	225.0	237.5	239.6
globus pallidus	191.0	198.3	—	225.0	237.5	239.6
hippocampus	191.2	198.3	—	225.0	237.5	239.6
hypothalamus	191.0	198.3	—	225.0	237.5	239.6
internal capsule	191.0	198.3	—	225.0	237.5	239.6
medulla oblongata	191.7	198.3	—	225.0	237.5	239.6
meninges	192.1	198.4	—	225.2	237.6	239.7
midbrain	191.7	198.3	—	225.0	237.5	239.6
occipital lobe	191.4	198.3	—	225.0	237.5	239.6
parietal lobe	191.3	198.3	—	225.0	237.5	239.6
peduncle	191.7	198.3	—	225.0	237.5	239.6
pons	191.7	198.3	—	225.0	237.5	239.6
stem	191.7	198.3	—	225.0	237.5	239.6
tapetum	191.8	198.3	—	225.0	237.5	239.6
temporal lobe	191.2	198.3	—	225.0	237.5	239.6
thalamus	191.0	198.3	—	225.0	237.5	239.6
uncus	191.2	198.3	—	225.0	237.5	239.6
ventricle (floor)	191.5	198.3	—	225.0	237.5	239.6
branchial (cleft) (vestiges)	146.8	198.89	230.0	210.6	235.1	239.0
breast (connective tissue) (female) (glandular tissue) (soft parts)	174.9	198.81	233.0	217	238.3	239.3
areola	174.0	198.81	233.0	217	238.3	239.3
male	175.0	198.81	233.0	217	238.3	239.3
axillary tail	174.6	198.81	233.0	217	238.3	239.3
central portion	174.1	198.81	233.0	217	238.3	239.3
contiguous sites	174.8	—	—	—	—	—
ectopic sites	174.8	198.81	233.0	217	238.3	239.3
inner	174.8	198.81	233.0	217	238.3	239.3
lower	174.8	198.81	233.0	217	238.3	239.3

FIGURE 5-14

The Neoplasm Table, in part.

CASE STUDY

Stephen Mathis is a 44-year-old male who has been seen by his regular primary care physician. After the radiological and laboratory test results came back, Mr. Mathis was diagnosed with a benign neoplasm of the ascending colon.

Can you find the correct ICD-9-CM code?

_____

_____

First turn to the neoplasm table in the alphabetic listing (Volume 2). The listings are in alphabetical order by the anatomical site (part of the body where the neoplasm is located). Go down the descriptive list until you get to *Colon*. There is a notation that directs you to look under *Intestine, large*. Continue through the descriptions in this neoplasm table until you get to *Intestine, intestinal*. Under *Intestine,* you find an indentation labeled *Large,* and indented under *Large* is *Colon.* Indented under *Colon* is *Ascending*—finally the correct descriptive listing of the neoplasm! Now you must go across the table to the right to the fourth column (the column titled Benign). There you find code 211.3. Now go to the numerical listing (Volume 1) to make certain this is the best code. There you find

> ✓4th 211 Benign neoplasm of other parts of digestive system
>
> 211.3 Colon

Ta da! Good job.

Neoplasms and Morphology (M) Codes

In addition to the code for a neoplasm, the alphabetic index may also include an M code. The M stands for Morphology, and this additional code identifies the behavior and histological (cell structure) type of the neoplasm.

> Craniopharyngioma (M9350/1) 237.0

The histology is described by the first four digits of the M code.

The behavior is described by the number shown after the slash of the M code.

Behavior classifications are

0 Benign

1 Uncertain behavior

2 Carcinoma in situ

3 Malignant, primary site

6 Malignant, secondary site

9 Malignant, uncertain whether primary or metastatic site

Refer to Appendix A of the ICD-9-CM book Volume 1, immediately after the E codes tabular (numerical) listings, for a complete listing of the M codes.

Table of Drugs & Chemicals

Directly located after the alphabetic listing in Volume 2 is Section 2. This portion of the first part of the ICD-9-CM book contains the Table of Drugs & Chemicals and the alphabetical listing for E codes.

The Table of Drugs & Chemicals has nothing to do with prescriptions that the physician may write for a patient during an encounter. The only time that a drug or chemical comes into the picture of ICD-9-CM coding is when that drug or chemical has caused an **adverse reaction**—in other words, when the patient has been harmed and/or put in jeopardy because of the ingestion of (entering the body) or exposure to a drug or chemical. When this happens, a *poisoning* code should be used, with one exception. If the drug or chemical was properly prescribed by a licensed health care professional and given to the correct person in the correct dosage and the patient has an adverse reaction, this is not a poisoning and does not get a poisoning code.

The first column of this table lists the names of drugs and chemicals, in alphabetical order. This list includes prescription medications, over-the-counter medications, household chemicals, and any other items with a chemical basis. Aspirin, indigestion relief medication, drugstore-brand allergy relievers, window cleaner, battery acid, and the like are all included, as are medications prescribed by the physician. Some of these drugs and chemicals are listed by their brand, or common, names such as Metamucil. Others are shown by their chemical, or generic, names such as barbiturates (sedatives). If you are not certain, consult a *Physicians' Desk Reference* (PDR), which lists all of these drugs by brand name as well as chemical name.

Depending on which drug or chemical caused the adverse reaction to the patient, the six titled columns will help you find the correct code(s) to identify the intent of a bad or unexpected reaction (Figure 5-15). The column titles are

- *Poisoning*. For coders, the word *poisoning* indicates that the patient's body reacted negatively to a drug or chemical. This is the first code you will use to identify the cause of the poisoning.

Note: The following columns in this table lead you to the E code that will identify the *intent* of the poisoning or the adverse reaction to the drug or chemical. The intent of a poisoning or an adverse reaction identifies the reasoning behind the incident.

- *Accident*. This E code will be added to the poisoning code to indicate that the adverse reaction was caused by an accidental overdose, an accidental taking of the wrong substance, or an accident that happened during the use of drugs and chemical substances. Basically, this means that the ingestion of or exposure to this drug or this quantity of a drug that caused the problem was unintentional.

Key Term

Adverse reaction: When an individual is harmed or put in danger after interacting with a drug or chemical.

	Poisoning	External Cause (E Code)						Poisoning	External Cause (E Code)				
		Accident	Therapeutic Use	Suicide Attempt	Assault	Undeter-mined			Accident	Therapeutic Use	Suicide Attempt	Assault	Undeter-mined
1-propanol	980.3	E860.4	—	E950.9	E962.1	E980.9	Acetorphine	965.09	E850.2	E935.2	E950.0	E962.0	E980.0
2-propanol	980.2	E860.3	—	E950.9	E962.1	E980.9	Acetosulfone (sodium)	961.8	E857	E931.8	E950.4	E962.0	E980.4
2,4-D (dichlorophenoxyacetic acid)	989.4	E863.5	—	E950.6	E962.1	E980.7	Acetrizoate (sodium)	977.8	E858.8	E947.8	E950.4	E962.0	E980.4
2,4-toluene diisocyanate	983.0	E864.0	—	E950.7	E962.1	E980.6	Acetylcarbromal	967.3	E852.2	E937.3	E950.2	E962.0	E980.2
2,4,5-T (trichlorophenoxyacetic acid)	989.2	E863.5	—	E950.6	E962.1	E980.7	Acetylcholine (chloride)	971.0	E855.3	E941.0	E950.4	E962.0	E980.4
14-hydroxydihydromorph-inone	965.09	E850.2	E935.2	E950.0	E962.0	E980.0	Acetylcysteine	975.5	E858.6	E945.5	E950.4	E962.0	E980.4
ABOB	961.7	E857	E931.7	E950.4	E962.0	E980.4	Acetyldigitoxin	972.1	E858.3	E942.1	E950.4	E962.0	E980.4
Abrus (seed)	988.2	E865.3	—	E950.9	E962.1	E980.9	Acetyldihydrocodeine	965.09	E850.2	E935.2	E950.0	E962.0	E980.0
Absinthe	980.0	E860.1	—	E950.9	E962.1	E980.9	Acetyldihydrocodeinone	965.09	E850.2	E935.2	E950.0	E962.0	E980.0
beverage	980.0	E860.0	—	E950.9	E962.1	E980.9	Acetylene (gas) (industrial)	987.1	E868.1	—	E951.8	E962.2	E981.8
Acenocoumarin, acenocoumarol	964.2	E858.2	E934.2	E950.4	E962.0	E980.4	incomplete combustion of — see Carbon monoxide, fuel, utility						
Acepromazine	969.1	E853.0	E939.1	E950.3	E962.0	E980.3	tetrachloride (vapor)	982.3	E862.4	—	E950.9	E962.1	E980.9
Acetal	982.8	E862.4	—	E950.9	E962.1	E980.9	Acetyliodosalicylic acid	965.1	E850.3	E935.3	E950.0	E962.0	E980.0
Acetaldehyde (vapor)	987.8	E869.8	—	E952.8	E962.2	E982.8	Acetylphenylhydrazine	965.8	E850.8	E935.8	E950.0	E962.0	E980.0
liquid	989.89	E866.8	—	E950.9	E962.1	E980.9	Acetylsalicylic acid	965.1	E850.3	E935.3	E950.0	E962.0	E980.0
Acetaminophen	965.4	E850.4	E935.4	E950.0	E962.0	E980.0	Achromycin	960.4	E856	E930.4	E950.4	E962.0	E980.4
Acetaminosalol	965.1	E850.3	E935.3	E950.0	E962.0	E980.0	ophthalmic preparation	976.5	E858.7	E946.5	E950.4	E962.0	E980.4
Acetanilid(e)	965.4	E850.4	E935.4	E950.0	E962.0	E980.0	topical NEC	976.0	E858.7	E946.0	E950.4	E962.0	E980.4
Acetarsol, acetarsone	961.1	E857	E931.1	E950.4	E962.0	E980.4	Acidifying agents	963.2	E858.1	E933.2	E950.4	E962.0	E980.4
Acetazolamide	974.2	E858.5	E944.2	E950.4	E962.0	E980.4	Acids (corrosive) NEC	983.1	E864.1	—	E950.7	E962.1	E980.6
Acetic							Aconite (wild)	988.2	E865.4	—	E950.9	E962.1	E980.9
acid	983.1	E864.1	—	E950.7	E962.1	E980.6	Aconitine (liniment)	976.8	E858.7	E946.8	E950.4	E962.0	E980.4
with sodium acetate (ointment)	976.3	E858.7	E946.3	E950.4	E962.0	E980.4	Aconitum ferox	988.2	E865.4	—	E950.9	E962.1	E980.9
irrigating solution	974.5	E858.5	E944.5	E950.4	E962.0	E980.4	Acridine	983.0	E864.0	—	E950.7	E962.1	E980.6
lotion	976.2	E858.7	E946.2	E950.4	E962.0	E980.4	vapor	987.8	E869.8	—	E952.8	E962.2	E982.8
anhydride	983.1	E864.1	—	E950.7	E962.1	E980.6	Acriflavine	961.9	E857	E931.9	E950.4	E962.0	E980.4
ether (vapor)	982.8	E862.4	—	E950.9	E962.1	E980.9	Acrisorcin	976.0	E858.7	E946.0	E950.4	E962.0	E980.4
Acetohexamide	962.3	E858.0	E932.3	E950.4	E962.0	E980.4	Acrolein (gas)	987.8	E869.8	—	E952.8	E962.2	E982.8
Acetomenaphthone	964.3	E858.2	E934.3	E950.4	E962.0	E980.4	liquid	989.89	E866.8	—	E950.9	E962.1	E980.9
Acetomorphine	965.01	E850.0	E935.0	E950.0	E962.0	E980.0	Actaea spicata	988.2	E865.4	—	E950.9	E962.1	E980.9
Acetone (oils) (vapor)	982.8	E862.4	—	E950.9	E962.1	E980.9	Acterol	961.5	E857	E931.5	E950.4	E962.0	E980.4
Acetophenazine (maleate)	969.1	E853.0	E939.1	E950.3	E962.0	E980.3	ACTH	962.4	E858.0	E932.4	E950.4	E962.0	E980.4
Acetophenetidin	965.4	E850.4	E935.4	E950.0	E962.0	E980.0	Acthar	962.4	E858.O	E932.4	E950.4	E962.0	E980.4
Acetophenone	982.0	E862.4	—	E950.9	E962.1	E980.9	Actinomycin (C) (D)	960.7	E856	E930.7	E950.4	E962.0	E980.4
							Adalin (acetyl)	967.3	E852.2	E937.3	E950.2	E962.0	E980.2
							Adenosine (phosphate)	977.8	E858.8	E947.8	E950.4	E962.0	E980.4
							Adhesives	989.89	E866.6	—	E950.9	E962.1	E980.9

FIGURE 5-15
The Table of Drugs and Chemicals.

- *Therapeutic Use.* This code is used when the right drug is taken in the right dose by the right person, but an unexpected reaction occurred. The guidelines direct coders not to use a poisoning code when the intent was proper therapeutic use, as prescribed.
- *Suicide attempt.* This code indicates that the overdose or incorrect substance was taken with the full intent of causing one's own death. The E code shown in this column accompanies the poisoning code on the same line.
- *Assault.* This code specifies that one person caused the poisoning on purpose to inflict illness, injury, or death upon another person. This code implies attempted murder. The E code shown in this column accompanies the poisoning code on the same line.
- *Undetermined.* The same as unspecified used elsewhere in the ICD-9-CM book, this code is to be used only when the record does not state what caused the poisoning. The E code shown in this column accompanies the poisoning code on the same line.

Examples

Joe looks into a barrel he has found in the back of the warehouse where he works. Fumes from the industrial solvent being stored in that barrel overcome Joe and he passes out. He is taken to the doctor immediately. He has been adversely affected by a chemical, but it is an accident.

> 982.8 Poisoning, solvent industrial
>
> 780.09 Unconsciousness
>
> E 862.9 Accidental poisoning by industrial solvent.

Mrs. Smith fills the new prescription for naproxen given to her by her physician. By the second day of taking the drug, her whole body is covered with a rash. She has been taking the drug as prescribed, in the proper dosage. However, she is allergic to it, but no one could have foreseen that. She has had an adverse reaction to a drug given to her for therapeutic use.

> 693.0 Dermatitis due to drugs
>
> E 935.6 Adverse effect, therapeutic use

Memory Tip

When coding an encounter involving a poisoning—think PEE for Poison:
P = Poisoning code
E = Effect or reaction code
E = E code showing intent

TOO MUCH TO REMEMBER?

Using the ICD-9-CM book to identify diagnoses is like going on a treasure hunt. Sometimes it is very easy to find the best, most appropriate code in accordance with the physician's notes. Other times, it seems as though the code just isn't there. However, you must remember that, if the health care provider can diagnose it, it's in the book somewhere!

Multiple resources, such as the following, can help you in your search for the best, most appropriate code.

- A medical dictionary and/or *The Merck Manual of Medical Information*, if you don't understand the provider's notes or if you need further clarification to find an alternate term that might be easier to find in the ICD-9-CM book
- A *Physicians' Desk Reference* (PDR), if you are not certain of alternate or generic names for drugs or other chemicals
- Publications including *Coding Clinic* and *Correct Coding Initiative*, as well as *CodeWrite*
- Official guidelines focusing on the sections that relate directly to your workplace's health care specialty
- Many websites, including www.ahima.org, www.aapc.org, and www.cms.gov

Of course, if you need to, ask the provider who saw the patient.

CHAPTER SUMMARY

E codes, V codes, three digits, four digits, five digits, major complications, underlying diseases, and so on—don't worry; as you look back over this chapter, you should notice one very important thing—the ICD-9-CM book will almost always guide you to the correct code. The book will tell you when you need a fourth or a fifth digit. The alphabetic listing will guide you to the correct page in the numerical (tabular) listings, so you can find the best, most appropriate code. And, if the code's description doesn't match the physician's notes, just go back and keep looking.

IMPORTANT NOTE

There are two primary things you need to remember to be a good coder:

1. Remember how to identify the key words in the physician's notes, so that you can look up the best, most appropriate code(s).
2. Remember that when a patient has a case of poisoning or an injury you will need to add an E code.

The ICD-9-CM book will guide you through the rest of the coding process with its notations and instructions. It can point you in the right direction toward the best, most appropriate code. Just look and read.

Chapter Review

Find the best diagnosis code(s) for the following patients.

1. A 35-year-old female comes into the physician's office for an elective sterilization (to have her tubes tied). V25.2

2. A 27-year-old female is seen in the physician's office for a checkup. Her pregnancy has been complicated by a case of gonorrhea. 647.1

3. A 5-year-old male is seen by the physician for a Rubella screening. V73.3

4. A 65-year-old male is seen in the physician's office. The diagnosis is type I uncontrolled diabetes with circulatory problems. 250.7

5. A 47-year-old male is seen in the physician's office for stomach pains. The diagnosis is confirmed for a sigmoid colon carcinoma. 153.3

6. A 3-year-old male is seen by the physician because he has gotten a jelly bean stuck up his nose. 932

7. A 29-year-old female is brought into the emergency room diagnosed with anaphylactic shock caused by eating peanuts. 995.61

8. A 43-year old female is seen by the physician and diagnosed with an endometrial ovarian cyst. 617.1

9. A 32-year-old male is seen by the physician, complaining that he cannot stay awake. The diagnosis of narcolepsy is confirmed. 347.0

10. An 18-year-old male is seen by the physician and diagnosed with a seizure disorder. 345.8

11. An infant is born in a hospital, single birth, with no mention of cesarean delivery or section. V30.0

12. A 25-year-old male sees the physician for a checkup due to a family history of epilepsy. The patient has no evidence of seizures. V17.2

13. A 55-year-old male is diagnosed with a malignant neoplasm of the mandible. 170.1

14. A 79-year-old female is diagnosed by the physician with cardiorenal hypertension, benign. 404.10

15. A 49-year-old female sees the physician for a routine annual physical. V70.0

16. A 41-year-old female is diagnosed as HIV positive. She has no symptoms and does not exhibit any manifestations of AIDS. V08

The following patients will need more than one ICD-9-CM code.

17. A 21-year-old female is seen by the physician for headaches. The confirmed diagnosis is temporal lobe epilepsy and migraine headaches. _____ _____

18. A 37-year-old female is seen by the physician, complaining of morning sickness. This is a regularly scheduled 16-week appointment for the physician to supervise her high-risk pregnancy. _____ _____

19. A 5-month-old male is seen by the physician after evidence of being shaken. The diagnosis was confirmed for shaken infant syndrome with an intracranial contusion of the brainstem, with no loss of consciousness. _____ _____ _____

20. A 9-year-old female is seen by the physician for malnutrition, caused by her negligent mother. _____ _____

21. A 15-year-old male is brought into the emergency room and diagnosed with third-degree burns on his back, 18% body surface. He was caught in a house fire. _____ _____ _____

22. A 23-year-old male is seen by the physician, suffering from edema in his legs and hypertension, both caused by his morbid obesity. _____ _____ _____

23. A 32-year-old male is seen by the physician for a brain concussion, having been unconscious for five minutes. The man is an employee of NASA and was hurt while training in a weightlessness simulator. _____ _____

24. A 60-year-old male was brought in to see the physician with a simple fracture of the tibia. The patient stated that he had fallen off a ladder at home. _____ _____

25. A 28-year-old male is seen by the physician with a dislocated temporomandible (closed). The patient states that he was involved in a fist fight and was punched. _____ _____

26. A 34-year-old female is seen by the physician with wrist pain. She is diagnosed with carpal tunnel syndrome due to overexertion and strenuous movements. _____ _____

27. A 41-year-old male is seen by the physician with organic pneumonia, a complication of the patient's HIV-positive status. _____ _____

28. A 12-year-old female is seen by the physician with a closed fractured femur, (unspecified part). She fell off her bicycle. _____ _____

29. A 23-year-old female is seen by the physician with a crushed wrist, caused by her involvement in an automobile accident. _____ _____

30. A 57-year-old male is seen by the physician and diagnosed with gastritis due to taking tetracycline, as prescribed by the physician the week before. _____ _____

31. A 35-year-old male is brought into the physician's office and diagnosed with poisoning by an industrial-strength solvent he used at work. The patient states that he accidentally inhaled the solvent. _____ _____

32. A 90-year-old male is seen by the physician due to signs of malnutrition. This is the result of his daughter's neglecting him on a continued basis. _____ _____

33. A 29-year-old male is seen by the physician. He is diagnosed with Kaposi's sarcoma, a manifestation of his HIV-positive status. _____ _____

6

Coding Diagnoses: ICD-10-CM

KEY TERMS

etiology
Excludes1
Excludes2
health-related risk factors
laterality
morbidity
mortality

OBJECTIVES

- Distinguish between ICD-9-CM and ICD-10-CM.

- Recognize the similarities between ICD-9-CM and ICD-10-CM.

- Identify accurate and correct diagnostic codes using ICD-10-CM.

- Find the best, most appropriate code for billing purposes using ICD-10-CM.

Health care professionals have been using the *International Classification of Diseases*—9th revision—Clinical Modification (ICD-9-CM) since the late 1970s. Even though the terms and codes are updated each year (on October 1), the ICD-9-CM book was not designed to grow and change in the manner that our society has required. However, the next revision is ready to come in and replace ICD-9-CM, with more up-to-date terms, more specific descriptions, and more room to grow—enter ICD-10-CM.*

---

*Enhance the learning process by pairing this chapter with a current version of ICD-10-CM. Download it from www.cdc.gov/nchs/icd9.htm.

INTRODUCTION TO ICD-10-CM

When ICD-10-CM officially replaces ICD-9-CM, you will no longer use the ICD-9-CM book. However, you will have no problem finding the best, most appropriate code in ICD-10-CM when the time comes. The process of finding the best diagnosis code is the same with both books. It is just that the code you determine to be best will look a little different. Most students learning to code from ICD-10-CM actually prefer it. We believe you will like it better, too. Typically, it is the veteran coders, who have been using ICD-9-CM for decades, that are resistant to the change.

The *International Classification of Diseases—10th revision* (ICD-10) was designed to allow health care professionals to create a collection of medical terms used by physicians, medical examiners, and coroners around the world. This permits the organizations involved, including the World Health Organization (WHO), to create statistical evaluations as they pertain to global health care. This is important to us all as we become a more global society every day. Countries now share cures, treatments, diseases, and germs more than ever before.

There are actually two versions of ICD-10: ICD-10 and ICD-10-CM.

- The *International Classification of Diseases* (ICD-10) is the version used to code and organize data from death certificates for analyzing causes of **mortality**. This information is then used to assess the number of deaths that occurred due to a particular cause, to members of a specific group, or at a particular time.
- ICD-10-CM (*International Classification of Diseases—10th revision—Clinical Modification*) is used to code and categorize information from inpatient and outpatient files and physician's notes, in order to appraise the basis of various types of **morbidity**. This is the measurement of how regularly a specific disease occurs in a particular area or segment of the population. Then, this information is used to direct health care facilities and programs, so they can increase the use of certain procedures and/or therapies or reduce other areas based on the actual need of the people they serve.

The *International Classification of Diseases—10th revision—Clinical Modification* (ICD-10-CM) is a major redesign of the entire diagnostic coding system and is more efficient than ICD-9-CM. ICD-10-CM offers many improvements over ICD-9-CM, including the following:

1. More specific codes, including conditions that were not distinctly described in ICD-9-CM
2. A more logical grouping of codes
3. More thorough descriptions of each code
4. Extensions that provide additional, important information
5. Identification of **health-related risk factors** beyond the disease and injury classifications

Key Terms

Mortality: The proportion of deaths to the population as a whole, also known as the death rate.

Morbidity: The study of disease and the causes of disease in a given population or society.

Health-related risk factors: Lifestyles and behaviors, such as alcohol intake, cigarette smoking, and dietary issues (high-fat, high cholesterol) that affect one's well-being.

Memory Tip

Mor**T**ality—Think of the **T** in the middle like the cross on a grave to remind you that this relates to death.

Morbi**D**ity—**D** is for **D**isease.

6. Listing of injuries organized by site (e.g., head, knee, foot), then by type (e.g., fracture, burn), so they are easier to find
7. More clinical information to assist the coding process
8. More information that is relevant to ambulatory and managed care encounters
9. Built-in room for future expansion in the coding system

THE LOOK OF ICD-10-CM CODES

ICD-10-CM codes look completely different from ICD-9-CM codes.

Length of Codes

- ICD-9-CM codes are three, four, or five digits long.
- ICD-10-CM codes can be as long as seven characters (including letters and numbers).

Types of Characters

- ICD-9-CM codes are composed of numbers, with the exception of V and E codes.
- ICD-10-CM codes are all alphanumeric. This means that every code has both a letter and a sequence of numbers (Figure 6-1).

Example

ICD-9-CM shows   354.0 Carpal tunnel syndrome
ICD-10-CM shows   G56.0 Carpal tunnel syndrome

FIGURE 6-1
Alphanumeric ICD-10-CM codes.

> **G56   Mononeuropathies of upper limb**
> Excludes 1:current traumatic nerve disorder - see nerve injury by body region
> G56.0 Carpal tunnel syndrome
>> **G56.00   Carpal tunnel syndrome, unspecified side**
>> **G56.01   Carpal tunnel syndrome, right side**
>> **G56.02   Carpal tunnel syndrome, left side**

ICD-10-CM CODE DESCRIPTIONS

Key Term

Laterality: The location of the condition, such as right, left, upper, lower, anterior, and posterior. Bilateral means "both sides."

More Detailed Descriptions

- ICD-9-CM codes often do not provide certain details about the condition, such as **laterality**.
- ICD-10-CM offers additional codes to more fully describe not only the condition itself, but the location of the condition as well (Figure 6-2).

M79.6 Pain in limb, hand, foot, fingers and toes
Excludes2:pain in joint (M25.5-)
M79.60 Pain in limb, unspecified

M79.601 Pain in right arm
Pain in right upper limb NOS
M79.602 Pain in left arm
Pain in left upper limb NOS
M79.603 Pain in arm, unspecified
Pain in upper limb NOS
M79.604 Pain in right leg
Pain in right lower limb NOS
M79.605 Pain in left leg
Pain in left lower limb NOS
M79.606 Pain in leg, unspecified
Pain in lower limb NOS
M79.609 Pain in unspecified limb
Pain in limb NOS

FIGURE 6-2
ICD-10-CM codes specify laterality.

You will easily be able to see the inclusion of additional information in other sections of ICD-10-CM. For example, in the section having to do with pregnancy, codes specify the trimester. In the section regarding diabetes, you will find codes which specify whether or not insulin therapy is being used by the patient.

You can see that the change in the way the codes look and the additional information provided by the extended, more specific codes will certainly make your job coding encounters easier.

Example

ICD-9-CM shows   729.5 Pain in limb
ICD-10-CM shows   M79.6 Pain in limb, hand, foot, fingers and toes
and adds   M79.60 Pain in limb, unspecified
M79.601 Pain in right arm
M79.602 Pain in left arm
M79.603 Pain in arm, unspecified
M79.604 Pain in right leg
M79.605 Pain in left leg
M79.606 Pain in leg, unspecified
M79.609 Pain in unspecified limb
M79.62   Pain in upper arm

Combination Codes

- ICD-9-CM offers some combination codes.

Example

ICD-9-CM shows	290.3 Senile dementia with delirium
ICD-9-CM shows	049.1 Meningitis due to adenovirus

Key Term

Etiology: The identification of the disease or the cause of the disease.

FIGURE 6-3
ICD-10-CM combination codes provide more detail.

- ICD-10-CM has even more combination codes, incorporating some of the most common symptoms, diagnoses, **etiology** (the identification of the disease or cause), and/or manifestations. Again, this gives you the opportunity to show more details with fewer codes (Figure 6-3).

K50.00	**Crohn's disease of small intestine without complications**	
K50.01	Crohn's disease of small intestine with complications	
	K50.011	**Crohn's disease of small intestine with rectal bleeding**
	K50.012	**Crohn's disease of small intestine with intestinal obstruction**
	K50.013	**Crohn's disease of small intestine with fistula**
	K50.014	**Crohn's disease of small intestine with abscess**
	K50.018	**Crohn's disease of small intestine with other complication**
	K50.019	**Crohn's disease of small intestine with unspecified complications**

Example

ICD-9-CM shows	555.0 Crohn's disease of small intestine
	569.81 Fistula of intestine
ICD-10-CM shows	K50.013 Crohn's disease of small intestine with fistula

Z Codes—Formerly Known as V Codes

- ICD-9-CM assigns V codes to identify the circumstances under which individuals have contact with the health care system for reasons other than illness or injury. This information is included in the main alphabetic index and has its own section in the tabular (numerical) list.
- ICD-10-CM has Z codes to indicate when a person goes to see a provider for circumstances other than an illness or injury. All of these key words are included in the alphabetic index, just as they are in ICD-9-CM.

Example

ICD-9-CM shows	V22.0 Supervision of normal first pregnancy
ICD-10-CM shows	Z34.01 Encounter for supervision of normal first pregnancy, first trimester

E (External) Codes

- ICD-9-CM uses E codes for descriptions of external causes of injury or poisoning. These circumstances are listed in a separate alphabetic index, as well as a separate section in the tabular (numerical) list.
- ICD-10-CM breaks up these circumstances into several sections, which add a great deal of detail to the descriptions:

S codes are used for traumatic injuries.

T codes are used for burns, corrosions, poisonings, or toxic effects.

V codes identify that a transportation accident caused the injury.

W codes identify external causes that are accidental injuries.

X00–X58 codes continue to identify the causes of accidental injuries.

X92–Y08 codes identify the cause as assault.

Y21–Y33 codes show a cause of undetermined intent.

Y35–Y38 codes are used when the cause is legal intervention, war, military operations, or terrorist acts.

Y62–Y84 codes identify complications that are the result of medical and surgical care, including misadventures (*misadventures* is the official word for medical errors).

Y92 codes expand the descriptions of the location where the injury happened. This is an expansion of the codes offered in ICD-9-CM under E849 Place of Occurrence.

Y93 codes are activity codes that are to be used
(1) only with Y92 codes and
(2) only on the claim form for the initial encounter (the first time the individual sees the provider for that injury).

Example

Little Johnny is taken to his physician's office because he got hurt falling off the jungle gym in his backyard.

ICD-9-CM shows   E884.0 Fall from playground equipment
ICD-10-CM shows   W09.2xxa Fall on or from jungle gym, initial encounter

Notations and Explanations

Just as in ICD-9-CM, there are directions provided to you in ICD-10-CM. These directions appear throughout the book: sometimes in the alphabetic index, sometimes in the tabular (numerical) list, and sometimes in both. These directions include the following:

1. Punctuation
   - [ ] Brackets are used in the alphabetic index to identify manifestation codes and in the tabular (numerical) list to indicate symptoms, alternative wording, and/or explanatory phrases.

- ( ) Parentheses offer the coder additional words or phrases that may be included in the physician's statement that would be considered a part of this code.
- : Colons come before additional words or phrases that are typically necessary to complete an accurate description.

2. Abbreviations
   - *NEC* (*Not Elsewhere Classifiable*) means the same as it does in ICD-9-CM, that the physician was very specific in his or her notes and the ICD does not offer a more specific code to match. *Other* and *Other Specified* are alternate versions of this notation.
   - *NOS* (*Not Otherwise Specified*) indicates that the physician's notes contained insufficient detail to use a more specific code, just as it does in ICD-9-CM. *Unspecified* is another version of this same notation.

3. Terms
   - *And*. Used in ICD-10-CM, this means *and* as well as *and/or*.
   - *With* and *Without*. These offer you options for the last character for a set of codes. If there is no detail provided in the documentation, the implied choice is always *without*.
   - *Code first*. This is the notation below a category or a code, just as it is in ICD-9-CM, that directs you to not only code the underlying condition but also to place the code for the underlying condition before the manifestation (sign, symptom, or side effect) code on the claim form. This indicates that the underlying condition code is the principle diagnosis. For example, see the following notation (Figure 6-4):

     F02 Dementia in other disease classified elsewhere

         Code first the underlying physiological condition such as:

             Alzheimer's (G30.-)

             cerebral lipidosis (E75.-)

             . . .etc. . . .

     This notation tells the coder that, if the physician's notes, for example, diagnose the patient with dementia as a result of Gaucher disease, you should code them in the following order:

     E75.22 Gaucher disease

     F02 Dementia in other disease classified elsewhere

F02   Dementia in other diseases classified elsewhere
Code first the underlying physiological condition, such as:
Alzheimer's (G30.-)
cerebral lipidosis (E75.-)
dementia with Lewy bodies (G31.83)
epilepsy (G40.-)
frontotemporal dementia (G31.09)
hepatolenticular degeneration (E83.0)
human immunodeficiency virus [HIV] disease (B20)
hypercalcemia (E83.52)
hypothyroidism, acquired (E00-E03.-)
intoxications (T36-T65)
multiple sclerosis (G35)
neurosyphilis (A52.17)
niacin deficiency [pellagra] (E52)
Parkinson's disease (G20)
Pick's disease (G31.01)
Polyarteritis nodosa (M30.0)
systemic lupus erythematosus (M32.-)
trypanosomiasis (B56.-, B57.-)
vitamin B deficiency (E53.8)

FIGURE 6-4
Example of a Code First notation.

- *Use secondary code/use additional code.* This instructs you to use a separate diagnosis code for the manifestation of the condition and to place it after the code for that condition (Figure 6-5).

    E84.0 Cystic fibrosis with pulmonary manifestations

    Use additional code to identify any infectious organism present, such as:

    Pseudomonas (B96.5)

E84   Cystic fibrosis
Includes: mucoviscidosis
E84.0 Cystic fibrosis with pulmonary manifestations
Use additional code to identify any infectious organism present, such as:
Pseudomonas (B96.5)

FIGURE 6-5
Example of a Use Additional Code notation.

Therefore, if the physician's notes indicated that this patient has pseudomonas as a result of having cystic fibrosis, your claim form would show, in this order:

E84.0 Cystic fibrosis with pulmonary manifestations

B96.5 Pseudomonas

This notation is the same as the Use Additional Code notation in ICD-9-CM.

- *In diseases classified elsewhere.* This identifies codes that are designated as manifestation codes. These codes are *never* to be first-listed, or shown as a principle diagnosis, because they identify health conditions or illnesses that are the result of another disease or condition.

Example

F02.80 Dementia *in other diseases classified elsewhere* without behavioral disturbance

- *Code also.* This is a notation that alerts you to a situation that may require two codes to describe the condition completely (Figure 6-6). In this circumstance, the order of the two codes is determined by the reason WHY the patient saw the provider for this encounter, as well as the severity of the conditions (with the more severe condition being placed first on the claim form).

FIGURE 6-6
Example of an ICD-10-CM Code Also notation.

H05.32	Deformity of orbit due to bone disease
	Code also associated bone disease
H05.321	**Deformity of right orbit due to bone disease**
H05.322	**Deformity of left orbit due to bone disease**
H05.323	**Deformity of bilateral orbits due to bone disease**
H05.329	**Deformity of unspecified orbit due to bone disease**

- **Includes.** This adds further definition for the code above the word. Some of this additional definition may appear only in the alphabetic index, not the tabular section.
- **Excludes.** In ICD-10-CM, Excludes means more than it does in ICD-9-CM. There are actually two Excludes notations—Excludes1 and Excludes2.

    Excludes1 means that the code shown above the notation cannot ever be used with the code listed after the Excludes1 note (Figure 6-7).

Key Term

Excludes1: This notation identifies codes that are mutually exclusive with the code listed above.

As shown in our example, this means that you are not permitted to include A18.32 and A04.0 on the same claim form. The Excludes1 notation is used to tell you that these two codes:

1. are contradictory to each other,
2. could not coexist in the same person at the same time, or
3. are redundant (repeat the same information).

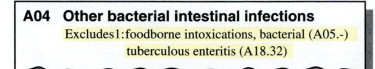

FIGURE 6-7
Example of an ICD-10-CM
Excludes1 notation.

Excludes2 explains that (Figure 6-8)

1. the conditions listed below the notation are not a part of the code shown above the notation.
2. it is a warning to be careful that you do not mistakenly use the code above when the code below might be more accurate.
3. an additional code may be needed. You can see how helpful this note is. It may direct you to a better, more specific code.

Key Term

Excludes2: This notation identifies conditions that are specifically not included in the description of the code.

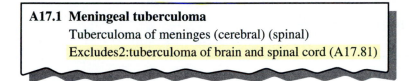

FIGURE 6-8
Example of an ICD-10-CM
Excludes2 notation.

ICD-10-CM Dummy Place Holders and Additional Characters

As you have learned, ICD-10-CM codes can have as few as three characters and as many as seven characters. However, in some cases, due to built-in room for the addition of even more specificity in the future, a sixth or seventh digit is required for a code that has no fifth or sixth digit. Therefore, an *x* is used to fill in the space. The letter *x* is always the letter used as the dummy place holder.

Throughout the ICD-10-CM book, you will find that fifth, sixth, and seventh characters are added with consistent meaning in different chapters. You will need to keep looking for them, much in the same way that you look for indications that a fourth or fifth digit is required in ICD-9-CM. A good example of this can be seen in the following:

T60 Toxic effect of pesticides

T60.3 Toxic effect of herbicides and fungicides

There is no fifth character, however, the sixth character is needed to identify the circumstances causing the adverse effect. Therefore, a dummy place holder is used in the fifth place.

T60.3x1 Toxic effect of herbicides and fungicides, accidental

T60.3x2 Toxic effect of herbicides and fungicides, intentional self-harm

T60.3x3 Toxic effect of herbicides and fungicides, assault

T60.3x4 Toxic effect of herbicides and fungicides, undetermined

The final character (seventh character) extension explains how many times the provider has seen the patient regarding this concern.

a	initial encounter
d	subsequent encounter
q	sequela

CASE STUDY

Let's look at Mary Lou Dawson. She is seen for the first time, complaining of a reaction to a herbicide, after she accidentally sprayed herself in the face while tending to her garden.

What is the correct code?

_____

_____

T60.3x1a

   T60   Toxic effect of pesticides

   Add the point 3 for herbicides and fungicides

   Add the x as a dummy place holder

   Add the 1 to indicate the adverse effect was an accident

   Add the a to indicate this was the patient's first encounter with the provider for this condition

COMPLETE ICD-10-CM CODING GUIDELINES

You will find that coding patient encounters using ICD-10-CM is overall exactly the same process as using ICD-9-CM. Although the codes look different, and you have more codes to choose from, you will still

1. Find the key words in the physician's notes or other documentation.
2. Look for those diagnostic descriptions in the alphabetic index.
3. Confirm the code(s) in the tabular (numerical) list.

The official government version of the *ICD-10-CM Guidelines for Coding and Reporting* appears on the following websites:

ICD-10 web page	www.cdc.gov/nchs/icd9.htm
NCHS mortality web page	www.cdc.gov/nchs/about/major/dvs/mortdata.htm
NCHS website	www.cdc.gov/nchs

CHAPTER SUMMARY

ICD-10-CM will be instituted very soon; when it is in place, it will take over the system very quickly. However, don't worry—you are prepared because you know how to code, and it won't matter which book you use. The changes make it easier for you to find the best, most appropriate code, not more difficult. Just remember what you learned in Chapter 5 and apply it. Then, double-check your codes and you will be a great coder!

IMPORTANT NOTE

If you are able to download the latest version of ICD-10-CM, and would like to practice using this new system, assign ICD-10-CM codes to the patient scenarios in the Chapter 5 chapter review.

Chapter Review

For the following multiple-choice questions, please choose the best answer.

1. Mortality is the assessment of

    a. Causes of injuries

    b. Causes of illnesses

    c. Causes of death

    d. Causes of poisonings

2. Morbidity is the assessment of the

    a. Basis of types of disease

    b. Basis of types of population growth

    c. Basis of types of procedures

    d. Basis of types of insurance

3. ICD-10-CM codes are

    a. Up to 3 characters long

    b. Up to 5 characters long

    c. Up to 7 characters long

    d. Up to 10 characters long

4. The term that refers to the location of a condition or injury is

    a. Global placement

    b. Laterality

    c. Trimester

    d. Encounter

5. A combination code might include the etiology as well as the

    a. Circumstances

    b. External cause

    c. Name of the disease

    d. Manifestations

6. NOS (Not Otherwise Specified) is the same as

   a. Not Elsewhere Classified

   b. Unspecified

   c. Other Specified

   d. Underlying Condition

7. When a seventh character is required, but the best most appropriate code is only five characters long, one must use a dummy place holder, shown by the use of the letter

   a. *d*

   b. *x*

   c. *s*

   d. *y*

8. *Alphanumeric* means that a code has

   a. Only letters

   b. Only numbers

   c. Letters and numbers

   d. Numbers and special symbols

9. Brackets [ ] are used to identify manifestation codes in

   a. ICD-10-CM only

   b. Both ICD-9-CM and ICD-10-CM

   c. ICD-9-CM only

   d. Neither ICD-9-CM nor ICD-10-CM

10. ICD-9-CM V codes are identified in ICD-10-CM with

    a. Z codes

    b. X codes

    c. E codes

    d. V codes

7 Coding Procedures: CPT

OBJECTIVES

- Find the best, most appropriate code(s) in the CPT book for procedures and services delivered during a patient encounter.

- Apply the rules and guidelines relating to CPT coding.

- Interpret the physician's notes accurately to code appropriately.

- Understand the laws and regulations as they pertain to CPT coding and billing.

Procedures and treatments are the key to the health care system. After all, not only is it about discovering what is wrong with the individual (the diagnosis); it's also about *what* the health care provider is going to *do* about it (the procedures and treatments).

Health care providers are not paid by the diagnosis code. The ICD-9-CM diagnosis codes are included to provide an explanation as to *why* the provider performed the services (the CPT codes) shown on that health claim form. The ICD-9-CM diagnosis codes are the reasons, or the rationale, for doing what was done—the procedures. The Current Procedural Terminology (CPT)* codes tell the insurance company specifically WHAT was done and, therefore, how much the provider should be paid.

IMPORTANT NOTE

Certain features, such as the color of pages and notations or the page references by code series, may differ by publisher. Please do not permit these design elements to confuse you as you learn to code procedures.

---

*Enhance the learning process by pairing this chapter with a current copy of the AMA's Current Procedural Terminology (CPT) book.

All CPT codes are five-digit numbers that simplify the reporting of the procedures and services provided to each patient. These CPT codes are presented in the *Current Procedural Terminology* (CPT) book.

> **IMPORTANT NOTE**
>
> Many hospitals use Volume 3 of the ICD-9-CM book for coding inpatient procedures, rather than the CPT book. You will learn how to code using ICD-9-CM, Volume 3 procedure codes in Chapter 8.

Memory Tip

CPT codes = WHAT the provider did for the patient

NUMERICAL LISTINGS OF CPT CODES

The chief portion of the *Current Procedural Terminology* (CPT) book contains the listing of every CPT code, in numerical order, from 00100 to 99602. This portion of the book is divided into six sections:

Evaluation and Management (E/M) 99201–99499

Anesthesia 00100–01999, 99100–99140

Surgery 10021–69990

Radiology 70010–79999

Pathology and Laboratory 80048–89356

Medicine 90281–99199, 99500–99602

Key Terms

Evaluation and Management: The section that includes codes for face-to-face time spent with patients.

Anesthesia: The section that includes codes for services for administering anesthetics.

Surgery: The section that includes codes for surgical procedures.

CODING AND REPORTING GUIDELINES

At the beginning of each of the six sections, you will find a few gray pages with guidelines for that section (e.g., "Surgery Guidelines"). These gray pages review specific information that relates to coding using the procedures described in that section. Be certain to spend some time reading through this information. It will be very helpful when you are trying to find the best correct code.

Key Term

Radiology: The section that includes codes for X-rays, nuclear medicine, and diagnostic ultrasound.

ALPHABETIC INDEX

At the back of the book, you will find the index. The CPT index is the alphabetic listing of all procedures and services. Just like the alphabetic index in ICD-9-CM, you will look up the key terms from the physician's notes in this part of the book to point you to the correct part of the numerical listing of CPT. Also like ICD-9-CM, you must *never* code out of the alphabetic index. Even when there is only one code shown in the index, you still must go to the numeric listings and confirm that this is the best code available.

Key Terms

Pathology and Laboratory: The section that includes codes for lab tests and analyses.

Medicine: The section that includes codes for other medical services.

> **IMPORTANT NOTE**
>
> *Never* code out of the alphabetic index. ALWAYS confirm the code in the numeric listing.

You can look up the procedure and/or service in the index using any of the four types of descriptors listed alphabetically.

1. *Procedure or service itself,* such as bypass graft, cast, or fitting
2. *Anatomical site,* such as colon, face, or hand
3. *Condition,* such as fracture, dislocation, or hematoma
4. *Synonyms, eponyms, and abbreviations,* such as EKG, Heller procedure, or LDH

Example

You have a patient who has had an open treatment of a bimalleolar ankle fracture. You can look under the condition, *Fracture,* or you can look under the anatomical site, *Ankle.* Either way, you will get to the correct code of 27814.

EVALUATION AND MANAGEMENT CODES

Evaluation and Management (E/M) is the first section in CPT; it lists codes numbered 99201 through 99499. Although this is the first section, these codes are near the highest numbers. The numeric listing of the book is in numerical order, but not from front to back. The codes are shown in numerical order section by section; however, you should be able to find your way around.

The Evaluation and Management (E/M) section contains the codes assigned to the visit between provider and patient. These codes are used to pay the provider for meeting face-to-face with the patient and his or her family, evaluating the situation, and determining the correct procedures and services to help the patient in the best way. The various codes measure three key aspects of this encounter:

1. *Location of the encounter.* Did the provider see the patient in their office or another outpatient location, in the hospital, or in a skilled nursing facility?
2. *Relationship.* Is this individual a new patient of the provider, is the person an established patient, or is this a one-time visit for a consultation?
3. *Complexity/time spent.* How much time did the encounter require of the provider? How complex was the situation or concern?

In order to assign the best code for this portion of the encounter, you will need to know the answers to all these components, to determine the appropriate level.

Memory Tip

Evaluation and Management Codes compensate physician's for their knowledge and expertise.

BOX 7-1	CPT E/M Location Headings

- ❑ Office or Other Outpatient Services
- ❑ Hospital Observation Services
- ❑ Hospital Inpatient Services
- ❑ Consultations
- ❑ Emergency Department Services
- ❑ Pediatric Critical Care Patient Transport
- ❑ Critical Care Services
- ❑ Inpatient Neonatal and Pediatric Critical Care Services
- ❑ Inpatient Pediatric Critical Care
- ❑ Inpatient Neonatal Critical Care
- ❑ Intensive (Non-Critical) Low Birth Weight Services
- ❑ Nursing Facility Services
- ❑ Domiciliary, Rest Home (e.g., Boarding Home), or Custodial Care Services
- ❑ Home Services
- ❑ Prolonged Services
- ❑ Case Management Services
- ❑ Care Plan Oversight Services
- ❑ Preventive Medicine Services
- ❑ Newborn Care
- ❑ Special Evaluation and Management Services
- ❑ Other Evaluation and Management Services

Location

Let's go to the Evaluation and Management (E/M) section of the CPT book. You will see on the very first page the heading

Office or Other Outpatient Services

Such headings identify the **location** of the encounter. Other headings in the E/M section are shown in Box 7-1.

Relationship

Continue down the page under *Office or Other Outpatient Services* and you will see the first subheading. This subheading identifies the relationship between the provider and the individual—**new patient** or **established patient**.

Key Terms

Location: Where the provider met with the patient.

New patient: A person who has not received any professional services from this provider, or another provider of the same specialty who belongs to the same group practice, within the past three years.

Established patient: A person who has received professional services from this provider within the past three years.

FIGURE 7-1
E&M New Patient listings.

> # New Patient
>
> **99201** **Office or other outpatient visit** for the evaluation and management of a new patient, which requires these three key components:
>
> ■ **a problem focused history;**
>
> ■ **a problem focused examination; and**
>
> ■ **straightforward medical decision making.**
>
> Counseling and/or coordination of care with other providers or agencies are provided consistent with the nature of the problem(s) and the patient's and/or family's needs.
>
> Usually, the presenting problems are self limited or minor. Physicians typically spend 10 minutes face-to-face with the patient and/or family.

Complexity/Time

Next you see that there are only five codes in the section *Office or Other Patient Services: New Patient:* 99201 through 99205. How can you know which is the correct code? How can you tell them apart?

There are two ways you can tell which is the best code. Look at the bullet points in the description of each code (Figure 7-1). You will notice a difference immediately in the description of the **complexity** of the encounter:

> 99201 is described as problem-focused history and examination with straightforward medical decision making.
>
> 99202 is described as expanded problem focused with straightforward medical decision making.
>
> 99203 is described as detailed with medical decision making of low complexity.
>
> 99204 is described as comprehensive with medical decision making of moderate complexity.
>
> 99205 is described as comprehensive with medical decision making of high complexity.

Next look at the time measurement described in the last paragraph under each code.

> 99201 is 10 minutes face-to-face with the patient and/or family.
>
> 99202 is 20 minutes face-to-face with the patient and/or family.
>
> 99203 is 30 minutes face-to-face with the patient and/or family.
>
> 99204 is 45 minutes face-to-face with the patient and/or family.
>
> 99205 is 60 minutes face-to-face with the patient and/or family.

Key Term

Complexity: The measure of how complicated the issue is.

When we attempt to evaluate the amount of time the provider spent face-to-face with the patient, it is not expected that you stand outside the examination room with a stopwatch. Guidelines direct you to use the number of minutes only when more than 50% of the time was spent counseling the patient. Otherwise, time is an approximate measurement of how long it took for the physician to

1. document the appropriate level of patient history,
2. perform the appropriate level of physical examination, and
3. determine the best course of service or treatment (the appropriate level of medical decision making).

There are four **levels of patient history.** They are

1. Problem-focused: a brief history of the present health concern (the chief complaint)
2. Expanded problem-focused: a brief history of the present health concern as well as a review of the body system(s) related to this specific concern
3. Detailed: an extended history of the present health concern, an extended review of body systems, as well as concern-related past, family, and/or social history (PFSH)
4. Comprehensive: an extended history of the present health concern, a complete review of body systems, and a complete PFSH

There are four **levels of physical examination.** They are

1. Problem-focused: a limited examination of the body area related to the concern
2. Expanded problem-focused: a limited examination of the related body area and any other related body area(s) or organ system(s)
3. Detailed: an extended examination of the related body area(s) or organ system(s) and any other related body area(s) or organ system(s)
4. Comprehensive: a general, multisystem examination, or a complete examination of a single organ system and other related body area(s) or organ system(s)

There are four **levels of medical decision making.** They are

1. Straightforward: a minimal number of diagnoses, management options, and risks for complications; and little-to-no data to be reviewed
2. Low Complexity: a limited number of diagnoses, management options, and data to be reviewed; and low risk for complications
3. Moderate Complexity: a multiple number of diagnoses and/or management options, a moderate amount of data to be reviewed and a moderate level of risk for complications
4. High Complexity: an extensive number of diagnoses and/or management options, an extensive amount of data to be reviewed and a high level of risk for complications

Key Term

Levels of Patient History: The amount of detail involved in the documentation of patient history.

Key Term

Levels of Physical Exams: The extent of the patient's body systems investigated during the encounter.

Key Term

Medical decision making (MDM): The description of how difficult it was for the provider to decide what to do next.

CASE STUDY

Bart, a 35-year-old patient comes to see Dr. Morgan for the first time for treatment of a sprained wrist, a very specific concern. After taking a problem-focused history and performing a problem-focused examination, Dr. Morgan decided the next step is to have an X-ray taken of the problem area. That is very straightforward medical decision making.

Can you find the best, most appropriate E/M code?

_____

_____

Given the level of complexity, the correct answer is CPT code 99201.

In comparison, another new patient's chart contains physician's notes indicating information on the health of the patient's parents, siblings, and other family members, along with details about the individual's past medical conditions. The notes include a social history as well. This is a rather comprehensive history. In addition, the notes indicate that the physician did a very thorough physical examination, head to toe, of the patient due to a chief complaint of extreme lethargy. These notes indicate an appropriate E/M code of 99205 comprehensive history, comprehensive examination, high complexity, spending 60 minutes face-to-face.

Continue down the page under *Office or Other Outpatient Services* and you will see the second subheading Established Patient. This next section, codes 99211 through 99215, uses the same description of service levels, as those for a new patient. The only difference is that these services are being provided to an established patient.

IMPORTANT NOTE

E/M Guidelines direct you to choose the code at which the required components are met or exceeded. Therefore, if you have a new patient in the office with a problem-focused history, a problem-focused exam, and a low complexity level of decision making, you must choose code 99201.

Some of the subsections within the E/M section of the CPT book differentiate between a new patient and an established patient, but others do not. You must read the descriptions at the beginning of each subsection to be certain whether or not this is a criterion for a particular E/M code.

In a medical office environment, every time you work toward completing a health claim form, you should have an Evaluation and Management code. How could any procedure or service be performed without a face-to-face meeting with the provider?

Get very familiar with this section of the CPT book. You may find it easier not to use the index (the alphabetic listing) to find your way around it. Don't get overwhelmed. Once you get a job, you will find that one portion of this section will become your main focus.

- If you work for a provider in a private medical office, most of your E/M codes will be found under the Office heading on the first two pages of the section.
- If you go to work in conjunction with a hospital, you will find most of your E/M codes under Hospital Observation Services, Hospital Inpatient Services, or Emergency Department Services.

Most of the time, you will be using the same, small set of codes over and over again. But because you don't know where you will be working, you should learn about the entire section.

Example

In the E/M section, under the subheading Emergency Department Services, the same codes are offered whether the individual is a *new* or an *established patient*.

Reading the Physician's Notes

Let's look at some statements from patients' charts and identify the key words that will help you find the correct E/M code.

1. A 65-year-old male is seen for the <u>first time</u> by the physician in the <u>office</u> for a <u>contusion of his hand</u>.
   a. Location: <u>office</u> tells us where the encounter took place.
   b. Relationship: <u>first time</u> tells us this is a new patient.
   c. Complexity/time: <u>contusion of his hand</u> tells us this is problem focused. Therefore, the correct code is 99201.
2. The physician performs an <u>initial observation at the hospital</u> of a <u>current patient</u>, a 27-year-old female. A <u>detailed examination</u> reveals lower right quadrant pain accompanied by nausea, vomiting, and a low-grade fever. <u>Overnight admission to the hospital</u> is suggested to rule out appendicitis.
   a. Location: <u>initial observation at the hospital</u> tells us this code is in the Hospital Observation Services section.
   b. Relationship: <u>current patient</u> tells us this is an established patient.
   c. Complexity/time: <u>detailed examination</u> and <u>overnight admission to the hospital</u> all lead us to the correct code of 99218.
3. A general surgeon saw a 37-year-old female <u>in his office</u> for a <u>second opinion</u> regarding a lump in her right breast. An <u>expanded problem-focused history</u> is positive for breast cancer on her maternal side. After reviewing existing mammogram and physical examination, the physician made a <u>straightforward decision</u> to advise a lumpectomy.
   a. Location: <u>in his office</u> tells us where the encounter took place.
   b. Relationship: <u>second opinion</u> tells us this is a consultation.
   c. Complexity/time: <u>expanded problem-focused history</u> and <u>straightforward decision</u> lead us directly to the correct code of 99242.

4. A 15-year-old male presents at the <u>emergency department</u> with a painful, swollen wrist. The patient states he was hurt at a softball game. An <u>expanded problem-focused history</u> and <u>physical examination</u> are performed and X-rays taken.
    a. Location: <u>emergency department</u> tells you the location.
    b. Relationship: You will note that the codes in the Emergency Department Services section do not differentiate between new and established patients.
    c. Complexity/time: <u>expanded problem-focused</u> history and <u>physical examination</u> tell you the extent of the encounter. The correct code is 99282.

CASE STUDY

A physician arrives at a nursing facility to do an annual assessment of her patient, an 80-year-old female. A detailed interval history is taken and a comprehensive physical examination performed. Decision making is extremely complex, as the patient has senile dementia, hypertension, and hypothyroidism. A new treatment plan is created due to changes in the patient's condition.

Can you find the best, most appropriate E/M code?

- Determine the location.
- What is the relationship?
- What level of complexity was the decision making?

_____

_____

The location is a nursing facility, and all codes in this section are for both new and established patients. In addition, the detailed interval history, comprehensive physical examination, and extremely complex decision making lead to the correct code, 99302.

If you would like to look at some additional examples of physician's notes that translate into various E/M codes, you will find them in Appendix C of the CPT book. In addition, in Appendix C of this textbook, you will find the most recent published guidelines for Evaluation and Management coding from the Centers for Medicare & Medicaid Services.

THE NUMERIC LISTINGS IN CPT

The chief portion of the CPT book contains the numerical listing of all procedures and services. This portion of the book is made up of the other five sections—Anesthesia, Surgery, Radiology, Pathology and Laboratory, and Medicine.

These sections are in numerical order. On each page, in the upper, outside corner, you will see the range of codes covered on that page, along with the name of the section.

Once you find the code, or range of codes, in the index for the procedure you are looking for, you can easily find the correct page in the numeric listing. Just as in ICD-9-CM, you will see that the numeric listing not only shows a more detailed description of the procedure or service represented by that code but also includes directions and information *not* contained in the index. This is why you *never* code from the index.

Example

If you go to any page of some CPT books, and look at the top of the page, you will notice something that looks like the following:

Anesthesia   00796–00938

This tells you that this page contains information on procedures and services coded with numbers from 00796 through 00938.

CPT Formatting

As you read the numeric listings, you will see that parts of the columns are indented. The indented portion is an adjustment, an additional version, or additional information attached to a previous code (found at the margin). The description written next to the previous code, up to the semicolon (;), is to be repeated along with the description of the indented portion. This is printed this way to save space in the book. For example,

84106 <u>Porphobilinogen, urine;</u> qualitative

84110   <u>quantitative</u>

The actual description for code 84110 is

84110 <u>Porphobilinogen, urine; quantitative</u>

The description of the previous code is repeated, up to the semicolon (;), and completed with the additional information shown at the indented description (Figure 7-2).

| 84106 | Porphobilinogen, urine; qualitative |
| 84110 | quantitative |

FIGURE 7-2
Example of CPT formatting.

Here's another example:

> 31820 Surgical closure tracheostomy or fistula; without plastic repair
> 31825   with plastic repair

The complete description for 31825 is

> 31825 Surgical closure tracheostomy or fistula; with plastic repair

Now you can read the book and find the correct code more easily.

Example

(See Figure 7-3.)

> 31800 Suture of tracheal wound or injury; cervical
> 31805   intrathoracic

Can you identify the complete description of code 31805? If you said

> 31805 Suture of tracheal wound or injury; intrathoracic

you are correct. Great job!

FIGURE 7-3
Another example of CPT formatting.

31800	Suture of tracheal wound or injury; cervical
31805	intrathoracic
31820	Surgical closure tracheostomy or fistula; without plastic repair
31825	with plastic repair
	(For repair tracheoesophageal fistula, see 43305, 43312)

CPT Directional Symbols

The numeric listing includes instructions regarding when to use a different code or to use an additional code. You may see the instruction as a symbol in front of the code and/or in parentheses with or below the code and its description (Figure 7-4).

> + 35681 Bypass graft; composite, prosthetic and vein (List separately in addition to code for primary procedure)
>
> (Do not report 35681 in addition to 35682, 35683)

FIGURE 7-4
Example code with three sets of instructions.

+ 35681	Bypass graft; composite, prosthetic and vein (List separately in addition to code for primary procedure)
	(Do not report 35681 in addition to 35682, 35683)

In this example, there are three sets of instructions with this code and its description. Let's dissect this entry in the CPT book. First, the code with its description is

> 35681 Bypass graft; composite, prosthetic and vein

Now let's look at the directions given to us by the book. The complete listing shown is

> **+** 35681 Bypass graft; composite, prosthetic and vein (List separately in addition to code for primary procedure)
>
> (Do not report 35681 in addition to 35682, 35683)

The symbol in front of the code number—*the* **+** *sign*—tells you that this is an *add-on code,* to be used with other codes that further describe the complete procedure or service. If you look along the bottom edge of the page, you will see a legend that will remind you of this symbol's meaning.

You will see that other symbols used throughout the book are also in the legend across the bottom of both facing pages. These symbols include the following

- ● A bullet indicates a new code, added to this edition for the first time.

- ▲ A triangle indicates a revised code. This means that an existing code shown in previous editions has had its description changed to this new description.

- ⊙ A dot with a circle around it indicates that this procedure code <u>includes</u> the administration of conscious sedation.

- ⊘ A circle with a line through it indicates a code that is exempt from using **modifier** *-51*. Modifier *-51* is used to indicate multiple procedures performed at the same session with other procedures. (More on modifiers later in this chapter.)

CPT Directional Notations

Using our same example, we can review the directional notations in CPT's numerical listings. These notations, included within code descriptions, direct you to more accurate coding.

> **+** 35681 Bypass graft; composite, prosthetic and vein
>
> **(List separately in addition to code for primary procedure)**
>
> (Do not report 35681 in addition to 35682, 35683)

The instruction in the first set of parentheses, included as a part of the code's description (Figure 7-5)—(*List separately in addition to code for primary procedure*)—instructs you to be certain to include another code for the primary procedure on the claim form. In other words, this code represents only a portion of this health care service and cannot stand by itself. As the **+** sign tells you, this code, 35681, is an add-on code and should be *added to* the code for the primary procedure. This notation is very similar to the *Code First* instruction in ICD-9-CM.

Memory Tip

These symbols, along with their meanings, are printed across the bottom of each page throughout most CPT books.

Key Term

Modifier: A code added to a CPT code to provide more detail or an explanation of an unusual circumstance affecting a service.

FIGURE 7-5
This code directs you to also use a primary procedure code.

+ 22328	each additional fractured vertebrae or dislocated segment (List separately in addition to code for primary procedure)

+ 35681 Bypass graft; composite, prosthetic and vein

(List separately in addition to code for primary procedure)

(Do not report 35681 in addition to 35682, 35683)

This instruction, shown below the main description for code 35681, tells you to be certain that you don't make the mistake of including either code 35682 or 35683 on the same claim form. These are called **mutually exclusive codes.**

Other instructions commonly seen in the CPT book include the following:

(Use 78496 in conjunction with code 78472)

This instruction tells you the correct choice for a primary procedure code to use with this add-on code.

(For open procedure, use 37140)

This instruction tells you that, if this detail is specified (in this case, "open procedure") in the physician's notes, you should choose the different code indicated.

Key Term

Mutually exclusive codes: Two codes that are not permitted to be placed on the same claim form.

Example

43280 Laparoscopy, Surgical, esophagogastric fundoplasty

(For open approach, use 43324)

(79420 has been deleted. To report, use 79445)

This instruction is really for experienced coders, professionals who have been coding for so long that they already know the correct code. This instruction is reminding them that this code has been changed as a part of the updating that the CPT book goes through each year. If you are a new coder, you don't have to worry about this instruction. However, it should serve as a reminder that changes occur to the codes in the book every year. It is important that you use the most up-to-date edition.

(separate procedure)

This instruction tells you that this procedure was performed independently and is considered unrelated or specifically different from other procedures and/or services provided at the same time to that patient but is nonetheless necessary and appropriate. This code may be reported by itself or along with the modifier -59 (if reported with other procedure codes).

(Do not report modifier -63 in conjunction with 33786)

Here you are told directly that a specific modifier may not be used with this code. See page 151 for more on modifiers.

CPT Instructional Notations

You may find instructional notations regarding the correct reporting of certain codes and modifiers shown at the beginning of subsections within each area of the CPT book. These are in addition to the pages at the beginning of each of the six sections, and appear throughout the numerical listings.

If you go to the first page for the subsection of the Musculoskeletal System in the Surgery section, you will see a long list of instructions to be used when coding from this portion of the book. Definitions of terms, and additional coding guidelines are also included in these notes. The following is an example from these instructions:

> Manipulation is used throughout the musculoskeletal fracture and dislocation subsections to specifically mean the attempted reduction or restoration of a fracture or joint dislocation to its normal anatomic alignment by the application of manually applied forces.

The instructional notations are there to remind you of alternate terms, such as manipulation, attempted reduction and restoration, that might be used in the physician's notes, and/or code descriptions so you can find the best code more easily. Sometimes these instructional paragraphs also include examples to help you better understand the best way to use the information in the book. Consider the following example:

> The physician's notes reveal a closed treatment of a vertebral fracture was performed by *manually restoring the fracture to its normal alignment,* followed by the application of a brace. No anesthesia was required.

Because you read the instructional notation, you know that the phrase *"manually restoring the fracture to its normal alignment"* shown in the physician's notes means the same as the code description phrase *"by manipulation"* in the CPT book (Figure 7-6), and therefore the correct code is

> 22315 Closed treatment of vertebral fracture(s) and/or dislocation(s) requiring casting or bracing, with and including casting and/or bracing, with or without anesthesia, *by manipulation* or traction

Carefully reading all instructional notations both in the pages at the beginning of each section, as well as the in-column notations at the beginning of some of the subsections, is essential if you are just beginning your coding career. Again, once you get settled in a job, you will begin to know these guidelines from experience and from your work with the information day after day.

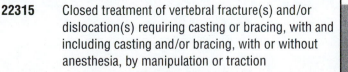

22315 Closed treatment of vertebral fracture(s) and/or dislocation(s) requiring casting or bracing, with and including casting and/or bracing, with or without anesthesia, by manipulation or traction

(For spinal subluxation, use 97140)

FIGURE 7-6
Note the phrase "by manipulation" is different than the phrase used in the physician's notes, but it means the same.

USING DOCUMENTATION TO DETERMINE PROCEDURE CODES

As you know, you need to review the physician's notes, pull out the key words regarding the procedures and services performed, and match them to the best, most appropriate code(s) in the CPT book. This process is very similar to the way you code diagnoses.

As discussed in Chapter 5, you will often receive a superbill in your office. On this superbill, you will find that the provider has circled or checked off the best code available for what occurred during the encounter with the patient. Then all you have to do is copy those codes onto the health claim form and your work is done, right? You know better than that by now. Remember that the provider will circle the best code available on the superbill. The superbill is printed with the codes *most often used* in that health care facility. That does not necessarily include the *best possible* of all codes in the CPT book. Therefore, you must look at the physician's notes as well as look in the CPT book and make certain that the code circled by the provider is, indeed, the best of all possible codes. In this section, we are going to focus only on the procedure coding, not on the E/M codes, which we practiced earlier in this chapter. (We will put them all together later on in Chapter 9.)

Remember our patient with the family history of colon cancer from Chapter 5? Harvey Practice had come to see his regular physician for a colonoscopy. He has a family history of colon cancer, so he is very diligent about getting his regular checkup. A colonoscopy was performed in the ambulatory surgical center and, using a snare technique, one polyp was removed and sent to pathology. As you can see from the superbill (Figure 7-7), the physician checked off the code

45378 Colonoscopy, diagnostic

Let's go to the CPT index and look up Colonoscopy. As you read down the column, you can see that Diagnostic is not listed as a description nor is the code 45378. Let's try looking under Colon, where you find

Endoscopy
    Exploration . . . 44388, 45378, 45381, 45386

Therefore, if you were to code directly from the superbill, you would end up with the actual description of

45378 Colon, endoscopy, exploration

FAMILY DOCTORS ASSOCIATES
123 Main Street
Anytown, FL 32711
(407) 555-1200

Date: *March 3, 2005*   Attending Physician: *John Healer, MD*

Patient Name: *Harvey Practice*

CPT DESCRIPTION	CPT DESCRIPTION	CPT DESCRIPTION
OFFICE/HOSPITAL	**PATHOLOGY/LAB/RADIOLOGY**	**PROCEDURES/TESTS**
☐ 99201 OFFICE-NEW; FOCUSED	☐ 73100 X-RAY WRIST TWO VIEWS	☐ 12011 SIMPLE SUTURE, FACE
☐ 99202 OFFICE-NEW; EXPANDED	☐ 73590 X-RAY TIBIA/FIBULA, TWO	☐ 29125 SPLINT-SHORT ARM
☐ 99203 OFFICE-NEW; DETAILED	☐ 73600 X-RAY ANKLE TWO VIEWS	☐ 29355 WALKER CAST-LONG LEG
☐ 99204 OFFICE-NEW; COMPREHEN	☐ 76085 MAMMOGRAM-COMP DET	☐ 29540 STRAPPING-ANKLE
☐ 99205 OFFICE-NEW; COMPREHEN	☐ 76092 MAMMOGRAM SCREENING	☒ 45378 COLONOSCOPY-DIAGNOSTIC
☐ 99211 OFFICE-ESTB; MINIMAL	☐ 80050 BLOOD TEST-GEN HEALTH	☐ 45391 COLONOSCOPY-ULTRASOUND
☐ 99212 OFFICE-ESTB; FOCUSED	☐ 80061 BLOOD TEST-LIPID PANEL	☐ 50390 ASPIRATION, RENAL CYST
☐ 99213 OFFICE-ESTB; EXPANDED	☐ 82947 BLOOD TEST-GLUCOSE	☐ 90703 TETANUS INJECTION
☒ 99214 OFFICE-ESTB; DETAILED	☐ 83718 BLOOD TEST-HDL	☐ 92081 VISUAL FIELD EXAM
☐ 99215 OFFICE-ESTB; COMPREHEN	☐ 85025 BLOOD TEST-CBC	☐ 93000 ECG, 12 LEADS, W/RPT
☐ 99281 EMER DEPT; FOCUSED	☐ 86403 STREP TEST, QUICK	☐ 93015 TREADMILL STRESS TEST
☐ 90844 COUNSELING—50 MIN.	☐ 87430 ENZY IMMUNOASSAY-STREP	☐ 99173 VISUAL ACUITY SCREEN

ICD DESCRIPTION	ICD DESCRIPTION	ICD DESCRIPTION
☐ 034.0 STREP THROAT	☐ 522 LOW RED BLOOD COUNT	☐ V01.5 RABIES EXPOSURE
☐ 042 HUMAN IMMUNO VIRUS	☐ 538.8 STOMACH PAIN	☒ V16.0 FAM HISTORY-COLON
☐ 250.51 DIABETES W/VISION	☐ 643 HYPEREMESIS	☐ V16.3 FAM HISTORY- BREAST
☐ 250.80 DIABETES, TYPE II	☐ 707.14 ULCER OF HEEL/MID FOOT	☐ V20.2 WELL CHILD
☐ 307.51 BULIMIA NON-ORGANIC	☐ 788.30 ENURESIS	☐ V22.0 PREGNANCY-FIRST NORM
☐ 354.0 CARPEL TUNNEL SYNDROME	☐ 815.00 FRACTURE, HAND	☐ V22.1 PREGNANCY-NORMAL
☐ 362.01 RETINOPATHY (DIABETIC)	☐ 823.2 FRACTURE, TIBIA	☐ E816.2 MOTORCYCLE ACCT
☐ 401.9 HYPERTENSION, UNSPEC	☐ 831.00 DISLOCATION, SHOULDER	☐ E826.1 FALL FROM BICYCLE
☐ 482.30 PNEUMONIA	☐ 845.00 SPRAINED ANKLE	☐ E849.0 PLACE OF OCCUR-HOME
☐ 490 BRONCHITIS, UNSPECIFIED	☐ 880.03 OPEN WOUND UPPER ARM	☐ E881.0 FALL FROM LADDER
☐ 493.92 ASTHMA, UNSPECIFIED	☐ 912.0 ABRASION, SHOULDER	☐ E906.0 DOG BITE

FOLLOW UP

PRN _____

WEEKS _____

NXT APPT. _____

TIME _____

FIGURE 7-7
Superbill showing procedure codes.

FIGURE 7-8
This code matches the superbill, but does it describe what was actually done?

⊙ **45378** Colonoscopy, flexible, proximal to splenic flexure; diagnostic, with or without collection of specimen(s) by brushing or washing, with or without colon decompression (separate procedure)

When you go to the numeric listing, you see (Figure 7-8)

> 45378 Colonoscopy, flexible, proximal to splenic flexure; diagnostic, with or without collection of specimen(s) by brushing or washing, with or without colon decompression (separate procedure)

This matches the superbill but is it the best, most appropriate code? When you look at the physician's notes, you see that the colonoscopy included the removal of a polyp by snare technique. First, let's identify the key words for coding the procedure according to the notes.

> The colonoscopy included the removal of a polyp by snare technique.

If you go back to the index and look under Colonoscopy again, you will see

> Removal
>   Polyp................45384–45385

There is no mention of snare technique in the index, so let's go into the numeric listing and find codes 45384 and 45385 to see if either of those is better than 45378. You see (Figure 7-9)

> 45378 Colonoscopy, flexible, proximal to splenic flexure; diagnostic, with or without collection of specimen(s) by brushing or washing, with or without colon decompression (separate procedure)

Continuing down the column at the indented descriptions below 45378, we see . . .

> 45384   with removal of tumor(s), polyp(s), or other lesion(s) by hot biopsy forceps or bipolar cautery
> 45385   with removal of tumor(s), polyp(s), or other lesion(s) by snare technique

The complete description for code 45385, reads as

> 45385 Colonoscopy, flexible, proximal to splenic flexure; with removal of tumor(s), polyp(s), or other lesion(s) by snare technique

This matches the physician's notes exactly. You have found your best code—one that was not listed on the preprinted superbill.

In addition, the fact that the physician found and removed a polyp from Harvey Practice's colon during the procedure means that we should add the diagnosis code 211.3 colon polyps to the claim. Another element that is not available on the superbill.

⊙ **45378**	Colonoscopy, flexible, proximal to splenic flexure; diagnostic, with or without collection of specimen(s) by brushing or washing, with or without colon decompression (separate procedure)	
⊙ **45379**	with removal of foreign body	
⊙ **45380**	with biopsy, single or multiple	
⊙ **45381**	with directed submucosal injection(s), any substance	
⊙ **45382**	with control of bleeding (eg, injection, bipolar cautery, unipolar cautery, laser, heater probe, stapler, plasma coagulator)	
⊙ **45383**	with ablation of tumor(s), polyp(s), or other lesion(s) not amenable to removal by hot biopsy forceps, bipolar cautery or snare technique	
⊙ **45384**	with removal of tumor(s), polyp(s), or other lesion(s) by hot biopsy forceps or bipolar cautery	
⊙ **45385**	with removal of tumor(s), polyp(s), or other lesion(s) by snare technique	

FIGURE 7-9
Code 45385 matches the physician's notes.

CASE STUDY

A 22-year-old female goes to the physician's office for a mammogram. She has a family history of malignant neoplasm of the female breast (breast cancer). In addition to the E/M code, you will need to code the mammogram. When you go to the index and look up Mammogram, you will see that Mammography, shown right below mammogram, actually has the better description.

Mammography 76090-76092

Screening 76092

with Computer-aided Detection 76082-76083

You know that a screening mammogram is used for a checkup, but do you know if the physician requested computer-aided detection? How will you know?

_____

_____

If your preprinted superbill does not have both codes as choices for the physician, you will have to go to the documentation to determine the correct code. However, you know the rule: *never code from the index.*

FIGURE 7-10

Two codes are needed, but you wouldn't have known it if you had looked only at the superbill.

76092	Screening mammography, bilateral (two view film study of each breast)
	(Use 76083 in conjunction with 76092 for computer aided detection applied to a screening mammogram)

Let's go to the numerical listing. Directly under 76092 is a notation that says you must use both 76092 and 76083 if the computer-aided detection is used. So, if the physician's notes or the lab report indicate the computer analysis, then you must first code 76092, then 76083 (Figure 7-10). This is why you must always check the numeric listing. If you had coded only from the index or the superbill, you would not have known to include both codes.

CASE STUDY

Carole Silhouette, a 35-year-old female, has hurt her ankle. She states that she jumped from the back of her friend's truck and landed on the side of her foot. Dr. Mason, her regular physician, examines her foot and lower leg and diagnoses a sprain. Dr. Mason then orders an X-ray of the ankle (two views) and, once it is confirmed that the ankle is not fractured, applies a strapping.

Can you find the best, most appropriate procedure codes?

_____

_____

This time, there are three codes. Can you find the key words? They are *regular physician, X-ray of the ankle,* and *applies a strapping.* Good job!

In the E/M section, we can go directly to Office or Other Outpatient Services. The key words *regular physician* tell us Carole is an established patient. The physician only examined Carole's foot and leg so this was a problem-focused encounter. Therefore, our correct E/M code is 99212.

Now, let's go to the CPT index and look up our next key word, *X-ray.*

X-Ray

Ankle...................................73600–73610

Turn to the numeric listing and find code 73600 (Figure 7-11).

73600 Radiologic examination, ankle; two views

73610   complete, minimum of three views

FIGURE 7-11

The code 73600 is correct, as only two views were taken.

73600	Radiologic examination, ankle; two views
73610	complete, minimum of three views

The physician's notes indicate that only two views were taken, so 73600 is the correct code.

Now, let's go back to the index to look up our next key word, *strapping*. You see

Strapping

Ankle............29540

Turn to the numeric listing and find code 29540. It is the only choice, and it is the best code. Good job!

MODIFIERS

Modifiers are used to explain unusual circumstances or situations, with regard to the performance of procedures. These two-digit numbers are added after a procedure code to indicate to the insurance carrier why something out of the ordinary occurred. You will find a description explaining how and when you might use that particular modifier. In Appendix A of the CPT book, you will find a listing of all approved modifiers for use with CPT codes (Figure 7-12). (Appendix A is located after the main text of the book and before the index.) Let's go through each modifier along with some additional explanation.

Memory Tip

A modifier *modifies*, or adjusts, the description of a code by explaining an unusual circumstance.

FIGURE 7-12
Modifiers as listed in the CPT Appendix A.

Appendix A

Modifiers

This list includes all of the modifiers applicable to *CPT 2005* codes.

21 **Prolonged Evaluation and Management Services:** When the face-to-face or floor/unit service(s) provided is prolonged or otherwise greater than that usually required for the highest level of evaluation and management service within a given category, it may be identified by adding modifier 21 to the evaluation and management code number. A report may also be appropriate.

22 **Unusual Procedural Services:** When the service(s) provided is greater than that usually required for the listed procedure, it may be identified by adding modifier 22 to the usual procedure number. A report may also be appropriate.

23 **Unusual Anesthesia:** Occasionally, a procedure, which usually requires either no anesthesia or local anesthesia, because of unusual circumstances must be done under general anesthesia. This circumstance may be reported by adding modifier 23 to the procedure code of the basic service.

IMPORTANT NOTE

Many modifiers refer to the "post-operative period." This is a specific amount of time, after surgery, that the patient is still officially under the surgeon's care. The amount of time varies with the particular procedure as determined by the standard of care.

Evaluation and Management Modifiers

-21   When the face-to-face time is more than the highest level of E/M service in that category, add modifier 21 to the E/M code. It may be appropriate to attach a report to your claim form to explain further.

-24   When a physician meets with a patient during the patient's postoperative period of time about a totally different health issue, modifier 24 should be added to the appropriate E/M code.

-25   When a physician must perform an E/M service totally separate from another service provided on the same day, modifier 25 should be added to the E/M service code.

-32   When the physician's services are required by an insurance carrier or legislative ruling, modifier 32 should be used.

-57   When a physician meets with a patient only to determine if a surgical procedure should be performed, modifier 57 should be added to the appropriate E/M code. This is only used for the initial decision for the surgery, not the preoperative visit.

Examples

A patient has a biopsy after a lump in her breast is found. During the post-operative period, the patient needs to meet with her physician because she sprained her ankle. This E/M code requires modifier 24.

A patient meets with his physician to have a mole removed from his hand. The physician spends about 20 minutes to do this. While he is there, test results on his blood work come back and show a problem with his cholesterol level. The physician takes time to discuss diet and exercise with the patient. This is time spent that has nothing to do with the time spent attending to the patient's hand. Therefore, the E/M code gets modifier 25.

A patient is diagnosed with lung cancer. The insurance company mandates a second opinion before approving any course of treatment. The physician providing the second opinion consultation uses modifier 32 with the E/M code for that consultation.

Surgical Modifiers

-23   A patient may require general anesthesia, even though the procedure usually needs only the use of a local or perhaps no anesthesia at all. In this case, modifier 23 is added to the CPT code for that procedure.

-47   In some instances, the surgeon, rather than an anesthesiologist, will administer regional or general anesthesia to a patient. In this case, modifier 47 should be appended to the procedure code.

-50   If a procedure is performed to both sides of an area or organ (bilaterally), and this distinction is not included in the CPT code description, then modifier 50 should be added to the code for the procedure.

-51   When more than one procedure is performed at the same time by the same provider, the additional procedures (other than the first code) should have modifier 51 added, unless the additional procedures are designated as add-on codes (shown in the CPT main text with a **+** next to the five-digit code). Add-on codes do not use this modifier.

-54   CPT codes for surgical procedures are packaged (we will review this in more detail on page 161). This means that the one code for the procedure includes the physician's time for preoperative and postoperative management services. However, one physician may perform the surgical procedure only, and another may handle the preoperative and/or postoperative care. In this case, the physician doing only the procedure adds modifier 54 to indicate that someone else took care of the patient pre- and postoperatively.

-55   This is the modifier to be used by a physician who saw the patient only for postoperative management and did not perform the surgery.

-56   Modifier 56 is used by the physician who works with the patient only for preoperative management.

-58   Modifier 58 is added to the code for a procedure that is planned to occur in stages, or for therapy that is previously planned to directly follow a surgical procedure. This modifier would not be used if the patient had to return to the operating room for a second procedure. That would use modifier 78 (see below).

-62   Some operations require two surgeons to work together. In this case, you need to attach modifier 62 to the procedure code, so the insurance carrier does not suspect that the second surgeon is billing in error.

-63   The code for any surgical procedure performed on an infant who weighs less than 4 kilograms should have modifier 63 attached to it to identify the increased complexity and work required on a baby this small.

-66   When a complex surgical procedure needs a team of surgeons of various specialties to complete the operation, each member of the team uses this modifier attached to the procedure code.

-78   If the patient must go back into surgery for a related procedure during the postoperative period following the original procedure, the code for the subsequent procedure should have modifier 78 included.

(continued)

-79   When a patient is in the period of time following a surgical procedure and this patient needs another surgical procedure for a condition having nothing to do with the first, the second procedure code should include the modifier 79.

-80   A surgeon assisting the primary surgeon during an operation must use modifier 80 on his or her claim for that procedure.

-81   Modifier 81 indicates that an assistant surgeon provided minimum assistance during the procedure.

-82   If a qualified resident surgeon is not available to assist the primary surgeon during a surgical procedure and therefore someone else must fill in, then that second person must use modifier 82 on his or her claim for this procedural service.

Examples

Bobby, a 5 year-old male, had been suffering from severe diarrhea and rectal bleeding, so the physician felt a flexible sigmoidoscopy was warranted. However, because of the patient's age, he would not lie still long enough. Being concerned about accidental puncturing of the child's colon, the physician gave the patient general anesthesia before performing the diagnostic test. The modifier 23 would be added to the code for the sigmoidoscopy.

Two surgeons work together, performing a surgical procedure on a patient. When the time comes, each surgeon's office submits a claim form for performing the same surgery on the same patient on the same day. The insurance carrier gets one claim form and pays it. Then, the same carrier receives the second claim form and wonders why another physician is claiming to have performed the same procedure on the same patient on the same day. Again, this needs some explanation in order to get both surgeons properly compensated. Therefore, the coder in each office will add modifier 62 to the correct surgical procedure code. This modifier explains that two surgeons worked together on one operation.

Procedure Modifiers

-22   On occasion, a procedure becomes more complicated or difficult than normally expected. In this case, the physician may have to work harder and/or spend more time. Modifier 22 indicates that this happened. It would be wise to attach a report to outline the special circumstances of the case to improve the chances of having an increased fee paid without requiring an appeal.

-26   Some procedures are paid based only on a technical component, such as certain X-rays. When a professional component is necessary—the need for a physician to interpret test results, for example—modifier 26 should be used along with the usual procedure code.

-52   A physician may determine that a reduced service or a portion of the service should be eliminated for the well-being of the patient. When this occurs, modifier 52 should be used.

-53   If a physician determines that a procedure that was started should not continue at all, and the procedure is discontinued for the well-being of the patient, the code for this discontinued procedure should have modifier 53 attached.

-59   When two distinct procedures are provided by the same physician on the same day to the same patient, the procedure codes are appended with modifier 59.

-76   If a physician needs to repeat the same procedure on a patient, modifier 76 should be used with the codes for the second time the service is provided.

-77   Modifier 77 is used for the same procedure being provided to a patient by a different provider.

Examples

Marshall, a two-year-old male, needed an assessment of tinnitus for both ears. After the first ear was assessed, he is so distraught that the physician decides to end the encounter and have him return another day to do the other ear. Modifier 52 should be added to the procedure code.

Annabelle goes into a physician's office to have a mole removed from her shoulder. While there, the physician also removes a cyst from her eyelid. The code for removing the cyst would be appended with modifier 59.

A chest X-ray is taken of Mrs. Jones. The film is clouded; therefore, the chest X-ray is repeated for clarity. On the claim form for the second X-ray, modifier 76 is included.

Shaun, a fifteen-year-old male, breaks his arm: Dr. Katzman X-rays it and applies a cast. The next day, something happens and the cast must be reapplied. Dr. Katzman is not in town, so Dr. Saunders applies the cast again. Dr. Saunders uses modifier 77 with the procedure code for application of a cast.

Laboratory Modifiers

-90   For pathology and laboratory work done by an outside lab, but reported on a claim form by the attending physician, modifier 90 must be attached to the procedure code for the testing to indicate this fact.

-91   When the same lab test must be done on the same day several times in order to get multiple results, modifier 91 should be used. This does *not* include rerunning a test to confirm original results or redoing a test because of a problem.

Multiple Modifiers

-99 If two or more modifiers are applicable to one procedure code, modifier 99 should be shown. A report or thorough description of the unusual circumstances affecting this procedure should be attached to the claim form.

Modifier Case Studies

CASE STUDY

A physician performs a routine ECG using 12 leads on Gail Sunshine in the office one morning. The interpretation and report indicate a normal reading. Ms. Sunshine leaves the office and goes to work. During lunch, she experiences chest pains and numbness in her left arm and immediately returns to the physician's office. The physician performs a second ECG in order to compare the two reports.

How will you report this on the claim form?

_____

_____

If you indicate that the same procedure was performed twice in one day, the insurance carrier is going to believe that the second procedure on the claim form is an error. Without further explanation, your claim will be rejected. You must find a way to indicate, clearly, to the insurance carrier that this procedure was actually performed twice in one day on the same patient with good reason. In order to do this, you will use modifier 76. So, the code for the second ECG will look like this on your claim form: 93000-76.

CASE STUDY

Byron Jules, a 12-year-old male, needs to get an abscess on his finger drained. Normally, the physician would apply a local anesthetic to the area and do the procedure with a scalpel in the office. However, Byron has cerebral palsy and therefore is unable to sit still for the duration of the procedure. Dr. Warren is concerned about the situation and therefore uses general anesthesia to sedate Byron during the procedure. The insurance carrier knows that, routinely, this procedure (code 26010) does not require anesthesia or at most would require only a local.

What should the coder do?

_____

_____

The coder must know to add the modifier 23 (Unusual anesthesia) to that procedure code, and attach a letter or report to explain the situation.

Anesthesia Physical Status Modifiers

When reporting an anesthesia service, a physical status modifier must be used in addition to the appropriate procedure code and any other necessary modifiers (Figure 7-13). This two-character modifier (one letter, one number) is used to identify the level of complexity of the anesthesia service provided, as defined by the American Society of Anesthesiologists (ASA).

The six Physical Status Modifiers are

P1: A normal, healthy patient

P2: A patient with mild systemic disease

P3: A patient with severe systemic disease

P4: A patient with severe systemic disease that is a constant threat to life

P5: A moribund patient who is not expected to survive without the operation

P6: A declared brain-dead patient whose organs are being removed for donor purposes

The physical status modifier should be placed immediately after the five-digit standard procedure code and before any regular modifiers that may be necessary.

Physical Status Modifier P1: A normal healthy patient

Physical Status Modifier P2: A patient with mild systemic disease

Physical Status Modifier P3: A patient with severe systemic disease

Physical Status Modifier P4: A patient with severe systemic disease that is a constant threat to life

Physical Status Modifier P5: A moribund patient who is not expected to survive without the operation

Physical Status Modifier P6: A declared brain-dead patient whose organs are being removed for donor purposes

FIGURE 7-13
CPT physical status modifiers.

Examples

An anesthesiologist administers anesthesia for a corneal transplant, being performed on a normal, healthy adult male. The correct code is 00144-P1.

> 00144 Anesthesia for procedures on eye; corneal transplant
>
> P1 A normal healthy patient

Two surgeons (a general surgeon and a gynecologist) perform a cesarean section for a live birth and a radical hysterectomy on a woman who is HIV positive. The codes are: 00846-P3; 59514-62; 59525-62.

> 00846 Anesthesia for intraperitoneal procedures in lower abdomen including laparoscopy; radical hysterectomy
>
> P3 A patient with severe systemic disease
>
> 59514 Cesarean delivery only
>
> 59525 Subtotal or total hysterectomy after cesarean delivery
>
> 62 Two surgeons

Modifiers Approved for Ambulatory Surgery Center (ASC) Hospital Outpatient Use

Level 1 modifier codes were created to meet the particular type(s) of services—and therefore the special circumstances—provided by an ambulatory surgery center or a hospital outpatient service department. These facilities use the same modifiers in Appendix A, with three additions:

-27 *Multiple outpatient hospital E/M encounters on the same date.* Used for hospital outpatient purposes, this modifier identifies "separate and distinct E/M encounters performed in multiple outpatient hospital settings on the same date."

-73 *Discontinued outpatient hospital/ambulatory surgery center (ASC) procedure prior to the administration of anesthesia.* The title is pretty self- explanatory, so let's look at an example. An individual goes to an ASC for a procedure. The staff begins to prepare the patient for surgery (taking vital signs, inserting an intravenous line, and moving the individual into the operating room outer area) when something happens that requires them to cancel the procedure for that patient on that day. If anesthesia has *not* been given to the patient yet, modifier 73 is used in conjunction with the correct CPT procedure code for the surgery that didn't happen.

-74 *Discontinued outpatient hospital/ambulatory surgery center (ASC) procedure after administration of anesthesia.* If the same situation occurs as shown above for modifier 73, but the procedure is canceled *after* the anesthesia has been given to the patient, modifier 74 is used.

Modifiers are a very good example of why a trained insurance coder is needed. Modifiers are not typically included on superbills. Therefore, it is the coder who must recognize the situations in which a modifier or two are required to avoid the claim being rejected or delayed.

Spend some time looking through the descriptions of each of the modifiers in Appendix A. The descriptions help you understand when to use each modifier. In addition, the pages at the beginning of each section of the numeric listings (Anesthesia, Surgery, Radiology, Pathology and Laboratory, and Medicine) include additional descriptions and examples for using modifiers that apply to each section.

Just like the ICD-9-CM and CPT codes, you will find that, after working in the same office for a while, you will use the same group of modifiers on a regular basis.

Example

Don Scotty sees Dr. Jacobson in a hospital outpatient clinic. As a result of that encounter, Mr. Scotty is sent to see Dr. Cheli in the emergency room for a consultation. This requires two separate E/M codes on the same date for the same patient in different areas of the same facility. These E/M codes require the use of modifier 27.

CATEGORY III CODES

Between the Medicine section of the main text of the CPT book and Appendix A-Modifiers, you will find a listing of Category III codes (Figure 7-14). These alphanumeric codes (four numbers followed by the letter *T*) are temporary codes used for measuring the use of new technology and procedures. These procedures, technologies, and services do not meet the standard requirements for procedures found in the numeric listings. They are separated and have a different style of code, so that it is easier to collect data on the frequency of their use by providers.

Memory Tip

Category III codes are four digit codes followed by the letter T. **T** is for **T**emporary.

0008T	Upper gastrointestinal endoscopy including esophagus, stomach, and either the duodenum and/or jejunum as appropriate, with suturing of the esophagogastric junction
	▶(0009T has been deleted. To report, use 58356)◀
0010T	Tuberculosis test, cell mediated immunity measurement of gamma interferon antigen response
	▶(0012T has been deleted. To report, use 29866)◀
	▶(0013T has been deleted. To report, see 29867, 27415)◀
	▶(0014T has been deleted. To report, use 29868)◀
0016T	Destruction of localized lesion of choroid (eg, choroidal neovascularization), transpupillary thermotherapy

FIGURE 7-14
Examples of CPT Category III codes.

Category III codes are to be used only to specifically match the procedure, technology, or service provided to the individual by the provider when

1. a regular CPT code is *not* available *and*
2. a Category III code is available.

New codes are released every six months by the American Medical Association and published on the AMA/CPT website. They are also published annually in each new updated printing of the CPT book.

If you are working in a health care facility that uses new and emerging technology, procedures, and/or services, and you cannot find an appropriate code in the numeric listings of the CPT book, be certain to look for a Category III code *before* choosing an unlisted code.

IMPORTANT NOTE

Category III (temporary) codes are *not* included in the alphabetical index.

Example

The following are a few Category III codes:

0003T Cervicography

0021T Insertion of transcervical or transvaginal fetal oximetry sensor

0084T Insertion of a temporary prostatic urethral stent

UNLISTED CODES

At the end of each subsection and section in the CPT book, you will find a code or codes for services in that category not specified anywhere else in that section. These codes are ONLY to be used when

1. a regular CPT code is *not* available *and*
2. a Category III code is *not* available.

Example

01999 Unlisted anesthesia procedure(s)

69799 Unlisted procedure, middle ear

78099 Unlisted endocrine procedure, diagnostic nuclear medicine

89399 Unlisted miscellaneous pathology test

99600 Unlisted home visit service or procedure

THE SURGICAL PACKAGE

There are certain services that, as a rule, are always performed when a physician provides a particular surgical service. Those services, therefore, are always included in the code for the surgery and do not require additional or separate codes (Figure 7-15). The services are

- The operation itself
- Local infiltration, metacarpal/metatarsal/digital block or topical anesthesia
- Subsequent to the decision for surgery, one related E/M encounter on the date immediately prior to or on the date of the procedure (including history and physical)
- Immediate postoperative care, including dictating operative notes and talking with the family and other physicians
- The writing of orders
- Evaluation of the patient in the postanesthesia recovery area
- Typical postoperative follow-up care

CPT Surgical Package Definition

The services provided by the physician to any patient by their very nature are variable. The CPT codes that represent a readily identifiable surgical procedure thereby include, on a procedure-by-procedure basis, a variety of services. In defining the specific services "included" in a given CPT surgical code, the following services are always included in addition to the operation per se:

- local infiltration, metacarpal/metatarsal/digital block or topical anesthesia;

- subsequent to the decision for surgery, one related E/M encounter on the date immediately prior to or on the date of procedure (including history and physical);

- immediate postoperative care, including dictating operative notes, talking with the family and other physicians;

- writing orders;

- evaluating the patient in the postanesthesia recovery area;

- typical postoperative follow-up care.

FIGURE 7-15
CPT surgical package definition.

Example

A physician performed a superficial needle bone biopsy on a 37-year-old female using a topical anesthesia. The encounter for patient history and preoperative physical the day before the procedure, the anesthesia, the procedure itself, the dictation of postoperative notes, a postoperative discussion with the patient and her family, the writing of follow-up orders, and a check of the patient in the recovery area are all included in the CPT code 20220. You do not need to have a separate E/M code or anesthesia code. The one code includes it all.

CHAPTER SUMMARY

Coding the procedures and services provided in your health care facility is done by using the same process as coding diagnoses. First, find the physician's description in the alphabetic index of the book. Then confirm this code as the best, most appropriate code available in the numerical listings of the book. Be careful to follow the guidelines, as outlined in the gray pages preceding that section. You will need to review physician's notes and operative notes carefully to determine, not only what procedure codes are needed, but also if any modifiers are required. Above all, make certain the codes accurately reflect what is documented.

Chapter Review

Find the best CPT procedure code(s) for the following patients.

1. A 35-year-old male comes into the urologist's office, referred by his family physician, for an elective sterilization procedure, unilateral vasectomy.

   _____

2. A 55-year-old female an established patient, comes into the physician's office, complaining of chest pain. An ECG with 10 leads is performed.

   _____

3. A 15-year-old female presents in the emergency room with a severe asthma attack. The physician gives her an injection for rapid desensitization after determining that it is an allergic reaction.

   _____

4. A 25-year-old male is seen in the physician's office for a preemployment drug testing, ordered for multiple drugs with a single analysis.

   _____

5. A 92-year-old male is given his annual checkup by his physician in his room at the rest home where he lives. The patient has been previously diagnosed with diabetes, rheumatoid arthritis, and emphysema. The patient is reported to be stable and is given an influenza virus vaccine injection, whole virus IM.

   _____

6. A 52-year-old female, home-bound due to two broken legs, is seen by her regular physician at her home for an infusion of medication for pain management, intravenously.

   _____

7. A 23-year-old female is seen by her OB/GYN for a regular checkup and a sonogram of her abdomen. She is approximately 12 weeks pregnant with her first child.

   _____

8. A 37-year-old male is referred to a gastroenterologist for a diagnostic flexible sigmoidoscopy. The patient has a history of colon cancer. The procedure is performed in the office.

   _____

9. A 43-year-old female, complaining of a sore throat, is seen by her family physician at his office. A strep test, quick, and a complete blood cell count are performed.

   _____

10. A 15-year-old male is seen in the physician's office with severe leg pain. The physician takes an X-ray of his femur (two views) and then applies a long leg cast.

_____

11. The surgeon performs a stereotactic biopsy, aspiration of a lesion on a patient's spinal cord.

_____

12. Thirty-one year-old male is brought into the ER after an explosion. Physicians take him to OR for the removal of a foreign body from his right eye and repair of corneal lacerations on both eyes.

_____

13. A large staghorn calculus was removed from patient's right kidney filling renal pelvis and calyces.

_____

14. A 73-year-old female receives training from a physical therapist on stair climbing for 30 minutes.

_____

15. A psychiatrist talks with an employer on behalf of his 24-year-old female patient who was diagnosed with mild schizophrenia, now controlled with medication.

_____

16. An 81-year-old male has a talectomy performed on his left side.

_____

17. A 2-year-old male is given a heart transplant due to a life-threatening congenital heart defect.

_____

18. A 47-year-old male is sent for imaging of his kidney with a function study.

_____

19. A 14-year-old female stepped on a rusty nail while walking in her bare feet. Her regular pediatrician performs a problem-focused history and problem-focused exam. His straightforward decision was to clean and perform a full thickness skin debridement of the wound before bandaging it. He also administered a tetanus shot for possible exposure.

_____

20. A 27-year-old male receives surgery to become a female.

_____

Coding Procedures: ICD-9-CM Volume 3 and ICD-10-PCS

8

OBJECTIVES

- Distinguish between CPT procedure codes and ICD-9-CM Volume 3 procedure codes.

- Determine when to apply ICD-9-CM Volume 3 procedure codes.

- Identify the best, most appropriate procedure code, as indicated by physician documentation, using ICD-9-CM Volume 3.

- Define the objectives that guided the development of ICD-10-PCS.

- Understand the structure of ICD-10-PCS.

- Recognize the differences between ICD-9-CM Volume 3 and ICD-10-PCS.

- Recognize the similarities between ICD-9-CM Volume 3 and ICD-10-PCS.

KEY TERMS

bilateral edit

non-covered procedure

non-specific OR procedure

operating room (OR)

procedure coding system (PCS)

root operation

Individuals are admitted into the hospital so that health care professionals can provide services and treatments—more commonly referred to as procedures and services. This is the WHAT in our coding process. In Chapter 7, we learned about coding procedures and services from the CPT book. However, most hospitals use ICD-9-CM* Volume 3 procedure codes to identify WHAT they have done for their patients, instead of CPT codes. The process of coding from ICD-9-CM Volume 3 is the same as you have already learned. But, there are certain particulars that you must know should you get a job coding in a hospital.

*Enhance the learning process by pairing this chapter with a current copy of the ICD-9-CM Volume 3 book. A copy of ICD-10-PCS can be downloaded from www.cms.hhs.gov/paymentsystems/icd9/icd10.asp.

As you learned in Chapter 6, there will come a time in the near future that ICD-9-CM will be replaced with ICD-10-CM. When that happens, the new coding system will not have a Volume 3 containing procedure codes. Instead, there will be a separate book entitled, ICD-10-PCS. This chapter will introduce you to the new procedure coding system of the future—ICD-10-PCS—so you will be ready when these codes are put into use.

Memory Tip

When ICD-10-CM replaces ICD-9-CM, ICD-10-PCS will replace ICD-9-CM Volume 3.

ICD-9-CM VOLUME 3

Volume 3 of ICD-9-CM can be found in the back of the ICD-9-CM book, after the appendices. There are important differences between ICD-9-CM procedure codes and CPT codes:

1. ICD-9-CM procedure codes use up to a two-digit number to the left of a dot and up to two digits to the right of the dot.
2. ICD-9-CM procedure code descriptions may use different terminology for the same procedures.
3. ICD-9-CM procedure codes do not have a separate section for Evaluation and Management codes.
4. ICD-9-CM procedure codes do not have anesthesia codes.
5. ICD-9-CM procedure codes do not use modifiers.

Examples

12.12 (ICD-9-CM Volume 3) vs. 12345 (CPT)

Radiology (ICD-9-CM Volume 3) vs. X-ray (CPT)

How Codes Are Structured

In Chapter 5, you learned that *ICD-9-CM diagnostic codes* are three digits followed by a dot, then possibly followed by a fourth or fifth digit (such as 123.45); in Chapter 7, you learned that *CPT procedure codes* are always five digits, sometimes followed by a two-digit modifier (such as 12345-12). *ICD-9-CM procedure codes* are two-digit numbers followed by a dot, then possibly followed by a third or fourth digit (such as 12.34). Now you can spot what kind of code it is as soon as you see it.

Memory Tip

ICD-9-CM Volume 3 codes
  12.34
ICD-9-CM diagnosis codes
  123.45
CPT procedure codes
  12345

Coding Procedures Using ICD-9-CM Volume 3

Coding from ICD-9-CM Volume 3 follows the same process as all the other coding we have discussed. First, look up the description in the alphabetical portion at the beginning of Volume 3—the Index to Procedures. This section is structured in the same way as Volume 2—Alphabetic Index to Diseases in the front of this book. You will find main terms for procedures in bold at the left margin of the column. Indented underneath that term are additional descriptors that apply to that main term.

IMPORTANT NOTE

ICD-9-CM Volume 3 books are produced by several publishers. Elements such as red notation boxes and legends are not used by all of them. However, whichever book you use, the notations to help you code will be there.

Let's bring back the patient who had a diagnostic colonoscopy in Chapter 7. In the CPT book, you found that the code 45385 matched the physician's notes that stated, "Colonoscopy, flexible, proximal to splenic flexure; with removal of tumor(s), polyp(s), or other lesion(s) by snare technique." Now let's look up the same procedure in the Alphabetic Index of ICD-9-CM Volume 3 (Figure 8-1). You see

Colonoscopy 45.23
  with biopsy 45.25
    rectum 48.24

Remember, just as in the other chapters, the indented portions of the column are additional descriptors or definitions that attach to the term immediately above at the margin. In other words, these three lines are read

Colonoscopy 45.23
Colonoscopy with biopsy 45.25
Colonoscopy with biopsy, rectum 48.24

Also, as with all the other coding sections, you *never code from the Alphabetic Index,* so let's turn to the section directly after this one to find the numerical listings for the ICD-9-CM procedure codes and find 45. We see the code

✓3rd 45 Incision, excision, and anastomosis of intestine

You are in the correct portion of the body—the intestine. Let's keep looking down the column to find a closer definition. The red box next to the 45 is telling you that you must have a third digit. Remember these red-boxed instructions from Volume 1-Tabular Listing of the ICD-9-CM diagnosis code section? They mean the same thing here—that the code requires an additional digit.

✓4th 45.2 Diagnostic procedures on large intestine

Colonoscopy 45.23
  with biopsy 45.25
    rectum 48.24
  fiberoptic (flexible) 45.23
  intraoperative 45.21
  through stoma (artificial) 45.22
  transabdominal 45.21

FIGURE 8-1
Alphabetical listing from Volume 3.

FIGURE 8-2

The listing for the colonoscopy procedure in Volume 3.

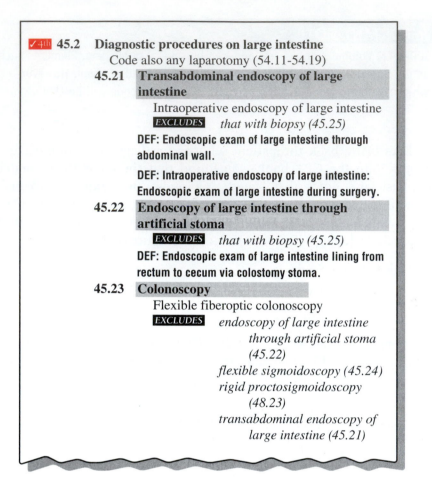

✓ 4th **45.2** **Diagnostic procedures on large intestine**
Code also any laparotomy (54.11-54.19)

45.21 **Transabdominal endoscopy of large intestine**
Intraoperative endoscopy of large intestine
EXCLUDES *that with biopsy (45.25)*
DEF: Endoscopic exam of large intestine through abdominal wall.
DEF: Intraoperative endoscopy of large intestine: Endoscopic exam of large intestine during surgery.

45.22 **Endoscopy of large intestine through artificial stoma**
EXCLUDES *that with biopsy (45.25)*
DEF: Endoscopic exam of large intestine lining from rectum to cecum via colostomy stoma.

45.23 **Colonoscopy**
Flexible fiberoptic colonoscopy
EXCLUDES *endoscopy of large intestine through artificial stoma (45.22)*
flexible sigmoidoscopy (45.24)
rigid proctosigmoidoscopy (48.23)
transabdominal endoscopy of large intestine (45.21)

That sounds very close to what you need. However, now the red box says that you need a fourth digit, so let's keep reading down the column (Figure 8-2).

45.21 Transabdominal endoscopy of large intestine

45.22 Endoscopy of large intestine through artificial stoma

45.23 Colonoscopy

This matches the physician's notes. You will see that, again, just like the diagnostic portion of ICD-9-CM, notations inform you of procedures that are *excluded* from this code. However, as you look down the rest of the column, you will notice that 45.23 is the best available code.

You can see clearly that the format of ICD-9-CM Volume 3 is very much like the diagnostic portion of the book—Volume 1-Tabular Listing. One difference is the color highlighting on some of the descriptions of the procedure codes in Volume 3.

As you can see in the legend across the bottom of the two pages,

- The blue-gray color ▉ indicates that the procedure is a Non-OR Procedure (not performed in the **operating room** [OR]).
- The gray color ▉ indicates that the procedure is a Valid OR Procedure (approved to be performed in the operating room).
- The gold color ▉ indicates that the procedure is a Non-specific OR Procedure (Not Otherwise Specified, but still performed in the operating room).

Memory Tip

Across the bottom of every page in many ICD-9-CM Volume 3 books, you will find reminders as to the meaning of the color highlights.

Key Terms

Operating room (OR): Sterile room for performing surgery.

Non-specific OR Procedure: A code that is recognized only when all operating room procedures performed during the same session are coded Not Otherwise Specified.

You already know that

- The red box with a check mark and 3 ✓3ʳᵈ indicates that a third digit is required for the correct code.
- The red box with a check mark and 4 ✓4ᵗʰ indicates that a fourth digit is required for the correct code.

Additionally, notations in this section include the following

- The red box with an NC NC indicates that this is a **Non-covered Procedure.**
- The dark gray box with a BI BI indicates that this is a **Bilateral Edit.**

There are a few instances in which a combination of color indicators is used. The following color combination indicates that this is a Non-specific Procedure that is valid (approved) to be done in the operating room.

45.00 Incision of intestine not otherwise specified

An additional note you may see in the Tabular (numeric) list is *Omit code.* This means that the procedure shown is not to be coded separately when performed at the same time as the code immediately above this notation.

Key Terms

Non-covered Procedure: A procedure that is not covered by Medicare.

Bilateral Edit: Procedures that, when coded twice, represent the same procedure performed on both of the same bilateral joints of the lower extremity. Otherwise, a code edit will cause a delay for verification that the two different procedures were performed on two different bilateral joints.

Example

37.75 Revision of lead [electrode] EXCLUDES *repositioning of temporary transvenous pacemaker system—Omit Code.*

In Chapter 7, while looking in the CPT book, you found the code and description for

Mammography

Screening..76092

with Computer-aided Detection...............76085

Now let's look for the proper ICD-9-CM procedure code. Just as in the CPT book, we have to look for Mammography, rather than Mammogram. In the Volume 3 Index to Procedures, we see the description

Mammography NEC 87.37

Remember *NEC* from the diagnostic section in Chapter 5? It stands for Not Elsewhere Classified. Even though there is only one choice, you know that you should *never* code from the Alphabetic Index, so let's turn to the numerical listings and find 87.37.

✓3ʳᵈ 87 Diagnostic radiology

Farther down the column, you see

✓4ᵗʰ 87.3 Soft tissue X-ray of thorax

87.37 Other mammography

Looking up and down the column (Figure 8-3), you can agree that this is the best code available.

FIGURE 8-3
ICD-9-CM procedure code for
mammogram.

✓ 4th **87.3   Soft tissue x-ray of thorax**
EXCLUDES   *angiocardiography (88.50-88.58)*
            angiography (88.40-88.68)

87.31   Endotracheal bronchogram
DEF: Radiographic exam of lung, main branch, with
contrast introduced through windpipe.

87.32   Other contrast bronchogram
Transcricoid bronchogram
DEF: Transcricoid bronchogram: Radiographic exam of
lung, main branch, with contrast introduced through
cartilage of neck.

87.33   Mediastinal pneumogram
DEF: Radiographic exam of cavity containing heart,
esophagus and adjacent structures.

87.34   Intrathoracic lymphangiogram
DEF: Radiographic exam of lymphatic vessels within
chest; with or without contrast.

87.35   Contrast radiogram of mammary ducts
DEF: Radiographic exam of mammary ducts; with
contrast.

87.36   Xerography of breast
DEF: Radiographic exam of breast via selenium-coated
plates.

87.37   Other mammography
AHA: 30, '89, 17; 20, '90, 28; N-D, '87, 1

CASE STUDY

Marion Alexander, a 35-year-old female, has hurt her ankle falling out of her hospital bed. Ms. Alexander was admitted for surgery to have her gallbladder removed. Her ankle shows some bruising and is swollen. She complains that it is very painful and she has difficulty putting her weight on it. Dr. Doverton, her attending physician, suspecting a sprain, orders X-rays of the ankle. After reviewing the radiology report, he concludes that the ankle is not fractured. Dr. Doverton applies a strapping and writes orders for a mild pain reliever.

How will you code this situation from ICD-9-CM Volume 3?

_____

_____

This time, there are two procedures to code. In Chapter 7, we found the CPT code for the X-ray of a man's sprained ankle and then the applied strapping. We used

73600 Radiologic examination, ankle, two views

29540 Strapping, ankle

Let's look it up in ICD-9-CM Volume 3.

First, let's code the X-ray of the ankle, which is a challenge already. When you turn to the letter *X* in the index, you'll find

X-ray

    chest (routine) 87.44

        wall NEC 87.39

    contrast—*see* Radiography, contrast

    diagnostic—*see* Radiography

    injection of radio-opaque substance—*see* Radiography, contrast

    skeletal series, whole or complete 88.31

    therapeutic—*see* Therapy, radiation

None of these are an exact match, so the closest is diagnostic, because the physician is looking to confirm that the ankle is not broken. Let's turn to Radiography, as the index directs. Under Radiography, you find (Figure 8-4)

Radiography (diagnostic) NEC 88.39

    Abdomen, abdominal (flat plate) NEC 88.19

        wall (soft tissue) NEC 88.09

    adenoid 87.09

    ankle (skeletal) 88.28

        soft tissue 88.37

There is no reason to go any farther here. You can see that the two choices for ankle are clear. However, you must now choose between the two codes. Let's go to the numerical listings.

88.28 Skeletal X-ray of ankle and foot

88.37 Other soft tissue X-ray of lower limb

> **Radiography** (diagnostic) NEC 88.39
>   abdomen, abdominal (flat plate) NEC 88.19
>   wall (soft tissue) NEC 88.09
>   adenoid 87.09
>   ankle (skeletal) 88.28
>   soft tissue 88.37
>   bone survey 88.31

FIGURE 8-4
ICD-9-CM Volume 3 Radiography codes.

You will need to look carefully at the physician's notes and the radiologist's report to determine if the X-ray was ordered to confirm there was no fracture (skeletal) or to confirm that it was a sprain (soft tissue). An examination of the notes clearly shows that the X-ray was ordered to confirm that the ankle was not fractured. Therefore, 88.28 is the best code. If you are not able to understand the physician's notes to be certain which code is the best, you must *not assume*. You *must ask*.

Again, to illustrate the differences in the terminology used by CPT and ICD-9-CM procedure code descriptions, let's look at the two X-ray codes side by side:

ICD-9-CM Volume 3	88.28 Skeletal X-ray of ankle and foot
CPT	73600 Radiologic examination, ankle; two views

In addition to the difference in terms (*X-ray* versus *radiologic*), there is a difference in the information you will need in order to code correctly. The ICD-9-CM procedure codes need you to know exactly what *type* of X-ray (skeletal or soft tissue), whereas the CPT procedure codes need you to know how many views were taken (two views or minimum of three views).

Now you need to turn to the strapping of the ankle. Turn to the letter *S* in the Volume 3's Index to Procedures. There is no listing for Strapping. What now? Well, a strapping is a kind of bandage, so let's try that. Under *B* you see

> Bandage 93.57
>> Elastic 93.56

Perhaps a splint would be more accurate (Figure 8-5).

> Splinting
>> dental (for immobilization) 93.55
>>> orthodontic 24.7
>> musculoskeletal 93.54
>> ureteral 56.2

Which do you think is the most accurate with regard to what the physician actually did? If you said 93.54, you are correct. Good job!

One thing is for certain—the terminology in this listing of procedure codes is not exactly the same as the CPT book. Therefore, if you get a job handling coding in a hospital that uses the ICD-9-CM procedure codes instead of the CPT codes, you will have to get familiar with the terms used in ICD-9-CM Volume 3. Until you get used to this set of terminology, you will need to ask for clarification.

FIGURE 8-5
ICD-9-CM Volume 3 code for applying a splint.

Splinting
    dental (for immobilization) 93.55
        orthodontic 24.7
    musculoskeletal 93.54
    ureteral 56.2

The bottom line is that, when you are coding, you must match the descriptions in whichever coding book you are using to the information you have in the documentation. As you know, a superbill or preprinted encounter form does not usually have enough information for you to choose the best available code. This can cause you to undercode—possibly resulting in your office being paid less monies to which it is entitled—or, worse, to overcode. Of course, you have already learned that overcoding constitutes fraud and is against the law.

> **IMPORTANT NOTE**
>
> Practice coding procedures from ICD-9-CM Volume 3 by recoding the scenarios in Chapter 7's Chapter Review using these codes instead of CPT. Then compare the results from both systems.

ICD-10-PCS

Just as ICD-10-CM is being developed to replace ICD-9-CM with a more precise and efficient diagnostic coding system, the new and improved ICD-10-PCS will eventually replace the ICD-9-CM Volume 3 procedure codes. ICD-10-PCS stands for International Classification of Diseases—10th revision—**Procedure Coding System.**

Since 1979, ICD-9-CM Volume 3, has been used for the reporting of inpatient procedures in the United States. Along with ICD-10-CM for the reporting of diagnoses, ICD-10-PCS will be adopted in order to provide more specificity for various procedures, as well as to make it easier to incorporate new procedures as they are developed and accepted by health care professionals. As you read through this overview, you should gain a clear perspective on why these changes are being made to the system.

Key Term

Procedure coding system (PCS): The new version of identifying services and treatments performed in a hospital.

The Objectives for ICD-10-PCS

One of the first tasks in the development of ICD-10-PCS was to establish specific objectives for the project. Four objectives were identified:

1. *Completeness:* The creation of a unique code for every identifiably different procedure performed and for any procedure that could possibly be performed
2. *Expandability:* An organization of the book that can easily accept new procedures and incorporate them logically into the existing list; this acknowledges the incredible speed with which technology and science are working to develop treatments and services to care more effectively for patients
3. *Multiaxial:* The use of consistency in the characters used to create codes within each section and, whenever possible, from section to section
4. *Standardized terminology:* The use of only one meaning for each term, even if multiple meanings are accepted in the industry, as well as specific definitions as they are intended for those terms

The successful accomplishment of these four objectives will help assure that ICD-10-PCS will make coding procedures more accurate, more efficient, and easier.

Notations in ICD-10-PCS

ICD-10-PCS has changed some of the notations that you are used to from either CPT or ICD-9-CM Volume 3:

1. *Procedure descriptions will no longer include diagnostic information.* Previously, some of the procedure codes included diagnostic statements or categories in the description of the procedure code. In ICD-10-PCS, the description of each procedure code is limited to the details of the procedure itself. The ICD-10-CM diagnostic codes will serve to explain the disease or condition.

2. *Not Otherwise Specified (NOS) options are omitted.* ICD-10-PCS requires you to have, at the very least, a minimum amount of detail regarding each portion of the procedure. When the documentation has no additional specifics available, ICD-10-PCS provides coding rules to guide you to the best, most appropriate code.

3. *Not Elsewhere Classified (NEC) options are reduced.* Due to the added levels of specificity throughout ICD-10-PCS, the need for the NEC option is lessened. You will find the most common inclusion of NEC in procedure descriptions is located in the sections regarding new devices and nuclear medicine, because these areas are more quickly affected by new technology and science.

Examples

ICD-9-CM Volume 3 shows
The repair of a rupture of an eyeball (16.82)

ICD-10-PCS shows
Repair, eye anterior chamber, right, open (08Q20ZZ)
The rupture will be identified by the diagnostic code.

The Structure of ICD-10-PCS Codes

Of course, the main purpose of creating ICD-10-PCS is to give you, the professional coder, an easier way and a more specific opportunity to find the best, most appropriate code. This purpose has led to a new structure for these codes with a higher level of specificity. In this book, a unique code is available for each procedure as well as each variation of that procedure.

You may remember that ICD-9-CM procedure codes use a two-digit number to the left of a dot and up to two digits to the right of the dot. ICD-10-PCS codes have seven characters and are alphanumeric. This means that the codes include both letters and numbers.

The first character in the seven-character sequence identifies the section of the ICD-10-PCS book to which the procedure belongs (Box 8-1).

BOX 8-1   *ICD-10-PCS Sections*

ICD-10-PCS contains 16 sections:

0	Medical and Surgical
1	Obstetrics
2	Placement
3	Administration
4	Measurement and Monitoring
5	Extracorporeal Assistance and Performance
6	Extracorporeal Therapies
7	Osteopathic
8	Miscellaneous
9	Chiropractic
B	Imaging
C	Nuclear Medicine
D	Radiation Oncology
F	Physical Rehabilitation and Diagnostic Audiology
G	Mental Health
H	Substance Abuse Treatment

IMPORTANT NOTE

ICD-10-PCS codes may include any letter of the alphabet *except* the letters *O* and *I*. This is done to avoid any confusion between the letter *O* and the number 0, as well as the letter *I* and the number 1. The codes use all numbers, including the numbers 0 and 1.

Example

An ankle X-ray is an *imaging* procedure—Section B.
A breech extraction is an *obstetrics* procedure—Section 1.
An amputation is a *surgical* procedure—Section 0.

The ICD-10-PCS Book

Just like the ICD-9-CM book and the CPT book, the ICD-10-PCS book is divided into two parts: the alphabetic index and the tabular (numerical) listing.

The alphabetic index's entries are primarily sorted by **root operation** terms which identify the specific service or type of procedure that is the basis of the entire treatment.

IMPORTANT NOTE

In ICD-10-PCS, the word *operation* has nothing to do with surgery.

Example

Root operation terms include *bypass, drainage, excision,* and *insertion.*

After you find the root operation term, as stated in the physician's notes, there are subentries listed by

- Body system—such as digestive system, musculoskeletal system
- Body part—such as arm, leg, hand, foot

In addition, the index also lists common terms for specific procedures.

A major difference between ICD-10-PCS and both ICD-9-CM Volume 3 and CPT is that the alphabetic index will give you only the first three or four characters of the seven-character procedure code. You then *must* go to the tabular (numerical) listing to find the additional characters. This means that, once ICD-10-PCS comes into full effect, you *won't be able to* code from the alphabetic index anymore. (Even though you don't do that because you know you're not supposed to, right?)

Example

Fragmentation
    Of the Bladder..........0TF8---

The tabular (numerical) list's entries are divided by body systems, similar to those in ICD-9-CM Volume 3. Of course, like all the other books, this section is in numerical order by the first character in the code.

You will note that each section is in order first by the body system that was the object of the procedure then, by the root operation term for that procedure.

Example

Hysterectomy is listed and then cross-referenced to
    Resection (a root operation term),
        Female Reproductive System (body system)

ICD-10-PCS Character Order and Place Holders

Each section of the tabular (numerical) list provides a grid, which specifies the assigned meaning to each letter or number, along with its position in the seven-character code.

Because this coding system is designed for future expansion, there will be cases in which a specific procedure does not have the details to require all seven characters. In these cases, the letter Z is used to indicate that nothing in that position was applicable to this procedure. (See Box 8-2.)

BOX 8-2   ICD-10-PCS Character Order and Place Holders

0: Medical and Surgical [FIRST CHARACTER]

2: Heart and Great Vessels [SECOND CHARACTER]

7: Dilation: Expanding the orifice or the lumen of a tubular body part [THIRD CHARACTER]

Body Part Character 4	Approach Character 5	Device Character 6	Qualifier Character 7
0 Coronary Artery, One	1 Open Intraluminal	D Intraluminal Device	Z None
1 Coronary Arteries, Two	2 Open Intraluminal Endoscopic	Y Device NEC	
2 Coronary Arteries, Three	5 Percutaneous Intraluminal	Z None	
3 Coronary Arteries, Four or more	6 Percutaneous Intraluminal Endoscopic		

To find the correct ICD-10-PCS code for a *Dilation, Coronary Artery, One, Open Intraluminal with Intraluminal device,* take the physician's procedure description in order:

1. The first character comes from the number or letter for the section. This is a surgical procedure, so use 0.
2. The second character is determined by the number or letter for the body system. This is heart and great vessels, so use 2.
3. The third character is determined by the number or letter for the type of procedure. This is a dilation, so use 7.
4. The fourth character is determined by the number or letter for the body part. This is one coronary artery, so when you look at the chart, you will see that the digit for Coronary Artery, One, is 0.
5. The fifth character is determined by the number or letter for the approach. This is an Open Intraluminal; therefore, use 1.
6. The sixth character is determined by the number or letter for the device. This is an Intraluminal Device; therefore, use D.
7. The seventh character is determined by the number or letter for the qualifier. There is no qualifier for this procedure; therefore, we will use Z.

This leads to the correct ICD-10-PCS code for *Dilation, Coronary Artery, One, Open Intraluminal with Intraluminal device:*

02701DZ

IMPORTANT NOTE

Practice coding procedures from ICD-10-PCS by recoding the scenarios in the Chapter Review in Chapter 7.

CHAPTER SUMMARY

Rather than use the CPT book for coding procedures that have been performed for inpatients at a hospital, you will use the procedure codes provided in Volume 3 of the ICD-9-CM book. These codes look different from those for the same procedures in the CPT book; however, the process of finding the correct code is basically the same.

Once ICD-10-CM replaces ICD-9-CM, you will discover that there is no Volume 3, nor does the book contain any procedure codes. Instead, you will have a separate book, the ICD-10-PCS, to use for coding procedures provided to inpatients in a hospital setting.

Again, the process of reviewing the physician's notes, looking up the description in the alphabetic listing, and confirming the code in the tabular (numerical) listing is the same, no matter which book you are using or how many characters the best, most appropriate code has.

Chapter Review

Find the best ICD-9-CM Volume 3 procedure code(s) for these patients.

1. A 52-year-old male is seen in the hospital with a concussion. A skull X-ray and brain MRI are both performed.

   _____

2. A 39-year-old female is seen in the hospital with suspected appendicitis. An angiography MRI of the abdomen is ordered, along with a comprehensive metabolic blood test and a general health panel.

   _____

3. A hospitalized 35-year-old male is given aerosol inhalation of pentamidine.

   _____

4. A 73-year-old female has a routine ECG in preparation for her surgery the following day.

   _____

5. A 45-year-old female has a laparoscopic cholecystectomy by laser. _____

6. A 39-year-old male goes to the hospital to have an operative esophageal endoscopy.

   _____

7. A 58-year-old female has a bunionectomy with a soft tissue correction performed. _____

8. An 8-year-old male is seen at the hospital for a suspected broken clavicle. An X-ray is taken. A plaster cast is applied. _____

9. A 5-year-old female is given a measles-mumps-rubella vaccine at the hospital.

   _____

10. After cutting his foot on the beach, a 19-year-old male gets an administration of a tetanus antitoxin in the emergency room. _____

Choose the best possible answer from these multiple-choice questions on ICD-10-PCS.

1. In ICD-10-PCS, the initials *PCS* stand for

   a. Popular Coding System

   b. Procedure Coding System

   c. Possible Coding Solutions

   d. Proper Coding System

2. Of the four objectives for ICD-10-PCS, the one that relates to the meanings of the words and terms used is

   a. Completeness

   b. Expandability

   c. Multiaxial

   d. Standardized terminology

3. The descriptions for procedures identified in ICD-10-PCS

   a. Include diagnostic information

   b. Define the disease or condition that caused the procedure

   c. Do not include diagnostic information

   d. Match those used in the CPT book exactly

4. The structure of ICD-10-PCS codes includes

   a. Three numbers

   b. Five numbers

   c. Seven characters

   d. Up to nine characters

5. ICD-10-PCS codes include

   a. Only numbers

   b. Only letters

   c. One letter followed by numbers

   d. Letters and numbers

6. An example of a root operation term is

   a. *Bypass*

   b. *X-ray*

   c. *Obstetrics*

   d. *Hysterectomy*

7. Digestive system is an example of a

    a. Body part

    b. Root operation term

    c. Medical procedure

    d. Body system

8. The sections of ICD-10-PCS are identified by

    a. Numbers 1–17

    b. Numbers 0–9 then letters *B–H*

    c. Letters *A–Z*

    d. The name of the section in alphabetical order

9. ICD-10-PCS place holders use

    a. The number 0

    b. The letter *X*

    c. The letter *Z*

    d. The number 9

10. ICD-10-PCS is designed to replace

    a. CPT

    b. ICD-9-CM Volume 3

    c. ICD-10-CM

    d. ICD-9-CM

9

Complete Coding Practice: ICD-9-CM and CPT

KEY TERMS

CMS-1500

code linkage

OBJECTIVES

- Abstract physician's notes to determine the best, most appropriate diagnosis codes.

- Abstract physician's notes to determine the best, most appropriate procedure codes.

- Properly link procedure codes to their appropriate diagnostic code(s) to show medical necessity.

The final step in coding is putting all the information together in order to complete the health insurance claim form. Those preparing claims for procedures and services performed in an outpatient setting (such as a physician's office, a clinic, or an ambulatory surgical center) will most often use a form called the **CMS-1500**. Chapter 10 will go over the entire form and teach you everything you need to know in order to complete the CMS-1500 properly.

Key Term

CMS-1500: The claim form used most often by outpatient facilities.

LINKING DIAGNOSIS AND PROCEDURE CODES

As we discussed previously, the diagnosis codes provide the information that explains the medical necessity (the *why*) for performing the procedures or services (the *what*) as identified by the procedure codes. Making the connection between a specific diagnosis code and a specific procedure code is called **code linkage**. In other words, every procedure code directly relates to a diagnosis code shown on the claim form. You will need to show this link in Box 24E on the CMS-1500 claim form.

After you find all of the best, most appropriate diagnosis codes and the best, most appropriate procedure codes for each patient encounter, the final step will be linking the codes together to assure medical necessity and accuracy. Every procedure must link to at least one diagnosis code shown on the same claim form. It is perfectly acceptable if one procedure code relates to more than one diagnosis code (for most insurers), but it must relate to at least one.

Key Term

Code linkage: The process of directly connecting each procedure code to at least one diagnosis code on an insurance claim form.

CASE STUDY

Keith Massenger, a 48-year-old male, is seen by his regular physician, Dr. Gayle Froint, because of a problem with a decubitus ulcer on his right midfoot. The patient has been previously diagnosed with type II diabetes, and has a history of bronchial asthma. Dr. Froint orders a blood glucose test to make certain Keith's diabetes is under control. In addition, she performs a debridement of the wound and applies a small bandage.

Can you determine the correct diagnosis codes? What are the best procedure codes? Which procedure codes link to which diagnosis codes?

_____

_____

To find the correct diagnosis codes,

1. Identify the key words in the notes relating to the diagnoses.
2. Look up those words in the ICD-9-CM alphabetic listing.
3. Confirm each code in the tabular (numerical) listing.

The diagnosis codes for Keith Massenger's recent encounter with Dr. Froint are

1. 250.80 Diabetes with other specified manifestations, type II, not stated as uncontrolled
2. 707.14 Ulcer of heel and midfoot

Next find the correct procedure codes:

1. Identify the key words in the notes relating to the procedures.
2. Look up those words in the CPT alphabetic index.
3. Confirm each code in the numerical listing.

The procedure codes for this patient encounter are

99213 Office visit, established patient, MDM low complexity

82947 Glucose; quantitative, blood

11042 Debridement; skin, and subcutaneous tissue

Last, you must link each of the procedure codes to at least one of the diagnostic codes. The procedure codes link to the diagnosis codes this way:

99213 .... 1, 2

82947 1

11042 2

You can see that this makes the entire encounter very clear.

- The E/M code (99213) relates to both the patient's diabetes (250.80) and the ulcer on his foot (707.14). Therefore, this CPT code links to both diagnosis codes.
- The glucose test (82947) was medically necessary for a patient with diabetes (250.80). This means that the CPT code for the glucose test links to just the first-listed diagnosis code.
- The debridement of the wound (11042) would be medically necessary for a patient with an open wound on his foot (707.14), linking this procedure code only to the second diagnosis code.

Now the insurance carrier can immediately identify this to be a valid claim and pay it immediately. Failing to link the codes or linking them incorrectly can cause your claim to be denied.

IMPORTANT NOTE

Procedure codes do not link to E codes.

CODING PRACTICE

On the following pages, you will find physician's notes for thirteen patients. (Sorry, no superbills. You have to do this from scratch! While it is true that most of you will be getting superbills to work from in your office, it is important that you practice your new coding skills.) Using your ICD-9-CM and CPT books, review the documentation you have and

1. Find the best, most appropriate diagnosis code(s)
2. Find the most accurate evaluation and management code(s)
3. Find the best, most appropriate procedure code(s) for each of the thirteen cases
4. Link each procedure code (including the E/M code) to at least one diagnosis code

In upcoming chapters, you will learn how to enter all of this information into the computer and create a CMS-1500 health insurance claim form for some of these patient visits.

Physician's Notes for Marvin Doe

41-year-old male is seen by his regular family physician in the office for a quarterly evaluation of his previous diagnosis of type I diabetes. His condition has been in good control with continued insulin therapy, as prescribed. Patient reports problems with his eyes.

History: Type I diabetes diagnosed and confirmed one year ago. Insulin therapy via patient's self-injection IM of insulin as indicated by glucose testing q.i.d.

PE: BP 138/85, P 100, T 98.6, R 20. Ht. 5'11", Wt. 255 lbs.

HEENT: Atraumatic. Lungs clear. Chest has no palpable tenderness. Heart rate regular and rhythm without murmur. No edema, erythema, or ecchymoses. No body tenderness. Abdomen: obese, nontender. Femoral pulses symmetrical. Extremities without acute trauma. Nervous system: unremarkable. (Comprehensive examination.)

Laboratory: Glucose quantitative blood test ordered. Glucose 224, BUN 11, creatinine 0.8, CK normal at 122. A visual field examination and a visual acuity screening performed.

Impression: Confirmed diabetic retinopathy.

The best, most appropriate diagnosis code(s) are _____.
The best, most appropriate E/M code is ___99214___.
The best, most appropriate procedure code(s) are _____.
Link the procedure codes to the diagnosis code(s). _____

Physician's Notes for Roger Samuels

History: This 55-year-old male came to see his regular physician for a follow-up treatment regarding prostate cancer. Pt was diagnosed with malignant neoplasm of the prostate six months ago, which was confirmed to have metastasized to the lung, lower lobe one week ago.

Surgical report: Complete PE was performed prior to the patient being taken to the ambulatory surgery center for a radical prostate excision with a lymph node biopsy. Anesthesia was administered via IV due to the patient's existing lung cancer. Before the patient's release, he was also given three hours of chemotherapy, IV infusion.

Prognosis: Encouraging.

Plan: It is recommended that the pt return in one week for a post-surgical checkup. Once the prostate situation is under control, a treatment plan will be discussed regarding the lung cancer.

The best, most appropriate diagnosis code(s) are _____.

The best, most appropriate E/M code is ___99214_____.

The best, most appropriate procedure code(s) are _____.

Link the procedure code(s) to the diagnosis code(s). _____

_____

Physician's Notes for Patience Loyal

63-year-old female is seen by her family physician in the office. Patient states that she was driving down the road to work and got dizzy. She pulled over to the side of the road and realized that her heart was beating rapidly and she was perspiring. She states that she was very anxious and came to the physician's office directly as soon as the dizziness subsided.

History: Patient has a family history of hypertension but has experienced only slightly elevated blood pressure in the past. Overall health has been fairly stable, with the exception of concerns regarding the patient's obesity.

Physical examination: BP 170/95, P 110, T 99.5, R 22. Ht. 5'2", Wt. 185 lbs.

HEENT: Atraumatic. Lungs clear. Chest has no palpable tenderness. Heart rate regular and rhythm without murmur. Edema evidenced in ankles. No erythema or ecchymoses. Femoral pulses symmetrical, extremities without acute trauma. Nervous system unremarkable. (Detailed examination.)

Testing: ECG with 12 leads and interpretation/report performed. Blood tests: general health panel and lipoprotein (HDL cholesterol) ordered.

Impression: Essential hypertension confirmed, unspecified.

The best, most appropriate diagnosis code(s) are _____401.9_____.

The best, most appropriate E/M code is _____99214_____.

The best, most appropriate procedure code(s) are _____.

Link the procedure codes to the diagnosis code(s). _____

Physician's Notes for Wayne Johns

S: This 33-year-old male was brought into his regular physician's office after banging his head and losing consciousness for about 20 minutes. He parachuted from an airplane and landed in a tree, where his head knocked against a tree limb.

O: BP 110/80, P 95, T 98.6, R19. After a problem-focused PE, a head CT was ordered. CT scan confirms a brain concussion, as well as a brain tumor in the patient's parietal lobe.

A: Brain concussion, with loss of consciousness <30 min.

   Brain tumor, parietal lobe, unknown

P: Referral to oncologist for treatment of brain tumor

The best, most appropriate diagnosis code(s) are ___850.1 / 191.3___   E884.9

The best, most appropriate E/M code is _____.

The best, most appropriate procedure code(s) are _____.

Link the procedure code(s) to the diagnosis code(s). _____

Physician's Notes for Mary Lou Sweet

18-year-old female is seen for the first time by the family physician for severe wrist pain.

History: Patient states that she is in overall good health with no concerns other than the severe pain in her right wrist. Patient works in a bank credit card processing center doing data processing and spends up to eight hours per day working on a computer.

PE: BP 125/70, T 98.6, P 95, R 20. Ht. 5'1". Wt. 110 lbs.

HEENT: Atraumatic. Lungs clear. Right hand slightly swollen, extreme tenderness at wrist.

Testing: X-ray, rt wrist, AP and lateral views.

Impression: Carpal tunnel syndrome confirmed. Static short arm splint applied.

The best, most appropriate diagnosis code(s) are _____.

The best, most appropriate E/M code is _____.

The best, most appropriate procedure code(s) are _____.

Link the procedure codes to the diagnosis code(s). _____

Physician's Notes for Naomi Morgan

S: This 89-year-old female is seen in her room at the Village Nursing Home for her regular annual checkup.

O: Pt is stable and doing well on her current regime of medications. PE shows age appropriate condition. HEENT is unremarkable.

A: Annual physical exam shows age appropriate condition.

P: Coordination with resident medical director to review and affirm medical plan of care.

The best, most appropriate diagnosis code(s) are _____.

The best, most appropriate E/M code is _____.

The best, most appropriate procedure code(s) are _____.

Link the procedure code(s) to the diagnosis code(s). _____

Physician's Notes for Harvey Practice

19-year-old male is seen in the university clinic for a severe sore throat.

History: Patient states he has been in good health until experiencing a scratchy feeling in his throat approximately one week ago. Condition developed into pain and difficulty swallowing in the last two days.

PE: BP 115/70, T 99.7, P 100, R 20. Ht. 6'1". Wt. 180 lbs.

HEENT: Atraumatic. Lungs clear. Throat red and swollen.

Testing: CBC with automated differential WBC count. Enzyme immunoassay for streptococcus, group A.

Impression: Streptococcal sore throat.

The best, most appropriate diagnosis code(s) are _____.

The best, most appropriate E/M code is _____.

The best, most appropriate procedure code(s) are _____.

Link the procedure codes to the diagnosis code(s). _____

Physician's Notes for Marion Maxwell

S: This 37-year-old female is seen by her regular physician. Pt was diagnosed two days earlier with an anterior longitudinal cervical sprain and given Rx for Vicodin (hydrocodone) 500mg po prn. Pt is now complaining of shortness of breath and tightness of the chest.

O: PE reveals labored breathing. Histamine release test (leukocytes) positive for anaphylactic shock, a reaction to the hydrocodone. IV injection of 1 mg/ml epinephrine hydrochloride is administered to counter the allergic reaction.

A: Anaphylactic shock due to medication

P: Rx codeine 15mg po q6h for pain

Pt to return in one week for followup

The best, most appropriate diagnosis code(s) are _____.

The best, most appropriate E/M code is _____.

The best, most appropriate procedure code(s) are _____.

Link the procedure code(s) to the diagnosis code(s). _____

Physician's Notes for Sarah Student

27-year-old female is seen in the emergency department with a suspected fracture of the lower rt leg.

History: Patient states she was driving a motorcycle on the highway when she lost control and failed to make a curve. The motorcycle overturned and slid along the shoulder of the road, with her leg underneath. She did not hit anything.

PE: BP 120/75, T 98.6, P 100, R 20. Ht. 5'4". Wt. 122 lbs.

HEENT: Atraumatic. Lungs clear. External abrasions upper arm and shoulder on the rt side. Swelling and tenderness of posterior lower leg.

Testing: X-ray, tibia and fibula, two views.

Impression: Closed fracture of the shaft of the tibia. Application of long leg walker cast (thigh to toes). Rx antibiotic ointment to prevent infection of abrasion.

The best, most appropriate diagnosis code(s) are _____.

The best, most appropriate E/M code is _____.

The best, most appropriate procedure code(s) are _____.

Link the procedure codes to the diagnosis code(s). _____

Physician's Notes for Paul Pepperstone

59-year-old male is seen in his physician's office with complaints of abdominal pain, diarrhea, and rectal bleeding, which began three weeks ago.

History: Patient has not been seen in this office in over five years. Patient states no previous problems or concerns with digestive system.

PE: BP 145/95, T 98.6, P 110, R 20. Ht. 6'1". Wt. 185 lbs.

HEENT: Atraumatic. Lungs clear. Nothing remarkable. Tense abdomen with some guarding LLQ.

Testing: Flexible sigmoidoscopy to r/o colon cancer.

Impression: Sigmoidoscopy inconclusive. Schedule colonoscopy for two weeks.

The best, most appropriate diagnosis code(s) are _____.

The best, most appropriate E/M code is _____.

The best, most appropriate procedure code(s) are _____.

Link the procedure codes to the diagnosis code(s). _____

Physician's Notes for Mitzi Cagwell

20-year-old female came in to this family practitioner's office for the first time, complaining of an earache in the right ear. Patient states that she has also experienced a ringing in the same ear with increasing severity for the past two days. There appears to be only minor distress.

History: Overall health history reviewed with particular focus on past ENT and sinus problems. Patient states general good health with occasional sinus infections and congestion.

Vitals: T 101, BP 120/80, P 100, R 20.

HEENT: Tympanic membrane red, fluid noted in right ear.

Dx: Otitis media.

The best, most appropriate diagnosis code(s) are _____.

The best, most appropriate E/M code is _____.

The best, most appropriate procedure code(s) are _____.

Link the procedure codes to the diagnosis code(s). _____

Physician's Notes for Tex T. Books

History: This 35-year-old male is seen in his regular physician's office for a preemployment health examination.

PE: Unremarkable. Urinalysis and CBC normal.

Impression: Patient is in good health, appropriate for his age.

Plan: Screening form completed and signed.

The best, most appropriate diagnosis code(s) are _____.

The best, most appropriate E/M code is _____.

The best, most appropriate procedure code(s) are _____.

Link the procedure codes to the diagnosis code(s). _____

Physician's Notes for Joan Smith-Doe

History: This 52-year-old female is seen today after falling off her bicycle and twisting her left ankle. She was a patient of Dr. Abernathy but has not seen him in seven years. She states that she is experiencing pain around the entire foot, which dramatically increases when she attempts to place weight on it.

PE: Foot is pink with some bruising around the medial malleolus. Swelling evident. X-ray of ankle, both anterior and posterior, negative for fracture.

Impression: Sprained medial malleolus, right extremity.

Plan: Rest. Application of ice pack prn. Ibuprofen b.i.d. prn.

The best, most appropriate diagnosis code(s) are _____.

The best, most appropriate E/M code is _____.

The best, most appropriate procedure code(s) are _____.

Link the procedure codes to the diagnosis code(s). _____

CHAPTER SUMMARY

Understanding how to find the best, most appropriate diagnosis and procedure codes and then linking them together completes the process of coding. Certainly, you can see how important accuracy is to the entire administration of health insurance claim submission and reimbursement for health care facilities.

Now you have practiced coding from beginning to end. The next step is to copy all of the patient's information, along with these codes and the links, onto the CMS-1500 health insurance claim form.

10

Health Insurance Claim Form CMS-1500

OBJECTIVES

- Understand the format of the CMS-1500 health insurance claim form.

- Determine the information required to complete the CMS-1500 correctly.

- Understand the importance of each piece of data.

- Complete a CMS-1500 claim form.

The health insurance claim form used most often by health care facilities to get paid for services provided to an individual is called the CMS-1500 (Figure 10-1). You may remember from earlier in this book that CMS stands for the Centers for Medicare & Medicaid Services.

> ### IMPORTANT NOTE
> The CMS-1500 was formerly called the HCFA-1500 ("Hic-Fah"). Although the name has changed, many professionals are in the habit of calling this form the Hic-Fah-1500. Either name should lead you to the form shown in Figure 10-1.

CMS-1500

Let's review every box on this form, so you can better understand the specific piece of **data** that should be placed there and why the information is essential to the process of submitting claims and receiving payment for services. This is what insurance coding and billing is all about—bringing in the revenue—the money that the health care professional has earned by providing services to a patient.

The form is divided into four sections. If you look carefully, you'll see a line going across the center of the form, between boxes 12 and 14, that is bolder or thicker than the other lines on the form. This divides the form into two sections, top and bottom. Now look at the form and find the bolder line that divides it vertically (top to bottom) into a left section and a right section. The two lines on the form create four sections: top left, top right, bottom left, and bottom right. As we go over the form, we will look at the **fields** in each section, rather than in numerical order. OK? Let's begin.

Key Terms
Data: Pieces of information.

Fields (form locators): The boxes of the CMS-1500.

Section 1: Top Left

Section 1 is primarily information about the patient (Figure 10-2).

Box 1. Type of Insurance Policy

Box 1 contains check boxes for you to indicate what type of health insurance plan is covering services to this patient. We discussed most of these plans in Chapter 1.

- Medicare
- Medicaid
- CHAMPUS
- CHAMPVA
- Group health plan (which is checked when the policyholder gets his or her insurance coverage through his or her job or another organization)
- FECA BLK LUNG (short for FECA Black Lung, as part of the Black Lung Benefits Act). This is coverage specifically created for coal miners who develop respiratory conditions related to their working in those mines).
- Other

PLEASE
DO NOT
STAPLE
IN THIS
AREA

MCGRAW INSURANCE CO.
P.O. BOX 5544
WILSON, OH 45533

P

| | PICA | | **HEALTH INSURANCE CLAIM FORM** | PICA | |

1. MEDICARE	MEDICAID	CHAMPUS	CHAMPVA	GROUP HEALTH PLAN	FECA BLK LUNG	OTHER	1a. INSURED'S I.D. NUMBER	(FOR PROGRAM IN ITEM 1)
(Medicare #)	(Medicaid #)	(Sponsor's SSN)	(VA File #)	[X] (SSN OR ID)	(SSN)	(ID)	998436627	

2. PATIENT'S NAME (Last Name, First Name, Middle Initial)	3. PATIENT'S BIRTH DATE	SEX	4. INSURED'S NAME (Last Name, First Name, Middle Initial)
DECKER, DIANE E.	MM 05 DD 21 YY 73	M F [X]	DECKER, DIANE E.

2nd Fold

5. PATIENT'S ADDRESS (No., Street)	6. PATIENT RELATIONSHIP TO INSURED	7. INSURED'S ADDRESS (No., Street)
876 PROGRESS AVENUE	Self [X] Spouse Child Other	876 PROGRESS AVENUE

CITY	STATE	8. PATIENT STATUS	CITY	STATE
CITYVILLE	FL	Single [X] Married Other	CITYVILLE	FL

ZIP CODE	TELEPHONE (Include Area Code)		ZIP CODE	TELEPHONE (INCLUDE AREA CODE)
32901	(407) 555 9987	Employed [X] Full-Time Student Part-Time Student	32901	(407) 555 9987

9. OTHER INSURED'S NAME (Last Name, First Name, Middle Initial)	10. IS PATIENT'S CONDITION RELATED TO:	11. INSURED'S POLICY GROUP OR FECA NUMBER
		PMI03

a. OTHER INSURED'S POLICY OR GROUP NUMBER	a. EMPLOYMENT? (CURRENT OR PREVIOUS) [X] YES NO	a. INSURED'S DATE OF BIRTH MM 05 DD 21 YY 73 SEX M F [X]

b. OTHER INSURED'S DATE OF BIRTH MM DD YY SEX M F	b. AUTO ACCIDENT? PLACE (State) YES [X] NO	b. EMPLOYER'S NAME OR SCHOOL NAME PRIME INCORPORATED

c. EMPLOYER'S NAME OR SCHOOL NAME	c. OTHER ACCIDENT? YES [X] NO	c. INSURANCE PLAN NAME OR PROGRAM NAME MCGRAW HMO

d. INSURANCE PLAN NAME OR PROGRAM NAME	10d. RESERVED FOR LOCAL USE	d. IS THERE ANOTHER HEALTH BENEFIT PLAN? YES [X] NO *if yes*, return to and complete item 9 a-d.

READ BACK OF FORM BEFORE COMPLETING AND SIGNING THIS FORM.

12. PATIENT'S OR AUTHORIZED PERSON'S SIGNATURE. I authorize the release of any medical or other information necessary to process this claim. I also request payment of government benefits either to myself or to the party who accepts assignment below.

SIGNED SIGNATURE ON FILE   DATE 12/27/05

13. INSURED'S OR AUTHORIZED PERSON'S SIGNATURE. I authorize payment of medical benefits to the undersigned physician or supplier for services described below.

SIGNED SIGNATURE ON FILE

1st Fold

14. DATE OF CURRENT: MM 12 DD 05 YY 05 ILLNESS (First symptom) OR INJURY (Accident) OR PREGNANCY(LMP) INJURY	15. IF PATIENT HAS HAD SAME OR SIMILAR ILLNESS GIVE FIRST DATE MM DD YY	16. DATES PATIENT UNABLE TO WORK IN CURRENT OCCUPATION FROM MM DD YY TO MM DD YY

17. NAME OF REFERRING PHYSICIAN OR OTHER SOURCE MARK C. WELBY MD	17a. I.D. NUMBER OF REFERRING PHYSICIAN 7766554	18. HOSPITALIZATION DATES RELATED TO CURRENT SERVICES FROM MM DD YY TO MM DD YY

19. RESERVED FOR LOCAL USE	20. OUTSIDE LAB? YES [X] NO	$ CHARGES

21. DIAGNOSIS OR NATURE OF ILLNESS OR INJURY (RELATE ITEMS 1,2,3 OR 4 TO ITEM 24E BY LINE)

1. 354.0   3. |___.___

2. |___.___   4. |___.___

22. MEDICAID RESUBMISSION CODE   ORIGINAL REF. NO.

23. PRIOR AUTHORIZATION NUMBER

24. A. DATE(S) OF SERVICE From MM DD YY	To MM DD YY	B. Place of Service	C. Type of Service	D. PROCEDURES, SERVICES, OR SUPPLIES (Explain Unusual Circumstances) CPT/HCPCS	MODIFIER	E. DIAGNOSIS CODE	F. $ CHARGES	G. DAYS OR UNITS	H. EPSDT Family Plan	I. EMG	J. COB	K. RESERVED FOR LOCAL USE
02 21 06	02 21 06	11		99201		1	46.00	1				HEALER
02 21 06	02 21 06	11	1	73100		1	63.00	1				HEALER
02 21 06	02 21 06	11		29125		1	63.00	1				HEALER

25. FEDERAL TAX I.D. NUMBER SSN EIN 3452331123 [X]	26. PATIENT'S ACCOUNT NO. DECDI000 3	27. ACCEPT ASSIGNMENT? (For govt. claims, see back) [X] YES NO	28. TOTAL CHARGE $ 172.00	29. AMOUNT PAID $	30. BALANCE DUE $ 172.00

31. SIGNATURE OF PHYSICIAN OR SUPPLIER INCLUDING DEGREES OR CREDENTIALS (I certify that the statements on the reverse apply to this bill and are made a part thereof.) SIGNATURE ON FILE SIGNED DATE 12/30/03	32. NAME AND ADDRESS OF FACILITY WHERE SERVICES WERE RENDERED (If other than home or office)	33. PHYSICIAN'S, SUPPLIER'S BILLING NAME, ADDRESS, ZIP CODE & PHONE# JAMES C. HEALER MD 123 MAIN STREET ANYTOWN, FL 32711 PIN# 6654321 GRP#

FIGURE 10-1

CMS-1500 health insurance claim form.

PLEASE
DO NOT
STAPLE
IN THIS
AREA
P

MCGRAW INSURANCE CO.
P.O. BOX 5544
WILSON, OH 45533

HEALTH INSURANCE CLAIM FORM

| | PICA | | | | | | | | PICA | |

1. MEDICARE	MEDICAID	CHAMPUS	CHAMPVA	GROUP HEALTH PLAN	FECA BLK LUNG	OTHER	1a. INSURED'S I.D. NUMBER (FOR PROGRAM IN ITEM 1)
(Medicare #)	(Medicaid #)	(Sponsor's SSN)	(VA File #)	[X] (SSN OR ID)	(SSN)	(ID)	998436627

2. PATIENT'S NAME (Last Name, First Name, Middle Initial)
DECKER, DIANE E.

3. PATIENT'S BIRTH DATE MM 05 DD 21 YY 73 **SEX** M F [X]

4. INSURED'S NAME (Last Name, First Name, Middle Initial)
DECKER, DIANE E.

5. PATIENT'S ADDRESS (No., Street)
876 PROGRESS AVENUE

6. PATIENT RELATIONSHIP TO INSURED
Self [X] Spouse [ ] Child [ ] Other [ ]

7. INSURED'S ADDRESS (No., Street)
876 PROGRESS AVENUE

CITY CITYVILLE STATE FL

8. PATIENT STATUS
Single [X] Married [ ] Other [ ]
Employed [X] Full-Time Student [ ] Part-Time Student [ ]

CITY CITYVILLE STATE FL

ZIP CODE 32901 TELEPHONE (Include Area Code) (407) 555 9987

ZIP CODE 32901 TELEPHONE (INCLUDE AREA CODE) (407) 555 9987

9. OTHER INSURED'S NAME (Last Name, First Name, Middle Initial)

10. IS PATIENT'S CONDITION RELATED TO:

11. INSURED'S POLICY GROUP OR FECA NUMBER
PMI03

a. OTHER INSURED'S POLICY OR GROUP NUMBER

a. EMPLOYMENT? (CURRENT OR PREVIOUS) [X] YES [ ] NO

a. INSURED'S DATE OF BIRTH MM 05 DD 21 YY 73 SEX M F [X]

b. OTHER INSURED'S DATE OF BIRTH MM DD YY SEX M [ ] F [ ]

b. AUTO ACCIDENT? [ ] YES [X] NO PLACE (State)

b. EMPLOYER'S NAME OR SCHOOL NAME
PRIME INCORPORATED

c. EMPLOYER'S NAME OR SCHOOL NAME

c. OTHER ACCIDENT? [ ] YES [X] NO

c. INSURANCE PLAN NAME OR PROGRAM NAME
MCGRAW HMO

d. INSURANCE PLAN NAME OR PROGRAM NAME

10d. RESERVED FOR LOCAL USE

d. IS THERE ANOTHER HEALTH BENEFIT PLAN? [ ] YES [X] NO *if yes*, return to and complete item 9 a-d.

READ BACK OF FORM BEFORE COMPLETING AND SIGNING THIS FORM.
12. PATIENT'S OR AUTHORIZED PERSON'S SIGNATURE. I authorize the release of any medical or other information necessary to process this claim. I also request payment of government benefits either to myself or to the party who accepts assignment below.

SIGNED SIGNATURE ON FILE DATE 12/27/05

13. INSURED'S OR AUTHORIZED PERSON'S SIGNATURE. I authorize payment of medical benefits to the undersigned physician or supplier for services described below.

SIGNED SIGNATURE ON FILE

14. DATE OF CURRENT ILLNESS (First symptom) OR INJURY (Accident) OR PREGNANCY (LMP) MM 12 DD 05 YY 05 INJURY

15. IF PATIENT HAS HAD SAME OR SIMILAR ILLNESS GIVE FIRST DATE MM DD YY

16. DATES PATIENT UNABLE TO WORK IN CURRENT OCCUPATION FROM MM DD YY TO MM DD YY

17. NAME OF REFERRING PHYSICIAN OR OTHER SOURCE
MARK C. WELBY MD

17a. I.D. NUMBER OF REFERRING PHYSICIAN
7766554

18. HOSPITALIZATION DATES RELATED TO CURRENT SERVICES FROM MM DD YY TO MM DD YY

19. RESERVED FOR LOCAL USE

20. OUTSIDE LAB? [ ] YES [X] NO $ CHARGES

21. DIAGNOSIS OR NATURE OF ILLNESS OR INJURY (RELATE ITEMS 1,2,3 OR 4 TO ITEM 24E BY LINE)
1. 354.0
2.
3.
4.

22. MEDICAID RESUBMISSION CODE ORIGINAL REF. NO.

23. PRIOR AUTHORIZATION NUMBER

24. A. DATE(S) OF SERVICE						B. Place of Service	C. Type of Service	D. PROCEDURES, SERVICES, OR SUPPLIES (Explain Unusual Circumstances) CPT/HCPCS	MODIFIER	E. DIAGNOSIS CODE	F. $ CHARGES	G. DAYS OR UNITS	H. EPSDT Family Plan	I. EMG	J. COB	K. RESERVED FOR LOCAL USE
From MM 02	DD 21	YY 06	To MM 02	DD 21	YY 06	11		99201		1	46.00	1				HEALER
02	21	06	02	21	06	11	1	73100		1	63.00	1				HEALER
02	21	06	02	21	06	11		29125		1	63.00	1				HEALER

25. FEDERAL TAX I.D. NUMBER 3452331123 SSN [ ] EIN [X]

26. PATIENT'S ACCOUNT NO. DECDI000 3

27. ACCEPT ASSIGNMENT? (For govt. claims, see back) [X] YES [ ] NO

28. TOTAL CHARGE $ 172.00

29. AMOUNT PAID $

30. BALANCE DUE $ 172.00

31. SIGNATURE OF PHYSICIAN OR SUPPLIER INCLUDING DEGREES OR CREDENTIALS (I certify that the statements on the reverse apply to this bill and are made a part thereof.)
SIGNED SIGNATURE ON FILE DATE 12/30/03

32. NAME AND ADDRESS OF FACILITY WHERE SERVICES WERE RENDERED (If other than home or office)

33. PHYSICIAN'S, SUPPLIER'S BILLING NAME, ADDRESS, ZIP CODE & PHONE#
JAMES C. HEALER MD
123 MAIN STREET
ANYTOWN, FL 32711
PIN# 6654321 GRP#

FIGURE 10-2
Top left portion of the CMS-1500.

You will note that there is an indicator next to each little check box, telling you exactly what type of number should be placed in Box 1a, to the right. (More on this later when we discuss Section 2, where Box 1a is located.) When you are using a computerized patient accounting software program, such as NDCMediSoft Advanced, Intergy, or Medical Manager, the program will have you indicate the answer to this when you enter the patient's insurance information. Then the software will place the ☒ in the correct check box.

Box 2. Patient's Name (Last Name, First Name, Middle Initial)

In this box, place the last name, followed by the first name, then the middle initial of the patient, the person who came to the provider's office for consultation, treatment, or other service. This information must be entered in this order, in all capital letters. It is also important that you understand that the person's name must appear in exactly the same way that it is shown on the health insurance policy.

The easiest way to make certain it is correct is to enter the name as it appears on the insurance card—*exactly*. No nicknames and no alternate spellings are permitted. Sometimes patients will complete your office's registration form with their common name, or nickname.

A computer cannot see that Kathi and Kathy are the same. To a computer, these are two totally different names. And chances are it is a computer that will be reviewing your claim form when it arrives at the insurance carrier's office.

Examples

DECKER, DIANE E.

- Elizabeth may be called Beth, and Anthony may be called Tony. Stuart may write in Stu. Others use a first initial and are referenced by their middle name, such as J. Mark Smith's being called Mark.
- Some people may look at Kathi and Kathy and say, "What's the difference, it's the same name; anyone can see that!" Not so.

Box 3. Patient's BirthDate   Sex

Enter the birthdate of the patient as MM DD CC YY. Use two numbers for the month (08), two numbers for the day (09), and four numbers for the year (1975).

Also, the patient's sex must be indicated. This may seem very obvious and basic to you, as it should. However, this data must be included on the form. If one of these boxes is not checked (left blank), your claim will be rejected.

Example

MM DD CC YY

MM = two digits representing the month

DD = two digits representing the date of the month

CC = two digits representing the century (i.e., 19 or 20)

YY = two digits representing the year

- May 1, 1973, is written as 05/01/1973.

Box 5. Patient's Address (No. Street), City, State, Zip Code, Telephone (Include Area Code)

These boxes, one on top of the other, show the address for the patient. Each piece of data must go separately in each box. The number and street name of the house or apartment where he or she lives should be placed in the first box.

Example

Patient's address (no. street) would be shown as 876 Progress Avenue.

Box 6. Patient Relationship to Insured

Recall from Chapter 3 that the insured is also known as the policyholder, the person who brings the health insurance policy to the family. This box is asking you to describe the connection of the patient to the insured.

- If the same person with the insurance policy is the patient, then the relationship is Self X.
- If a husband has insurance through his job and his wife is included on the policy as a dependent, when the wife goes to see the physician, the wife is the patient, the husband is the insured, and the relationship for Box 6 is Spouse X.
- If a mother has insurance and her son is included on the policy as a dependent, when the boy goes to see the physician, he is the patient, his mother is the insured, and the relationship for Box 6 is Child X.
- If a stepfather has legal guardianship of his stepdaughter, he has insurance coverage through his job, and his stepdaughter is included on the policy as a dependent, when the stepdaughter goes to see the physician, she is the patient, the stepfather is the insured, and the relationship for Box 6 is Other X.

Box 8. Patient Status

The first part of this box identifies the patient's marital status.

Single

Married

Other (divorced, separated, or widowed)

The second part of this box identifies whether or not the patient is

Employed

Full-Time Student

Part-Time Student

Box 9. Other Insured's Name (Last Name, First Name, Middle Initial)

Box 9a. Other Insured's Policy or Group Number

Box 9b. Other Insured's Date of Birth   Sex

Box 9c. Employer's Name or School Name

Box 9d. Insurance Plan Name or Program Name

These five boxes are for you to provide information regarding the patient's secondary health insurance policy, should he or she have one. These boxes must be completed in full, along with the checking of ⊠ Yes in Box 11D, if applicable.

Box 10. Is Patient Condition Related to:

A. Employment? (Current or Previous)

A check next to YES indicates that this claim is for a condition or an injury that occurred at the patient's place of employment and might be covered under workers' compensation, rather than the health insurance policy. If this is not the case, the NO box must be checked.

B. Auto Accident? Place (State)

A check next to YES indicates that this claim is for a condition or an injury due to the patient's involvement in a car accident and might be covered under the patient's automobile insurance rather than the health insurance policy. If the patient was not hurt in a car accident for this encounter, then the NO box must be checked.

> **IMPORTANT NOTE**
>
> The United States Postal Service's approved two-letter abbreviation must be used in this box to indicate the state in which the auto accident occurred.

C. Other Accident?

A check next to YES indicates that this claim is for a condition or an injury that is due to the patient's involvement in an accident (nonautomobile) and may be covered under a liability policy rather than the health insurance policy. If there was no accident, check the NO box.

The NO box must be checked if the patient's condition or injury is not related to either the patient's employment or involvement in an auto or other accident. If any of these three questions go unanswered (left blank), the claim may be rejected, or at least delayed in processing. So, remember that these areas must be addressed.

Box 12. Patient's or Authorized Person's Signature

This box reads

> I authorize the release of any medical or other information necessary to process this claim. I also request payment of government benefits either to myself or to the party who accepts assignment below.
>
> SIGNED_____ DATE_____

You probably have never actually signed a claim form, no matter how many times you have gone to see a physician. However, you have certainly signed this release on a separate piece of paper given to you when you first went to see that provider. The date shown in this box is the date the patient signed that piece of paper. The release with the original signature must be in the patient's health record. Without the original signature from the patient, the claims process cannot be completed and your health care office does not get paid.

Section 2: Top Right

Section 2 is primarily information about the policyholder for the primary insurance policy (Figure 10-3).

Box 1a. Insured's ID Number (for Program in Item 1)

In Chapter 3, we reviewed the fact that a policy number, an ID number, and a subscriber number can all be the same thing. And that key number, identifying a particular policy with a particular policyholder, is what should be entered in Box 1a. Different insurance carriers call it different things. Box 1 actually tells you which number to enter in Box 1a. This is a very important box—one incorrect digit and your claim is rejected.

- For Medicare patients, the individual's Medicare number (found on the patient's Medicare ID card) is to be entered here.
- For Medicaid patients, the individual's Medicaid number (found on the patient's Medicaid ID card) is to be entered here.
- For CHAMPUS (now TriCare), enter the sponsor's SSN (Social Security number) (found on the sponsor's military ID card).
- For CHAMPVA, enter the individual's VA (Veteran's Administration) file number (found on the patient's VA ID card).
- For a group health plan, FECA Black Lung, or other, enter the number on the identification card.

Sometimes the number is the same as the individual's Social Security number, sometimes it is the Social Security number plus a letter or two, and sometimes it is a totally different number. Do not assume it is the policyholder's Social Security number. To avoid any mistakes, copy the number carefully—directly from the patient's insurance card.

> **Memory Tip**
> The insured is the person who brings the INSURance policy to the family.

PLEASE
DO NOT
STAPLE
IN THIS
AREA

MCGRAW INSURANCE CO.
P.O. BOX 5544
WILSON, OH 45533

HEALTH INSURANCE CLAIM FORM

PICA						PICA

1. MEDICARE (Medicare #)   **MEDICAID** (Medicaid #)   **CHAMPUS** (Sponsor's SSN)   **CHAMPVA** (VA File #)   **GROUP HEALTH PLAN** [X] (SSN OR ID)   **FECA BLK LUNG** (SSN)   **OTHER** (ID)

1a. INSURED'S I.D. NUMBER (FOR PROGRAM IN ITEM 1)
998436627

2. PATIENT'S NAME (Last Name, First Name, Middle Initial)
DECKER, DIANE E.

3. PATIENT'S BIRTH DATE MM 05 DD 21 YY 73   **SEX** M [ ] F [X]

4. INSURED'S NAME (Last Name, First Name, Middle Initial)
DECKER, DIANE E.

5. PATIENT'S ADDRESS (No., Street)
876 PROGRESS AVENUE

6. PATIENT RELATIONSHIP TO INSURED
Self [X] Spouse [ ] Child [ ] Other [ ]

7. INSURED'S ADDRESS (No., Street)
876 PROGRESS AVENUE

CITY CITYVILLE   STATE FL

8. PATIENT STATUS
Single [X] Married [ ] Other [ ]

CITY CITYVILLE   STATE FL

ZIP CODE 32901   TELEPHONE (Include Area Code) (407) 555 9987

Employed [X] Full-Time Student [ ] Part-Time Student [ ]

ZIP CODE 32901   TELEPHONE (INCLUDE AREA CODE) (407) 555 9987

9. OTHER INSURED'S NAME (Last Name, First Name, Middle Initial)

10. IS PATIENT'S CONDITION RELATED TO:

11. INSURED'S POLICY GROUP OR FECA NUMBER
PMI03

a. OTHER INSURED'S POLICY OR GROUP NUMBER

a. EMPLOYMENT? (CURRENT OR PREVIOUS) [X] YES [ ] NO

a. INSURED'S DATE OF BIRTH MM 05 DD 21 YY 73   **SEX** M [ ] F [X]

b. OTHER INSURED'S DATE OF BIRTH MM DD YY   SEX M [ ] F [ ]

b. AUTO ACCIDENT? [ ] YES [X] NO   PLACE (State)

b. EMPLOYER'S NAME OR SCHOOL NAME
PRIME INCORPORATED

c. EMPLOYER'S NAME OR SCHOOL NAME

c. OTHER ACCIDENT? [ ] YES [X] NO

c. INSURANCE PLAN NAME OR PROGRAM NAME
MCGRAW HMO

d. INSURANCE PLAN NAME OR PROGRAM NAME

10d. RESERVED FOR LOCAL USE

d. IS THERE ANOTHER HEALTH BENEFIT PLAN? [ ] YES [X] NO *if yes,* return to and complete item 9 a-d.

READ BACK OF FORM BEFORE COMPLETING AND SIGNING THIS FORM.

12. PATIENT'S OR AUTHORIZED PERSON'S SIGNATURE. I authorize the release of any medical or other information necessary to process this claim. I also request payment of government benefits either to myself or to the party who accepts assignment below.
SIGNED SIGNATURE ON FILE   DATE 12/27/05

13. INSURED'S OR AUTHORIZED PERSON'S SIGNATURE. I authorize payment of medical benefits to the undersigned physician or supplier for services described below.
SIGNED SIGNATURE ON FILE

14. DATE OF CURRENT: MM 12 DD 05 YY 05   ILLNESS (First symptom) OR INJURY (Accident) OR PREGNANCY (LMP)   INJURY

15. IF PATIENT HAS HAD SAME OR SIMILAR ILLNESS GIVE FIRST DATE MM DD YY

16. DATES PATIENT UNABLE TO WORK IN CURRENT OCCUPATION FROM TO

17. NAME OF REFERRING PHYSICIAN OR OTHER SOURCE
MARK C. WELBY MD

17a. I.D. NUMBER OF REFERRING PHYSICIAN
7766554

18. HOSPITALIZATION DATES RELATED TO CURRENT SERVICES MM DD YY FROM TO

19. RESERVED FOR LOCAL USE

20. OUTSIDE LAB? [ ] YES [X] NO $ CHARGES

21. DIAGNOSIS OR NATURE OF ILLNESS OR INJURY (RELATE ITEMS 1,2,3 OR 4 TO ITEM 24E BY LINE)
1. 354.0
2.
3.
4.

22. MEDICAID RESUBMISSION CODE   ORIGINAL REF. NO.

23. PRIOR AUTHORIZATION NUMBER

24. A DATE(S) OF SERVICE From MM DD YY	To MM DD YY	B Place of Service	C Type of Service	D PROCEDURES, SERVICES, OR SUPPLIES (Explain Unusual Circumstances) CPT/HCPCS | MODIFIER	E DIAGNOSIS CODE	F $ CHARGES	G DAYS OR UNITS	H EPSDT Family Plan	I EMG	J COB	K RESERVED FOR LOCAL USE
02 21 06	02 21 06	11		99201 |	1	46.00	1				HEALER
02 21 06	02 21 06	11	1	73100 |	1	63.00	1				HEALER
02 21 06	02 21 06	11		29125 |	1	63.00	1				HEALER

25. FEDERAL TAX I.D. NUMBER 3452331123   SSN [ ] EIN [X]

26. PATIENT'S ACCOUNT NO. DECDI000   3

27. ACCEPT ASSIGNMENT? (For govt. claims, see back) [X] YES [ ] NO

28. TOTAL CHARGE $ 172.00

29. AMOUNT PAID $

30. BALANCE DUE $ 172.00

31. SIGNATURE OF PHYSICIAN OR SUPPLIER INCLUDING DEGREES OR CREDENTIALS (I certify that the statements on the reverse apply to this bill and are made a part thereof.)
SIGNATURE ON FILE
SIGNED   DATE 12/30/03

32. NAME AND ADDRESS OF FACILITY WHERE SERVICES WERE RENDERED (If other than home or office)

33. PHYSICIAN'S, SUPPLIER'S BILLING NAME, ADDRESS, ZIP CODE & PHONE#
JAMES C. HEALER MD
123 MAIN STREET
ANYTOWN, FL 32711
PIN# 6654321   GRP#

FIGURE 10-3
Top right portion of the CMS-1500.

Box 4. Insured's Name (Last Name, First Name, Middle Initial)

Just as in Box 2 regarding the patient, this box must show the name of the policyholder of the primary health insurance policy covering this patient's health care. Remember, the name must be entered last name first.

Example

Diane E. Decker is entered as Decker, Diane E.

Box 7. Insured's Address (No. Street), City, State, Zip Code, Telephone (Include Area Code)

These boxes, one on top of the other, must show the address for the insured, the person who brings the insurance policy to the family. Each piece of data must go separately in each box. The number and street name of the house or apartment where the insured lives should be placed in the first box.

Example

876 Progress Avenue

Box 11. Insured's Policy Group or FECA Number

On the insurance card, you will see a number identified as a group number or name. It is usually next to or immediately below the policy number, or ID number. Some individual policies do not have group numbers. Look for it. If there is one, that data is placed in Box 11. If that space on the card is blank, you are permitted to leave this box blank.

IMPORTANT NOTE

The group number is different from the policy number.

Box 11a. Insured's Date of Birth   Sex

Enter the date of birth for the insured in Box 11a in the MM DD CCYY format—that is, the month in two numbers (08), the day in two numbers (09), and the year in four numbers (1973). The same box asks for a $\boxed{X}$ indicating the policyholder's sex.

Example

May 21, 1973, would be entered as 05/21/1973.

Box 11b. Employer's Name or School Name

This is the name of the company through which the insured receives the health insurance policy (if this is a group policy). This company name must match the insurance carrier's records as being the sponsor of the health plan. If the insurance is for a child covered by a school policy, then the name of the school should be shown here.

Box 11c. Insurance Plan Name or Program Name

Many insurance carriers offer different health insurance plans with different names. Often, a **plan name**, or **program name**, designates whether the policyholder is participating in an HMO plan or a PPO plan. Therefore, take note that the name of the plan (which you will find on the insurance card) is separate information from the name of the insurance carrier itself and must be entered as such. In addition, it is important to confirm that your health care office is a participating provider for that plan.

Examples

Blue Cross/Blue Shield offers many plans, including Health Options and Blue Options.

A provider may participate with the PPO, but not the HMO, of a particular insurance carrier.

Box 11d. Is There Another Health Benefit Plan?

Is this patient covered by a secondary health insurance plan? You will see the notation on the form in Box 11d that, if YES is checked, Boxes 9–9d must be completed. We reviewed those boxes when we went over Section 1. If the patient is not covered under a secondary policy, the NO box must be checked.

Box 13. Insured's or Authorized Person's Signature

This box reads

> I authorize payment of medical benefits to the undersigned physician or supplier for services described below.
>
> SIGNED_____

Just as with the patient's signature, the policyholder will rarely actually sign this form. Instead, a separate piece of paper containing this release information will be signed by the policyholder and be kept in the patient's chart. That way, it is available for all claims.

IMPORTANT NOTE

When completing the Medicare version of the CMS-1500 form, much of the upper right portion of this form is omitted. This is due to the fact that, with the Medicare program, the policyholder, or insured person, and the patient are *always* the same person. There are no dependents available on this type of policy.

Section 3: Bottom Left

Section 3 contains information about the patient's reason for coming to see the provider for this encounter (Figure 10.4).

MCGRAW INSURANCE CO.
P.O. BOX 5544
WILSON, OH 45533

PLEASE
DO NOT
STAPLE
IN THIS
AREA
P

| | PICA | | | **HEALTH INSURANCE CLAIM FORM** | PICA | | |

1. MEDICARE	MEDICAID	CHAMPUS	CHAMPVA	GROUP HEALTH PLAN	FECA BLK LUNG	OTHER	1a. INSURED'S I.D. NUMBER	(FOR PROGRAM IN ITEM 1)
☐ (Medicare #)	☐ (Medicaid #)	☐ (Sponsor's SSN)	☐ (VA File #)	☒ (SSN OR ID)	☐ (SSN)	☐ (ID)	998436627	

2. PATIENT'S NAME (Last Name, First Name, Middle Initial)
DECKER, DIANE E.

3. PATIENT'S BIRTH DATE MM 05 DD 21 YY 73 **SEX** M ☐ F ☒

4. INSURED'S NAME (Last Name, First Name, Middle Initial)
DECKER, DIANE E.

5. PATIENT'S ADDRESS (No., Street)
876 PROGRESS AVENUE

6. PATIENT RELATIONSHIP TO INSURED
Self ☒ Spouse ☐ Child ☐ Other ☐

7. INSURED'S ADDRESS (No., Street)
876 PROGRESS AVENUE

CITY CITYVILLE STATE FL

8. PATIENT STATUS
Single ☒ Married ☐ Other ☐
Employed ☒ Full-Time Student ☐ Part-Time Student ☐

CITY CITYVILLE STATE FL

ZIP CODE 32901 TELEPHONE (Include Area Code) (407) 555 9987

ZIP CODE 32901 TELEPHONE (INCLUDE AREA CODE) (407) 555 9987

9. OTHER INSURED'S NAME (Last Name, First Name, Middle Initial)

10. IS PATIENT'S CONDITION RELATED TO:

11. INSURED'S POLICY GROUP OR FECA NUMBER
PMI03

a. OTHER INSURED'S POLICY OR GROUP NUMBER

a. EMPLOYMENT? (CURRENT OR PREVIOUS) ☒ YES ☐ NO

a. INSURED'S DATE OF BIRTH MM 05 DD 21 YY 73 **SEX** M ☐ F ☒

b. OTHER INSURED'S DATE OF BIRTH MM DD YY **SEX** M ☐ F ☐

b. AUTO ACCIDENT? PLACE (State) ☐ YES ☒ NO

b. EMPLOYER'S NAME OR SCHOOL NAME
PRIME INCORPORATED

c. EMPLOYER'S NAME OR SCHOOL NAME

c. OTHER ACCIDENT? ☐ YES ☒ NO

c. INSURANCE PLAN NAME OR PROGRAM NAME
MCGRAW HMO

d. INSURANCE PLAN NAME OR PROGRAM NAME

10d. RESERVED FOR LOCAL USE

d. IS THERE ANOTHER HEALTH BENEFIT PLAN? ☐ YES ☒ NO **if yes,** return to and complete item 9 a-d.

READ BACK OF FORM BEFORE COMPLETING AND SIGNING THIS FORM.

12. PATIENT'S OR AUTHORIZED PERSON'S SIGNATURE. I authorize the release of any medical or other information necessary to process this claim. I also request payment of government benefits either to myself or to the party who accepts assignment below.
SIGNED SIGNATURE ON FILE DATE 12/27/05

13. INSURED'S OR AUTHORIZED PERSON'S SIGNATURE. I authorize payment of medical benefits to the undersigned physician or supplier for services described below.
SIGNED SIGNATURE ON FILE

14. DATE OF CURRENT: MM 12 DD 05 YY 05 ILLNESS (First symptom) OR INJURY (Accident) OR PREGNANCY(LMP) INJURY

15. IF PATIENT HAS HAD SAME OR SIMILAR ILLNESS GIVE FIRST DATE MM DD YY

16. DATES PATIENT UNABLE TO WORK IN CURRENT OCCUPATION FROM MM DD YY TO MM DD YY

17. NAME OF REFERRING PHYSICIAN OR OTHER SOURCE
MARK C. WELBY MD

17a. I.D. NUMBER OF REFERRING PHYSICIAN
7766554

18. HOSPITALIZATION DATES RELATED TO CURRENT SERVICES FROM MM DD YY TO MM DD YY

19. RESERVED FOR LOCAL USE

20. OUTSIDE LAB? ☐ YES ☒ NO $ CHARGES

21. DIAGNOSIS OR NATURE OF ILLNESS OR INJURY (RELATE ITEMS 1,2,3 OR 4 TO ITEM 24E BY LINE)
1. 354.0
2. ____.__
3. ____.__
4. ____.__

22. MEDICAID RESUBMISSION CODE ORIGINAL REF. NO.

23. PRIOR AUTHORIZATION NUMBER

24. A DATE(S) OF SERVICE From MM DD YY	To MM DD YY	B Place of Service	C Type of Service	D PROCEDURES, SERVICES, OR SUPPLIES (Explain Unusual Circumstances) CPT/HCPCS	MODIFIER	E DIAGNOSIS CODE	F $ CHARGES	G DAYS OR UNITS	H EPSDT Family Plan	I EMG	J COB	K RESERVED FOR LOCAL USE
02 21 06	02 21 06	11		99201		1	46.00	1				HEALER
02 21 06	02 21 06	11	1	73100		1	63.00	1				HEALER
02 21 06	02 21 06	11		29125		1	63.00	1				HEALER

25. FEDERAL TAX I.D. NUMBER 3452331123 SSN ☐ EIN ☒

26. PATIENT'S ACCOUNT NO. DECDI000 3

27. ACCEPT ASSIGNMENT? (For govt. claims, see back) ☒ YES ☐ NO

28. TOTAL CHARGE $ 172.00

29. AMOUNT PAID $

30. BALANCE DUE $ 172.00

31. SIGNATURE OF PHYSICIAN OR SUPPLIER INCLUDING DEGREES OR CREDENTIALS (I certify that the statements on the reverse apply to this bill and are made a part thereof.)
SIGNATURE ON FILE
SIGNED DATE 12/30/03

32. NAME AND ADDRESS OF FACILITY WHERE SERVICES WERE RENDERED (If other than home or office)

33. PHYSICIAN'S, SUPPLIER'S BILLING NAME, ADDRESS, ZIP CODE & PHONE#
JAMES C. HEALER MD
123 MAIN STREET
ANYTOWN, FL 32711
PIN# 6654321 GRP#

FIGURE 10-4
Bottom left portion of the CMS-1500.

Key Term

Onset: The date the patient exhibited the first symptom of the illness, or the date the accident occurred that caused this injury, or, if the patient is pregnant, the date of the patient's last menstrual period **(LMP).**

Key Term

LMP: Acronym for **L**ast **M**enstrual **P**eriod.

Box 14.   Date of Current: Illness (First Symptom)
MM   DD   CCYY   or Injury (Accident)
                                   or Pregnancy (LMP)

If the reason the patient is seeing the provider this day is an illness, an injury, or a pregnancy, you must enter the date this patient first experienced this concern—in other words, the date of the **onset**. The information in Box 14 only relates to the diagnosis shown in Box 21.

Next, you need to check off which of the three (illness, injury, **LMP**) the date you entered represents.

If the reason this patient saw this provider for this visit is not an illness, an injury, or pregnancy, then leave these two parts of Box 14 blank.

Examples

Jason has a broken leg, which he received in an auto accident that happened on July 7, 2005. Box 14 will show

07/07/2005   INJURY

Suzette is pregnant. Her last menstrual period began on October 12, 2005. Box 14 will show

10/12/2005   LMP

Krystal has gastroenteritis from food poisoning. She ate raw oysters on March 16, 2006. She began vomiting and experiencing severe diarrhea on March 18, 2006. Box 14 will show

03/18/2006   ILLNESS

Julia came to see her provider for a flu shot. Box 14 is left blank.

Box 15. If Patient Has Had Same or Similar Illness Give First Date MM DD CC YY

Again, relating only to *this* health care encounter, only the diagnosis that is shown on *this* claim form in Box 21, Box 15 is asking if this patient has had the same diagnosis before. If the patient has, the date of the first time the patient suffered from this problem must be indicated.

There are some billers who feel that Box 15 is a waste of time and serves no purpose. However, in our example, we see that being pushed to answer this question may present the health care provider with information and insight that might not otherwise be obtained. The other purpose of Box 15 is to determine whether or not this claim is for a preexisting condition. This is a fact that may affect the insurance company's coverage of this health care encounter.

Example

Mrs. Martin came into the physician's office with a rash on both of her hands. The doctor's diagnosis is 692.5 *Dermatitis, due to contact with flour*, after finding out that Mrs. Martin had just baked bread for her annual church bake sale. The physician noticed that, exactly a year ago, this patient had the same symptoms diagnosed as 692.5 *Dermatitis, due to contact with flour*. In this case, enter the date of the diagnosis from last year in Box 15.

Box 17. Name of Referring Physician or Other Source
Box 17a. I.D. Number of Referring Physician

Critically important, especially on claims going to an HMO, Boxes 17 and 17a show information about the physician or other health care professional who referred a particular patient to the provider filing the insurance claim form. As we discussed in Chapter 3, many HMO insurance carriers require that the patient's primary care physician see the patient first, then make an official referral, complete with an authorization number from the insurance company, in order to assure that the visit is covered.

The referring physician ID number that should be keyed into Box 17a is the National Provider Identification Number, Unique Physician Identification Number, or, if a member of the same network, the insurance plan ID number for the referring provider. You will find this information on the Referral Form.

Box 21. Diagnosis or Nature of Illness or Injury (Relate Items 1, 2, 3, or 4 to Item 24E by Line)

1. _____.___   3. _____.___
2. _____.___   4. _____.___

In this box, you have room for up to four ICD-9-CM diagnosis codes. They must be placed in the correct order, according to the coding guidelines (as we discussed in Chapter 5).

CASE STUDY

Remember Keith Massenger who came to see Dr. Froint about an ulcer on his right midfoot? He had been previously diagnosed with type II diabetes. If you refer to your notes, you will see there were two diagnosis codes, the underlying condition that caused the ulcer, the diabetes (250.80), and the second code for the manifestation, the ulcer on his foot (707.14).

How will you place this information onto the CMS-1500?

_____

_____

We determined, with the help of the ICD-9-CM book, that the diabetes must be coded first, then the ulcer. For the encounter with this patient, Box 21 would look like this:

1. _250.80__   3. ____.__
2. _707.14__   4. ____.__

All the way across this next area of the form lie Boxes 24A through 24K. These boxes relate to the procedures, services, and treatments (CPT codes) that were provided to the patient during this encounter. Let's go over them, one at a time.

Box 24A. Date(s) of Service

From   To

MM DD YY   MM DD YY

These dates (From . . . To) indicate the *exact date or range of dates* that the treatment or procedure was *provided.* This date must match all of the documentation in the patient's health record. If this claim form is for one visit on one day only, then you will show the same date under From as you will under To.

Example

From 09/01/05 To 09/01/05

If, on the other hand, the same procedure was provided several times over the course of several days, you would indicate the first date under From and the last date under To.

Example

Eric Julia needs short-term bronchial therapy, just five treatments five days in a row. It is a test to see if the treatments improve his breathing. Therefore, you would probably wait until the end of the week and create one claim form, showing the range of dates.

From 09/01/05 To 09/05/05

Key Term

Place of service: A code that specifies the physical location where the procedure was performed.

Box 24B. Place of Service

Place of service is a two-digit code that identifies the location where the procedure was performed. The codes most frequently used are shown in Box 10-1.

BOX 10-1   Frequently Used Place of Service Codes

11. Office
12. Home
21. Inpatient Hospital
22. Outpatient Hospital
23. Emergency Room—Hospital
24. Ambulatory Surgical Center
25. Birthing Center
26. Military Treatment Facility
31. Skilled Nursing Facility
32. Nursing Facility
33. Custodial Care Facility
34. Hospice
41. Ambulance—Land
42. Ambulance—Air or Water
50. Federally Qualified Health Center
51. Inpatient Psychiatric Facility
52. Psychiatric Facility Partial Hospitalization
53. Community Mental Health Center
54. Intermediate Care Facility/Mentally Retarded
55. Residential Substance Abuse Treatment Facility
56. Psychiatric Residential Treatment Center
60. Mass Immunization Center
61. Comprehensive Inpatient Rehabilitation Facility
62. Comprehensive Outpatient Rehabilitation Facility
65. End-Stage Renal Disease Treatment Facility
71. State or Local Public Health Clinic
72. Rural Health Clinic
81. Independent Laboratory
99. Other Unlisted Facility

For the complete list, see the first page, just inside the front cover of the CPT book.

Box 24C. Type of Service

Some offices do not use this box anymore; however, you should still know what it is, in case you get a job in an office that does. **Type of service** is a one- or two-digit code that categorizes the procedure performed. The codes used in Box 24C are shown in Box 10-2.

Key Term

Type of service: A code that categorizes the procedure performed.

BOX 10-2   Types of Service

1. Medical
2. Surgery
3. Consultation
4. Diagnostic X-ray
5. Diagnostic Lab
6. Radiation Therapy
7. Anesthesia
8. Surgical Assistance
9. Other Medical
10. Blood Charges
11. Used DME
12. DME Purchase
13. ASC Facility
14. Renal Supplies in the Home
15. Alternate Method Dialysis Payment
16. CRD Equipment
17. Preadmission Testing
18. DME Rental
19. Pneumonia Vaccine
20. Second Surgical Opinion
21. Third Surgical Opinion
99. Other (e.g., used for prescription drugs)

Box 24D. Procedures, Services, or Supplies

(Explain Unusual Circumstances)

CPT/HCPCS   Modifier

In the left side of this box, you will enter the five-digit CPT code for the procedure or service. The two remaining portions of this box are to be used for modifiers (when necessary) and for physical status modifiers (for anesthesia).

The note ("explain unusual circumstances") tells you that, if there are special circumstances involved with any of the CPT codes shown on this claim form, in addition to adding the appropriate modifier, you may need to attach a letter or report to explain those circumstances in more detail. When you do this up front, along with the original claim form, you will save a great deal of time and get your office paid faster, because you won't have to wait for the insurance carrier to look at the form, decide it wants more explanation, and ask you for it before paying.

Box 24E. Diagnosis Code

In this box, you will not actually put the diagnosis code that identifies the medical reason that made performing the procedure necessary. Here, you will indicate the number of the line on which the correct diagnosis code is shown, in Box 21, to *link* each CPT code to at least one diagnosis code (as we discussed in Chapter 9).

If we go back to our patient, Keith Massenger, with the ulcer that resulted from his diabetic condition, the physician treats the ulcer and performs a blood glucose level test. See Table 10-1 for Box 24D and 24E results.

As you can see in Table 10-1, we begin with the Evaluation and Management code for an established patient seen in the physician's office:

> 99213—The patient is there to see the doctor about the ulcer on his foot, which is a manifestation of his previously diagnosed diabetes, so both diagnosis codes apply to this E/M code.

> 11042—The CPT code for the debridement of the ulcer, which, of course, relates only to the ulcer (diagnosis #2 in Box 21).

> 82947—The CPT code for the blood glucose test, which relates only to the diabetes (diagnosis #1 in Box 21).

Box 24D	Box 24E
99213	1, 2
11042	2
82947	1

TABLE 10-1
Box 24E indicates Diagnosis Code Links.

Box 25. Federal Tax I.D. Number,   SSN,   EIN

This box asks for a federal tax number for the physician providing the service. This is either the physician's Social Security number (in which case, the box under SSN will be checked ☒) or the physician's federal **employer identification number (EIN)**, which is very similar to an individual's Social Security number, except that it is assigned to a corporation. Some physicians are registered as professional corporations and therefore, would use their EIN instead of their personal Social Security number. If so, check the EIN box ☒.

Key Term

Employer identification number (EIN): To a corporation, the same as a Social Security number is to an individual.

Box 26. Patient's Account No.

Most often, this is simply the patient's chart number. The chart number is indicated in Box 26 for possible future reference. In case the claim form is rejected, or comes back with any queries, having this chart number on the claim form makes it easier for you to find the appropriate health care record and answer any questions that might arise. Some offices use this reference to properly credit the patient's account when payment is received from the insurance carrier.

Box 27. Accept Assignment?

Yes   No

When a physician's office, or another health care facility, files a claim with an insurance carrier, it is usually with the intention of ultimately receiving monies for the services it has provided. However, you must remember that the benefits of the insurance plan actually belong to the policyholder. Therefore, the benefits must be assigned to the provider, so the insurance carrier can send the money to that provider. Otherwise, the insurance carrier would be obligated to send the money to the policyholder.

> **IMPORTANT NOTE**
>
> The insurance benefits actually belong to the insured. The provider must *accept assignment* of those benefits to have the money sent directly to the provider.
>
> For claims going to Medicare, *accept assignment* also means that the provider agrees to the allowed charge(s) for the procedure codes shown.

Make certain that Box 27 has the YES box checked ☒ unless your office has a different stated policy.

Box 31. Signature of Physician or Supplier Including Degrees or Credentials

This box reads

(I certify that the statements on the reverse apply to this bill and are made a part thereof.)

SIGNED_____ DATE_____

Again, it is rare that the physician will actually sign this form. Generally, you will just indicate the provider's signature is on file in your office, or you can have the computer print his or her name here.

Box 32. Name and Address of Facility Where Services Were Rendered (If Other Than Home or Office)

If the procedures and services shown in Box 24 were provided in the physician's office, or at the patient's home, Box 32 should be left blank. However, if the procedures were provided somewhere else, this box would need to show that location.

> **Example**
>
> Flu shots offered at a supermarket require Box 32 to show the address of that supermarket.

Section 4: Bottom Right

Section 4 contains information about the patient's disability and/or hospitalization, outside lab work, authorization numbers, and the actual charges for the current procedures (Figure 10-5).

PLEASE
DO NOT
STAPLE
IN THIS
AREA
P

MCGRAW INSURANCE CO.
P.O. BOX 5544
WILSON, OH 45533

| | PICA | | | | | **HEALTH INSURANCE CLAIM FORM** | | | PICA | |

1. MEDICARE	MEDICAID	CHAMPUS	CHAMPVA	GROUP HEALTH PLAN	FECA BLK LUNG	OTHER	1a. INSURED'S I.D. NUMBER	(FOR PROGRAM IN ITEM 1)
[ ] (Medicare #)	[ ] (Medicaid #)	[ ] (Sponsor's SSN)	[ ] (VA File #)	[X] (SSN OR ID)	[ ] (SSN)	[ ] (ID)	998436627	

2. PATIENT'S NAME (Last Name, First Name, Middle Initial)	3. PATIENT'S BIRTH DATE			SEX	4. INSURED'S NAME (Last Name, First Name, Middle Initial)
DECKER, DIANE E.	MM 05	DD 21	YY 73	M [ ] F [X]	DECKER, DIANE E.

2nd Fold

5. PATIENT'S ADDRESS (No., Street)	6. PATIENT RELATIONSHIP TO INSURED	7. INSURED'S ADDRESS (No., Street)
876 PROGRESS AVENUE	Self [X] Spouse [ ] Child [ ] Other [ ]	876 PROGRESS AVENUE

CITY	STATE	8. PATIENT STATUS	CITY	STATE
CITYVILLE	FL	Single [X] Married [ ] Other [ ]	CITYVILLE	FL

ZIP CODE	TELEPHONE (Include Area Code)		ZIP CODE	TELEPHONE (INCLUDE AREA CODE)
32901	(407) 555 9987	Employed [X] Full-Time Student [ ] Part-Time Student [ ]	32901	(407) 555 9987

9. OTHER INSURED'S NAME (Last Name, First Name, Middle Initial)	10. IS PATIENT'S CONDITION RELATED TO:	11. INSURED'S POLICY GROUP OR FECA NUMBER
		PMI03

a. OTHER INSURED'S POLICY OR GROUP NUMBER	a. EMPLOYMENT? (CURRENT OR PREVIOUS) [X] YES [ ] NO	a. INSURED'S DATE OF BIRTH MM 05 DD 21 YY 73 SEX M [ ] F [X]

b. OTHER INSURED'S DATE OF BIRTH MM DD YY SEX M [ ] F [ ]	b. AUTO ACCIDENT? PLACE (State) [ ] YES [X] NO	b. EMPLOYER'S NAME OR SCHOOL NAME PRIME INCORPORATED

c. EMPLOYER'S NAME OR SCHOOL NAME	c. OTHER ACCIDENT? [ ] YES [X] NO	c. INSURANCE PLAN NAME OR PROGRAM NAME MCGRAW HMO

d. INSURANCE PLAN NAME OR PROGRAM NAME	10d. RESERVED FOR LOCAL USE	d. IS THERE ANOTHER HEALTH BENEFIT PLAN? [ ] YES [X] NO *if yes*, return to and complete item 9 a-d.

READ BACK OF FORM BEFORE COMPLETING AND SIGNING THIS FORM.

12. PATIENT'S OR AUTHORIZED PERSON'S SIGNATURE. I authorize the release of any medical or other information necessary to process this claim. I also request payment of government benefits either to myself or to the party who accepts assignment below.

SIGNED SIGNATURE ON FILE   DATE 12/27/05

13. INSURED'S OR AUTHORIZED PERSON'S SIGNATURE. I authorize payment of medical benefits to the undersigned physician or supplier for services described below.

SIGNED SIGNATURE ON FILE

1st Fold

14. DATE OF CURRENT: ILLNESS (First symptom) OR INJURY (Accident) OR PREGNANCY(LMP)	15. IF PATIENT HAS HAD SAME OR SIMILAR ILLNESS GIVE FIRST DATE	16. DATES PATIENT UNABLE TO WORK IN CURRENT OCCUPATION
MM 12 DD 05 YY 05 INJURY	MM DD YY	FROM MM DD YY TO MM DD YY

17. NAME OF REFERRING PHYSICIAN OR OTHER SOURCE	17a. I.D. NUMBER OF REFERRING PHYSICIAN	18. HOSPITALIZATION DATES RELATED TO CURRENT SERVICES
MARK C. WELBY MD	7766554	FROM MM DD YY TO MM DD YY

19. RESERVED FOR LOCAL USE	20. OUTSIDE LAB? $ CHARGES [ ] YES [X] NO

21. DIAGNOSIS OR NATURE OF ILLNESS OR INJURY (RELATE ITEMS 1,2,3 OR 4 TO ITEM 24E BY LINE)	22. MEDICAID RESUBMISSION CODE ORIGINAL REF. NO.
1. 354.0 3. ___.___	
2. ___.___ 4. ___.___	23. PRIOR AUTHORIZATION NUMBER

24. A. DATE(S) OF SERVICE		B. Place of Service	C. Type of Service	D. PROCEDURES, SERVICES, OR SUPPLIES (Explain Unusual Circumstances) CPT/HCPCS | MODIFIER	E. DIAGNOSIS CODE	F. $ CHARGES	G. DAYS OR UNITS	H. EPSDT Family Plan	I. EMG	J. COB	K. RESERVED FOR LOCAL USE
From MM DD YY	To MM DD YY										
02 21 06	02 21 06	11		99201 |	1	46.00	1				HEALER
02 21 06	02 21 06	11	1	73100 |	1	63.00	1				HEALER
02 21 06	02 21 06	11		29125 |	1	63.00	1				HEALER

25. FEDERAL TAX I.D. NUMBER SSN EIN	26. PATIENT'S ACCOUNT NO.	27. ACCEPT ASSIGNMENT? (For govt. claims, see back)	28. TOTAL CHARGE	29. AMOUNT PAID	30. BALANCE DUE
3452331123 [X] [ ]	DECDI000 3	[X] YES [ ] NO	$ 172.00	$	$ 172.00

31. SIGNATURE OF PHYSICIAN OR SUPPLIER INCLUDING DEGREES OR CREDENTIALS (I certify that the statements on the reverse apply to this bill and are made a part thereof.)	32. NAME AND ADDRESS OF FACILITY WHERE SERVICES WERE RENDERED (If other than home or office)	33. PHYSICIAN'S, SUPPLIER'S BILLING NAME, ADDRESS, ZIP CODE & PHONE#
SIGNED SIGNATURE ON FILE DATE 12/30/03		JAMES C. HEALER MD 123 MAIN STREET ANYTOWN, FL 32711 PIN# 6654321 GRP#

FIGURE 10-5
Bottom right portion of the CMS-1500.

Box 16. Dates Patient Unable to Work in Current Occupation

FROM   MM DD YY   TO   MM DD YY

If the patient's condition (identified in Box 21) caused the person to be unable to work at his or her regular job, these dates must be filled in accurately, as the dates may be required to support the patient's disability claim or may be related to a workers' compensation or liability claim.

Example

Margo Van Worker's hand was fractured in three places. Therefore, she was unable to do her job as a data processor for eight weeks. The dates that she was medically unable to work would be entered in Box 16 of her claim form for the treatment of her hand.

Box 18. Hospitalization Dates Related to Current Services

FROM   MM DD YY   TO   MM DD YY

If the patient spent time in the hospital for treatment, tests, observation, or any other reason related to the diagnosis shown in Box 21, then, the start and end dates of this hospital stay should be shown here, in Box 18. This alerts the third-party payer that a claim form will be filed by the hospital for those inpatient services.

Example

Jack Franklin was in the hospital for five days due to problems controlling his diabetes. The date he was admitted into the hospital, as well as his discharge date, would be entered into Box 18 of the claim form filed by his physician for the treatment of his diabetes.

Box 20.   Outside Lab? $Charges

If a laboratory that is not a part of the health care facility (an outside lab) provides services being charged for on this claim form, it must be indicated in this box, along with the net charges (the exact amount the provider paid that lab for these services). In addition, if an outside lab is used, and this box is checked YES, then the address of that laboratory should be entered into Box 32.

Example

If the blood glucose test that was performed on our diabetic patient was processed by an outside lab, the appropriate information should be entered in Box 20 as well as Box 32.

Box 22. Medicaid Resubmission

Code   Original Ref. No.

Sometimes claims get lost; sometimes they get rejected for certain reasons. If a problem with a Medicaid claim is cleared up or explained, then the provider may get permission from Medicaid to resubmit the claim. When that permission to resubmit is given, you will also be given a code, to be entered into Box 22 of the new version of the claim. The reference number from the original version of the claim should also be included here.

Box 23. Prior Authorization Number

This relates to Box 22 and the resubmission process. This will show the original authorization number, so Medicaid can connect the first claim to the resubmission.

The following three boxes are the continuation of Box 24 that began on the bottom left side of this form, in which we enter information about the procedures and services performed for this individual during this particular encounter with the provider.

Box 24F. $ Charges

Box 24F shows the amount of money your office is charging for the procedure or service. Most of the time, these prices will be preloaded into your computer. If not, the office in which you work will have an established price list for all CPT codes used.

Box 24G. Days or Units

How many times did your provider perform this procedure or service during this encounter for this patient? Most often, this number will be one.

Example

In our example from Box 24A, the provider gave Eric Julia five respiratory therapy treatments over the course of the dates shown for this line. In this case, the number in Box 24G would be 5.

Box 24K. Reserved for Local Use

Depending on the insurance carrier's requirements, this box may show the provider's name and provider identification number, or it may be left blank.

Box 28. Total Charge

The total charges for all of the procedures and services billed for on this claim form is shown in Box 28.

Box 29. Amount Paid

If a prepayment from the insurance carrier has been made, it is shown in this box. The box will not usually reflect any payments made by the patient, such as co-payments or co-insurance.

Box 30. Balance Due

This box shows the total balance due and the amount expected to be paid by the insurance carrier.

> **IMPORTANT NOTE**
> Co-payments made by the patient are not included in Boxes 29 and 30.

Box 33. Physician's, Supplier's Billing Name, Address, Zip Code & Phone

This box shows the name and address of the physician and/or the health care facility, along with the provider identification number and/or the group number as assigned to this practice by the insurance carrier.

UB-92 FORM

If you go to work in a hospital, you may use a form called the UB-92 (Figure 10-6) more often than you use the CMS-1500. Although the two forms do not really look alike, they both require essentially the same information, although in a different manner. Remember, earlier we reviewed the differences between CPT procedure codes (most often used by physician's offices) and ICD-9-CM procedure codes (most often used by hospitals). Now that you understand the CMS-1500 and what data are needed and why, you will be able to learn how to complete a UB-92 with less training. Take a look at the form and note the similarities and differences.

The National Uniform Billing Committee (NUBC) determines the data elements and design of the UB-92 claim form. The directions for completing the form are outlined in the NUBC specifications manual.

CHAPTER SUMMARY

Learning about all the boxes on the CMS-1500 claim form and understanding what data the third-party payer is looking for and why it may feel it needs the information will help you prepare and submit more complete and better-quality claims. A better claim will get your health care facility paid the amount of money earned in a timely fashion.

APPROVED OMB NO. 0938-0279

ST11843 1PLY UB-92

1

2 | 3 PATIENT CONTROL NO. | 4 TYPE OF BILL

5 FED. TAX NO. | 6 STATEMENT COVERS PERIOD FROM THROUGH | 7 COV D. | 8 N-C D. | 9 C-I D. | 10 L-R D. | 11

12 PATIENT NAME | 13 PATIENT ADDRESS

14 BIRTHDATE | 15 SEX | 16 MS | ADMISSION 17 DATE 18 HR 19 TYPE 20 SRC | 21 D HR | 22 STAT | 23 MEDICAL RECORD NO | CONDITION CODES 24 25 26 27 28 29 30 | 31

32 OCCURRENCE CODE DATE | 33 OCCURRENCE CODE DATE | 34 OCCURRENCE CODE DATE | 35 OCCURRENCE CODE DATE | 36 OCCURRENCE SPAN CODE FROM THROUGH | 37 A B C

a b

38 | 39 VALUE CODES CODE AMOUNT | 40 VALUE CODES CODE AMOUNT | 41 VALUE CODES CODE AMOUNT

a b c d

42 REV. CD. | 43 DESCRIPTION | 44 HCPCS / RATES | 45 SERV. DATE | 46 SERV. UNITS | 47 TOTAL CHARGES | 48 NON-COVERED CHARGES | 49

1 2 3 4 5 6 7 8 9 10 11 12 13 14 15 16 17 18 19 20 21 22 23

50 PAYER | 51 PROVIDER NO. | 52 REL INFO | 53 ASG BEN | 54 PRIOR PAYMENTS | 55 EST. AMOUNT DUE | 56

A B C

57 **DUE FROM PATIENT ▶**

58 INSURED'S NAME | 59 P. REL | 60 CERT. - SSN - HIC. - ID NO. | 61 GROUP NAME | 62 INSURANCE GROUP NO.

A B C

63 TREATMENT AUTHORIZATION CODES | 64 ESC | 65 EMPLOYER NAME | 66 EMPLOYER LOCATION

A B C

67 PRN. DIAG. CD. | 68 CODE | 69 CODE | 70 CODE | 71 CODE | 72 CODE | 73 CODE | 74 CODE | 75 CODE | 76 ADM. DIAG. CD. | 77 E-CODE | 78

79 P.C. | 80 PRINCIPAL PROCEDURE CODE DATE | 81 OTHER PROCEDURE CODE DATE A | OTHER PROCEDURE CODE DATE B | 82 ATTENDING PHYS. ID

OTHER PROCEDURE CODE DATE C | OTHER PROCEDURE CODE DATE D | OTHER PROCEDURE CODE DATE E | 83 OTHER PHYS. ID A a b

84 REMARKS a b c d | OTHER PHYS. ID B a b

85 PROVIDER REPRESENTATIVE X | 86 DATE

UB-92 HCFA-1450 | OCR/ORIGINAL | I CERTIFY THE CERTIFICATIONS ON THE REVERSE APPLY TO THIS BILL AND ARE MADE A PART HEREOF.

FIGURE 10-6
The UB-92 claim form.

Chapter Review

For the following multiple-choice questions, choose the best available answer.

1. The patient, shown in Box 1 of the CMS-1500, is the person who
   a. Pays the insurance premium
   b. Sees the provider for consultation and/or treatment
   c. Owns the insurance policy
   d. Has known the provider for at least three years

2. The insured, shown in Box 4 of the CMS-1500, is also called the
   a. Policyholder
   b. Subscriber
   c. Patient
   d. Both policyholder and subscriber

3. The insurance plan name is always the same exact name as the insurance company or the insurance carrier.
   a. Never
   b. Sometimes
   c. Always
   d. Only in Medicare

4. Improper completion of the required boxes on the CMS-1500 may cause the claim to be
   a. Paid more quickly
   b. Paid directly to the hospital or lab
   c. Rejected
   d. Paid at a lower rate

5. Boxes 9 through 9d of the CMS-1500 are for supplying information about a patient's
   a. Primary insurance policy
   b. Employer providing group insurance
   c. Secondary insurance policy
   d. Tertiary insurance policy

6. Box 14 of the CMS-1500 asks for the date of the
   a. Patient's first visit to the provider shown in Box 31
   b. Patient's birthday
   c. Patient's first time insured by the carrier shown in Box 1
   d. Patient's onset of the condition shown in Box 21

7. The person whose name should appear in Box 17 of the CMS-1500 is

   a. The attending physician

   b. The referring physician

   c. The primary care physician

   d. The specialist

8. You should enter the following information in Box 24E of the CMS-1500.

   a. The primary diagnosis ICD-9-CM code

   b. The CPT code's modifier

   c. The link to the line showing the related ICD-9-CM code

   d. The date the procedure was performed

9. Box 18 of the CMS-1500 should show the dates the patient

   a. Was ever in the hospital

   b. Was most recently in the hospital

   c. Will be admitted to the hospital

   d. Was admitted to the hospital for the condition identified in Box 21 during this term of treatment

10. When the physician accepts assignment, as checked in Box 27 of the CMS-1500, it means

    a. The physician will be sent the money directly by the insurance carrier

    b. The physician officially accepts the patient shown in Box 2 to be his or her patient

    c. The physician accepts responsibility for everything shown on the form

    d. The physician acknowledges that he or she treated this patient

11

Electronic Claims Management: Using Patient Accounting Software

KEY TERMS

alternate code

attending provider

case

diagnosis code set

Electronic Data Interchange (EDI)

health care clearinghouses

PINs

place of service (POS)

practice

procedure code set

type of service (TOS)

OBJECTIVES

- Understand how to enter patient information and coding data into the computer using NDCMedisoft™ Advanced Version 9.

- Know how to create insurance claim forms electronically.

- Know how to submit insurance claim forms electronically.

Technology is a part of just about everything that we do, so it's logical that it has become an important part of the health care system. In the past few years, technology has dramatically changed the way we create and submit health insurance claim forms.

---

*Please contact your McGraw-Hill Higher Education sales representative for a Medisoft demo disk.

BENEFITS AND CHALLENGES OF ELECTRONIC CLAIMS PROCESSING

Electronic claims can be processed, approved, and paid, with the money in the physician's office bank account, in less time than it takes a paper claim to be printed, mailed, and arrive in the insurance company's mailbox. This is a big benefit to the business side of the health care industry.

> **IMPORTANT NOTE**
>
> The average amount of time for a health care facility to be paid by an insurance carrier has gone from four to six months to two to three weeks, thanks to electronic claims processing.

One Mistake Can Equal a Thousand Errors

Electronic recordkeeping is incredibly efficient. With a computer, you enter the patient's name, address, and phone number just once, and it is available to you a thousand times or more. This not only saves time but also reduces the opportunity to make mistakes. Every time someone has to key in a piece of information (data) there is an opportunity to make a mistake. Now you can enter the patient's name once and it will be placed into the receipt, the health claim form, the patient statement, and multiple other forms. This also means one mistake will be repeated a thousand times! Press the wrong key and you get Hones instead of Jones, or 73001 instead of 73010. Either of those errors may cause an entire claim to be rejected. Therefore, you must be very diligent in entering every piece of data—every letter, every number.

> **IMPORTANT NOTE**
>
> Our rule for this chapter—as well as for the rest of your career—is *check your entries, double-check your entries,* and *triple-check your entries.*

A Name Is Not a Name—Spelling Matters

In most cases, electronic health claim forms are reviewed and analyzed by computers. The computer scans the form to check for accuracy and agreement with the insurance carrier's preentered information, such as matching an insured's name and policy number with the data in the electronic files. The computer does not make judgments. It can only blindly match letter to letter and number to number.

Example

The insured's name is Sarah Brown. This is how it is spelled and shown on all her paperwork. However, when the biller enters the information into the office computer, she enters *Sara*, accidentally leaving off the letter *h* at the end. She doesn't check or double-check her work, or she thinks it is no big deal: *Sarah* or *Sara*—what's the difference?

Anyone can see it's the same person, right?

Well, no, because, when the claim form arrives at the insurance company, the computer scans the form and rejects the claim. It sends the claim back as having an error, but with no explanation (which is typical). There is no human being reading the form and thinking, "Sara? Oh, I know they really meant Sarah; let it go through." The computer cannot think about what you may have meant. It does not read *Sarah* and *Sara* as the same. The computer just sees two pieces of data that do not match. It's as if it were looking at *xqkr* and *xqkrd*. They do not match, so, the computer will reject the claim.

One Number Off Is a Whole New Code

You already have learned from earlier chapters about the critical importance of making certain that the correct diagnosis and procedure codes are entered, whether that entry is made by pen or keyboard. Consider the following situation. After being diagnosed, Christy's physician recommended she take classes to learn how to live with diabetes. Her insurance carrier approved the recommendation over the phone and agreed to pay for those classes. However, the claim was rejected. After nine months of battling, Christy discovered that the CPT code for the classes had been entered incorrectly. Instead of 99078 *Physician educational services rendered to patients in a group setting, diabetic instruction,* the biller entered 99080, *Special reports such as insurance forms.*

IMPORTANT NOTE

If one digit is off, your claim may be rejected because medical necessity has not been substantiated.

One of the great things about a computer is that, once you are certain that your entry is correct, you will never have to worry about it again, whether it is a patient's name, phone number, or policy number. Don't forget the rule:

Check, double-check, and triple-check your entries!

TYPES OF PATIENT ACCOUNTING SOFTWARE PROGRAMS

There are three types of programs designed for use in health care facilities to assist in submitting electronic health insurance claims:

1. *Web-based software programs.* All of your patient information is entered into forms and stored on a secured, password-protected website. You must use an Internet connection (such as Earthlink or AOL) and browser software (such as Netscape or Internet Explorer) to access your patient account files, input data, create claims, and submit claims.

2. *Server-based software programs.* This software is installed directly onto your computer (or network's server). You open the software as you do any other program that is on your PC and get right to work entering information. Your office is also totally responsible for making certain that the files are secured and backed up (in case of power or system failure). In addition, you (or your office's technical support person) must set up the program, so that your electronic claims are submitted correctly.

3. *Internet-based software programs.* Somewhat of a combination of the other two types of programs, these applications enable you to enter all data into forms (software) on your desktop computer. Once you are done, all the information is uploaded and stored on a secured, password-protected website.

Due to the fact that Medicare, along with other third-party payers, strongly prefer (and soon will be mandated) to accept claim forms that are submitted electronically, you will surely be working with some type of software program to create and submit health insurance claim forms.

We are going to learn using one of the most popular brands of software in the country, NDCMedisoft Advanced. Although the health care facility you eventually work in may use a different brand of software, most of the programs work in a similar fashion, so, even if you learn NDCMedisoft Advanced in school and your new employer uses *Intergy*, you will be able to figure it out with just a small amount of on-the-job training. One thing you can count on is that all such programs are focused on having you input data with the goal of correctly completing a CMS-1500 or UB-92 health insurance claim form. Therefore, almost all of the data that the built-in forms will require will match the necessary information for the CMS-1500 we reviewed in Chapter 10. They may look different, but underneath they are basically the same.

Before continuing this chapter, I would like to call your attention to the information in Appendix D—NDCMedisoft Advanced Issues & Answers. This Appendix contains information and tips that may be helpful to you while you are setting up and working with this software application.

ENTERING PATIENT DATA USING NDCMEDISOFT™ ADVANCED

Now we are going to take some of the cases that we coded in previous chapters and enter them into the computer in order to create health insurance claim forms (CMS-1500).

To make certain you are all working with the same information as this book, so your work on the computer will exactly match the directions and illustrations, you are going to learn how to enter a new insurance carrier, an employer, diagnosis codes, procedure codes, a provider, and a referring provider. Then the computer will be set up and ready for you to practice creating claim forms. OK? Great, let's begin. Go ahead and open your NDCMedisoft Advanced program.

1. Double-click on the red M icon that should be showing on the desktop of your computer screen. If you do not see it,
   a. Click on the START button in the lower left portion of your screen.
   b. Click on PROGRAMS.
   c. Choose NDCMedisoft Advanced Version 9.
2. You should see the program open to the main NDCMedisoft Advanced desktop. Then go to the FILE Menu and click on NEW PRACTICE.

Creating a New Practice

As you watch the software program launch (open) you may see a dialog box that says Open **Practice** (Figure 11-1). In this box, you may see the name of a pretend medical office preloaded by the software manufacturer.

FIGURE 11-1
Open Practice dialog box.

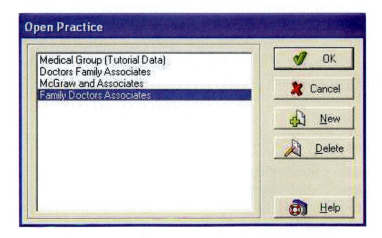

1. Look on the right side, in the middle, and click on the button that says New.

2. Once the program is fully open, if you do not see the Open Practice dialog box, go to the FILE Menu and click on NEW PRACTICE.

3. A dialog box will open, entitled Create a new set of data (Figure 11-2).

4. The first line says,

> Enter the practice or doctor's name to identify this set of data.

Key in the name of our health care office (Figure 11-3).

> Family Doctors Associates

Under that you will see

> Enter the data path:
> c:\medidata\▭

Key in the initials for our health care office.

> Enter the data path:
> c:\medidata\ fda ▭

5. Click on the button that says Create, on the right side of the dialog box.

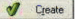

You will get a dialog box that will read:

> *Confirm: c:\MEDIDATA\fda does not exist.*
> *Do you want to create it?*

Click the YES button.

When you get to the main screen inside NDCMedisoft Advanced, you'll see a heading across the top in the blue title bar (Figure 11-4).

   NDCMedisoft Advanced - Family Doctors Associates

   File Edit Activities Lists Reports Tools Window Help Services

Excellent work!

You will then see a dialog box wanting you to enter information about our new practice. Enter this information in each field as appropriate.

Family Doctors Associates
123 Main Street
Anytown   FL   32711
Phone: 407-555-1200
Fax Phone: 407-555-1201
Type: Medical
Federal Tax ID: 59-0123456789

Extra 1 and Extra 2 may be left blank.
Click the SAVE button.

Entering a New Insurance Carrier

Again, to make certain all of the information on your screen is going to match this text, we are going to enter a new insurance company to use for our make-believe patients. Every one of our patients will have a policy with this company. This will help keep things simple.

1. Go to the LISTS Menu and click on Insurance Carriers from the drop-down menu. You will see a dialog box entitled Insurance Carrier List (Figure 11-5).

FIGURE 11-5
Insurance Carrier List dialog box.

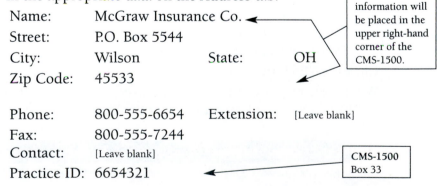

2. At the bottom of this dialog box, click on the button that says New.

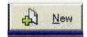

3. Allow the computer to assign a code for this carrier by clicking in the first blank field, next to the word Name (Figure 11-6).
4. Key in the appropriate data on the Address tab.

Name:	McGraw Insurance Co.		
Street:	P.O. Box 5544		
City:	Wilson	State:	OH
Zip Code:	45533		
Phone:	800-555-6654	Extension:	[Leave blank]
Fax:	800-555-7244		
Contact:	[Leave blank]		
Practice ID:	6654321		

All of this information will be placed in the upper right-hand corner of the CMS-1500.

CMS-1500 Box 33

The Practice ID is a number assigned to this health care facility by this insurance carrier.

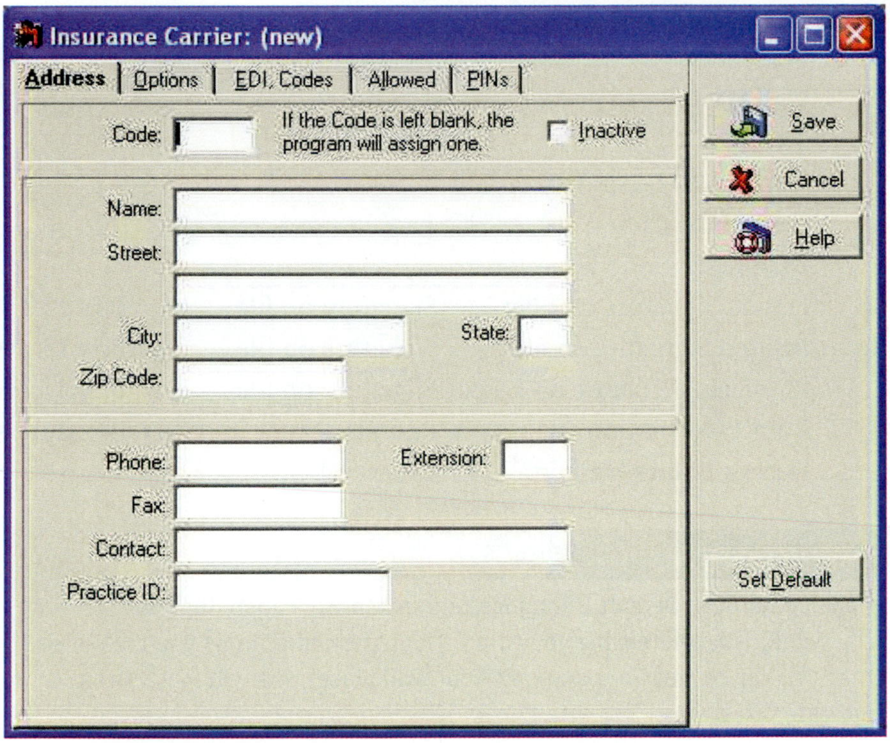

FIGURE 11-6
Insurance Carrier address tab screen.

5. Click on the Options tab and fill in the appropriate data (Figure 11-7).

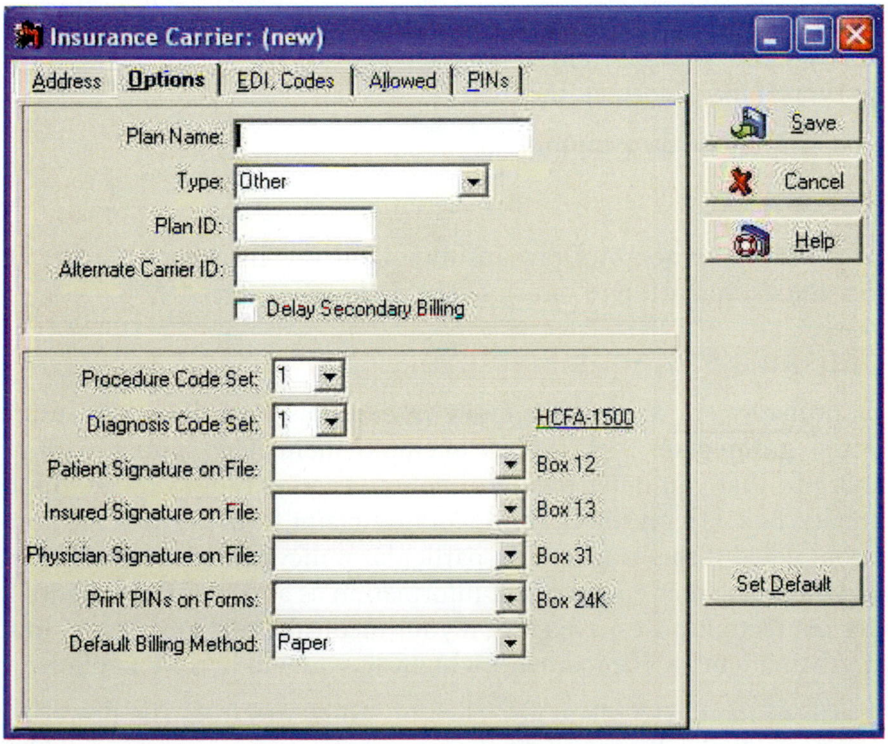

FIGURE 11-7
Insurance Carrier options tab screen.

Plan Name:	McGraw HMO	← CMS-1500 Box 11C
Type:	HMO	
Plan ID:	123432	
Alternate Carrier ID:	[Leave blank]	CMS-1500 Box 12
☐ Delay Secondary Billing	[Leave blank]	Box 13
		Box 31
Procedure Code Set:	1	Box 24K
Diagnosis Code Set:	1	
Patient Signature on File:	Signature on file	Box 12 ←
Insured Signature on File:	Signature on file	Box 13 ←
Physician Signature on File:	Signature on file	Box 31 ←
Print **PIN**s on Forms:	Provider Name and PIN	Box 24K ←
Default Billing Method:	Paper	

IMPORTANT NOTE

Make certain the Default Billing Method indicates "Paper" for your classwork. This will enable you to print out the claim forms you create, so that you can review your work. At your workplace, this will most often indicate "Electronic."

Now take a minute and *CHECK, DOUBLE-CHECK, and TRIPLE-CHECK* what you have entered into the computer on *both* the Address and the Options tab screens in comparison with what you see in this section of the book. Capitals, lowercase letters, numbers, punctuation, and spaces are all important. It must match *exactly*. When you are certain that everything is correct, then

Click on the Save button.

[Save]

You should now see McGraw Insurance on the Insurance Carrier list. Click the Close button to return to the desktop.

Entering a Patient's Employer

You probably are aware that many individuals have health insurance through group plans at their place of employment. This is one reason it is important that you enter this information accurately into the computer. Actually, Box 11b on the health insurance claim form (CMS-1500) must be completed if this is true for a particular policyholder. Another reason that you must enter employment information as a part of the patient's file is for contact purposes. This way, if your medical office must get in touch with the patient, or the insured, right away, you will be able to phone.

1. Go to the LISTS Menu and click on Addresses from the drop-down menu. You will see a dialog box entitled Address List (Figure 11-8). At the bottom of this dialog box, click on the button that says New.

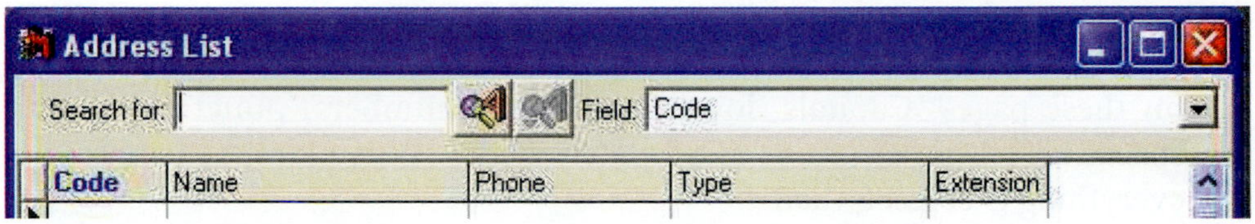

FIGURE 11-8
Address List screen.

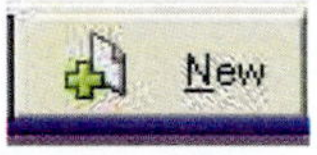

2. Allow the computer to assign a code for this employer by clicking in the first blank field, next to the word Name (Figure 11-9). Key in the appropriate data.

Name:	Prime Incorporated		
Street:	5580 Rehearsal Lane		
City:	Our Town	State:	FL
Zip Code:	32704		
Type:	Employer		
Phone:	(407) 555-1000	Extension:	1357
Fax Phone:	[Leave blank]		
Cell Phone:	[Leave blank]		
Office:	[Leave blank]		
Contact:	[Leave blank]		
E-mail:	[Leave blank]		
ID:	[Leave blank]		
Identifier:	[Leave blank]		
Extra 1:	[Leave blank]	Extra 2:	[Leave blank]

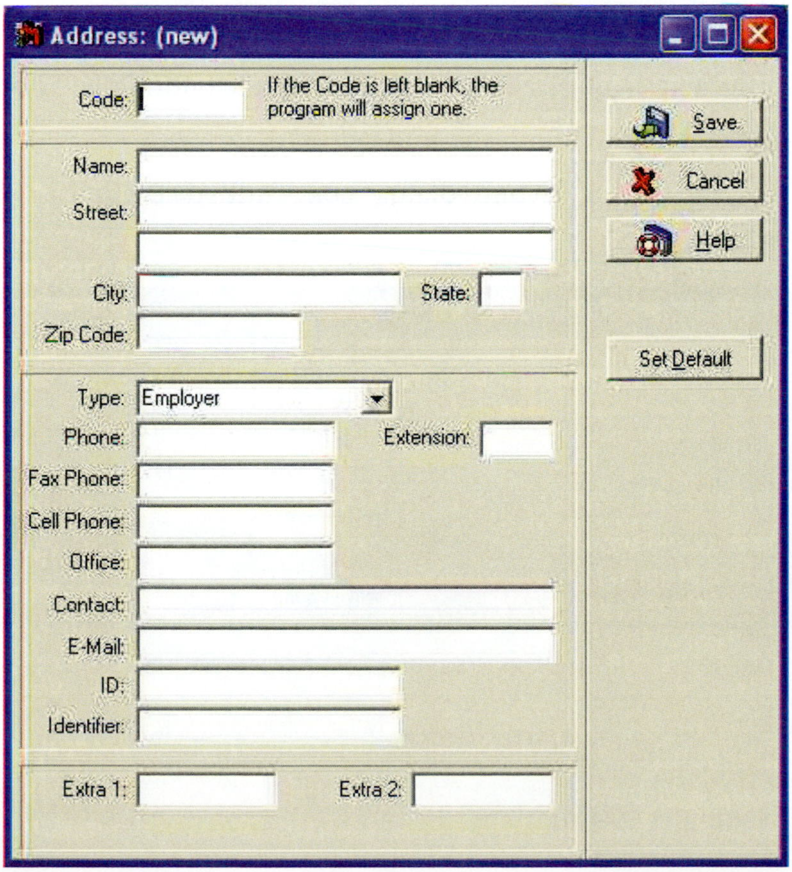

FIGURE 11-9
Address: (new) screen.

Now take a minute to *CHECK, DOUBLE-CHECK, and TRIPLE-CHECK* what you have entered into the computer in comparison with what you see on these pages. Capitals, lowercase letters, numbers, punctuation, and spaces are all important. It must match *exactly*. When you are certain that everything is correct, then

Click on the Save button.

You will now see Prime Incorporated in the Address List. Click the Close button in the lower right corner of the dialog box.

Entering Diagnosis Codes

In the real world, the computer will be preloaded with the diagnosis codes your office uses most often. However, as we have discussed before, there may be times when you find a different and more appropriate code than the one on the superbill. Therefore, it is important that you know how to enter diagnosis codes into the computer.

1. Go to the LISTS Menu and click on Diagnosis Codes from the drop-down menu. You will see a dialog box entitled Diagnosis List (Figure 11-10).

FIGURE 11-10
Diagnosis List.

![Diagnosis List dialog box showing Search for field, Field: Code 1, and columns Code 1, Description, Code 2, Code 3.]

2. At the bottom of this dialog box, click on the button that says New.

![New button]

3. You will see a second dialog box entitled Diagnosis: (new) (Figure 11-11).

FIGURE 11-11
Diagnosis: (new) box.

![Diagnosis: (new) dialog box with fields Code 1, Description, Alternate Code Sets (Code 2, Code 3), checkboxes HIPAA Approved and Inactive Code, and buttons Save, Cancel, Help.]

4. Key in the appropriate data.

Code 1:	V16.0
Description:	Family history of colon cancer
Alternate Code Sets	
Code 2: [Leave blank]	Code 3: [Leave blank]
☐ HIPAA Approved [Leave blank]	Inactive Code ☐ [Leave blank]

Now take a minute and *CHECK, DOUBLE-CHECK, and TRIPLE-CHECK* what you have entered into the computer in comparison with what you see here. Capitals, lowercase letters, numbers, punctuation, and spaces are all important. It must match *exactly*. When you are certain that everything is correct, then

Click on the Save button.

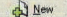

You now see this diagnosis code and its description in the diagnosis list. Click the Close button in the lower right-hand side of the dialog box.

Entering Procedure Codes

1. Go to the LISTS Menu and click on Procedure/Payment/Adjustment Codes from the drop-down menu. You will see a dialog box entitled Procedure/Payment/Adjustment List (Figure 11-12).

FIGURE 11-12
Procedure/Payment/Adjustment List.

2. At the bottom of this dialog box, click on the button that says New.

3. You will see a second dialog box entitled Procedure/Payment/Adjustment: (new) (Figure 11-13).
4. Key in the appropriate data.

Code 1:	45378
Description:	Colonoscopy-diagnostic
Code Type:	Procedure charge

You can choose other code types from the drop-down menu when entering other kinds of codes, such as payment codes.

Account Code:	[Leave blank]	**Alternate Code**	
Type of Service:	09	2:	45.25
Place of Service:	11	3:	01
Time to Do Procedure:	[Leave blank]		

CMS-1500 Boxes 24B and 24C

Key Terms

Type of Service (TOS): A one- or two-digit code that categorizes the procedure performed. This information is shown in Box 24C on the CMS-1500 form.

Place of Service (POS): A two-digit code that categorizes the location where the procedure was performed. This code is placed into Box 24B on the CMS-1500 form.

Alternate Code: This feature gives you the opportunity to enter at one time an alternate version of the same code, such as a CPT code and an ICD-9-CM procedure code, with the same description.

FIGURE 11-13
Procedure/Payment/Adjustment: (new) screen.

For our purposes in class, you can leave all the rest of these items blank as well. For Type of Service codes, see Box 11-1; Place of Service codes are in Box 11-2.

IMPORTANT NOTE

To assign a different code set to the insurance carrier's specifications, refer back to the entry for each insurance carrier under the LISTS Menu— Insurance Carrier—Options tab.

BOX 11-1   Types of Service

The following are the codes used to identify the Type of Service:

1	Medical	12	DME Purchase
2	Surgery	13	ASC Facility
3	Consultation	14	Renal Supplies in the Home
4	Diagnostic X-ray	15	Alternate Method Dialysis Payment
5	Diagnostic Lab	16	CRD Equipment
6	Radiation Therapy	17	Preadmission Testing
7	Anesthesia	18	DME Rental
8	Surgical Assistance	19	Pneumonia vaccine
9	Other Medical	20	Second Surgical Opinion
10	Blood Charges	21	Third Surgical Opinion
11	Used DME	99	Other (e.g., used for prescription drugs)

BOX 11-2   Place of Service Codes

The following are the codes used to identify the Place of Service:

11	Office	53	Community Mental Health Center
12	Home	54	Intermediate Care Facility/Mentally Retarded
21	Inpatient Hospital		
22	Outpatient Hospital	55	Residential Substance Abuse Treatment Facility
23	Emergency Room—Hospital		
24	Ambulatory Surgical Center	56	Psychiatric Residential Treatment Center
25	Birthing Center		
26	Military Treatment Facility	60	Mass Immunization Center
31	Skilled Nursing Facility	61	Comprehensive Inpatient Rehabilitation Facility
32	Nursing Facility		
33	Custodial Care Facility	62	Comprehensive Outpatient Rehabilitation Facility
34	Hospice		
41	Ambulance—Land	65	End-Stage Renal Disease Treatment Facility
42	Ambulance—Air or Water		
50	Federally Qualified Health Center	71	State or Local Public Health Clinic
51	Inpatient Psychiatric Facility	72	Rural Health Clinic
52	Psychiatric Facility Partial Hospitalization	81	Independent Laboratory
		99	Other Unlisted Facility

6. Now, click on the Amounts tab and key in the appropriate information (Figure 11-14).

      Charge Amounts

          A: 145.00

You can leave all the rest of the code boxes at zero. All of these code boxes, including the one at the bottom that reads Medicare Allowed Amount: gives you the ability to enter a procedure code once, along with all the possible charge versions. Do you remember our discussions about insurance carriers and their various programs to pay providers (remember fee-for-service and capitation plans from Chapter 1?)? There may be a difference in the agreed-upon amounts your office will receive for each procedure code. With this feature on the Amounts tab, you can enter all the information for a particular procedure code only once, and from then on, the computer will know exactly how much to bill for each service provided in your office. For your classwork, all patients will use charge code A. You will indicate this when you open a new case for a patient later on.

FIGURE 11-14
Amounts tab screen.

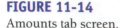

Now take a minute and *CHECK, DOUBLE-CHECK, and TRIPLE-CHECK* what you have entered into the computer in comparison with what you see here. Capitals, lowercase letters, numbers, punctuation, and spaces are all important. It must match *exactly.* When you are certain that everything is correct, then

Click on the Save button.

You will now see 45378 along with its description on the Procedure/ Payments/Adjustment List. Click the Close button in the lower right-hand side of this dialog box.

Examples

You own a medical billing service company. You have clients who are physicians and you have one client that is a hospital. The hospital prefers you to use ICD-9-CM procedure codes rather than CPT procedure codes. You can enter the procedure description and both codes at the same time. Then, when you enter particular patients and their information, you can tell the computer to use Code 1 (the CPT code) or Code 2 (the ICD-9-CM procedure code), and the computer will fill in the code from the correct list for you.

Medicare may pay $17 for a flu shot, whereas Blue Cross will pay $21 and Prudential $25 (these numbers are just being used for example and do not reflect any known actual charges from any of these companies). Now, you can enter the procedure code and each different amount. Then the computer will know which amount to use on which claim form.

Practicing What You've Learned on Your Computer

So that the textbook examples and your computer work will match, please input these diagnosis codes and procedure codes with the following charge amounts. Refer to your CPT book if you need descriptions. When you are done, return to your NDCMedisoft desktop.

Procedure Codes		Diagnosis codes	
99173	$ 29.00	250.51	Diabetes with vision problems
99201	46.00	354.0	Carpal tunnel syndrome
99212	56.00	362.01	Retinopathy (diabetic)
99214	76.00	401.9	Hypertension, unspecified
99215	115.00	785.0	Rapid heart beat
99281	103.00	823.20	Fracture, tibia
73100	63.00	912.0	Abrasion, shoulder
73590	43.00		
29125	63.00		
29355	531.00		
45378	145.00		
93000	55.00		
80050	61.00		
82947	15.00		
83718	25.00		
85025	23.00		
87430	35.00		
92081	33.00		

For procedure code descriptions, see the superbill (Figure 11-25) on page 245.

Entering Attending Providers

In NDCMedisoft Advanced, your Provider List is the record of all health care providers (e.g., physicians, therapists) in your particular facility. These are the professionals that will provide treatments and services (procedures) to your patients. As each new patient comes in, one of these providers will be designated as that patient's **attending provider**.

1. Go to the LISTS Menu and click on Providers from the drop-down menu. You will see a dialog box entitled Provider List (Figure 11-15).

Key Term

Attending provider: The physician in your office who has been assigned to this patient.

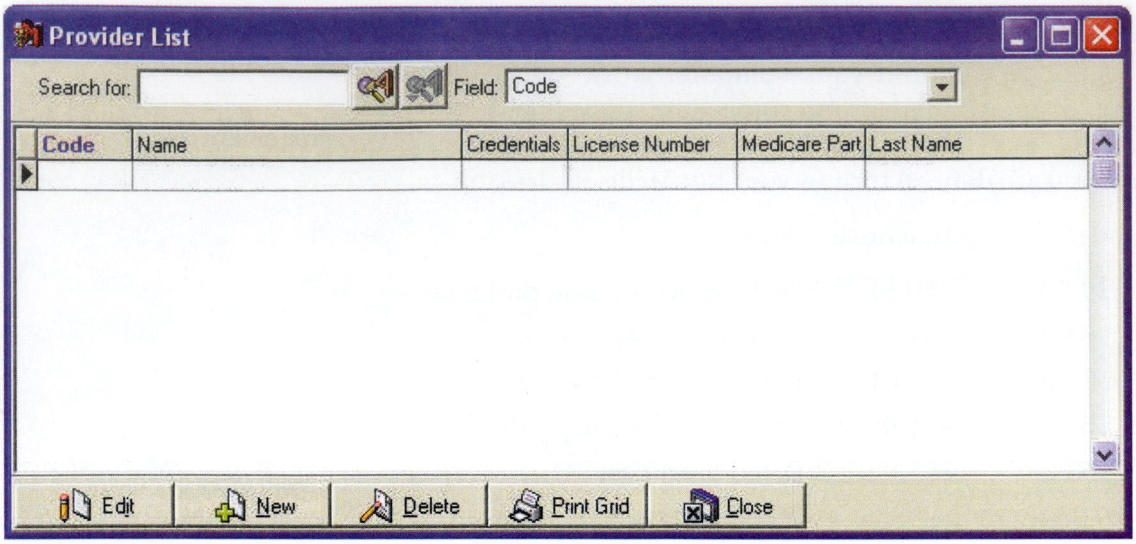

FIGURE 11-15
Provider List screen.

2. At the bottom of this dialog box, click on the button that says New.

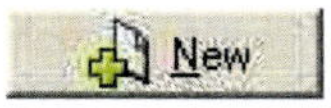

You will see a second dialog box entitled Provider: (new) (Figure 11-16).

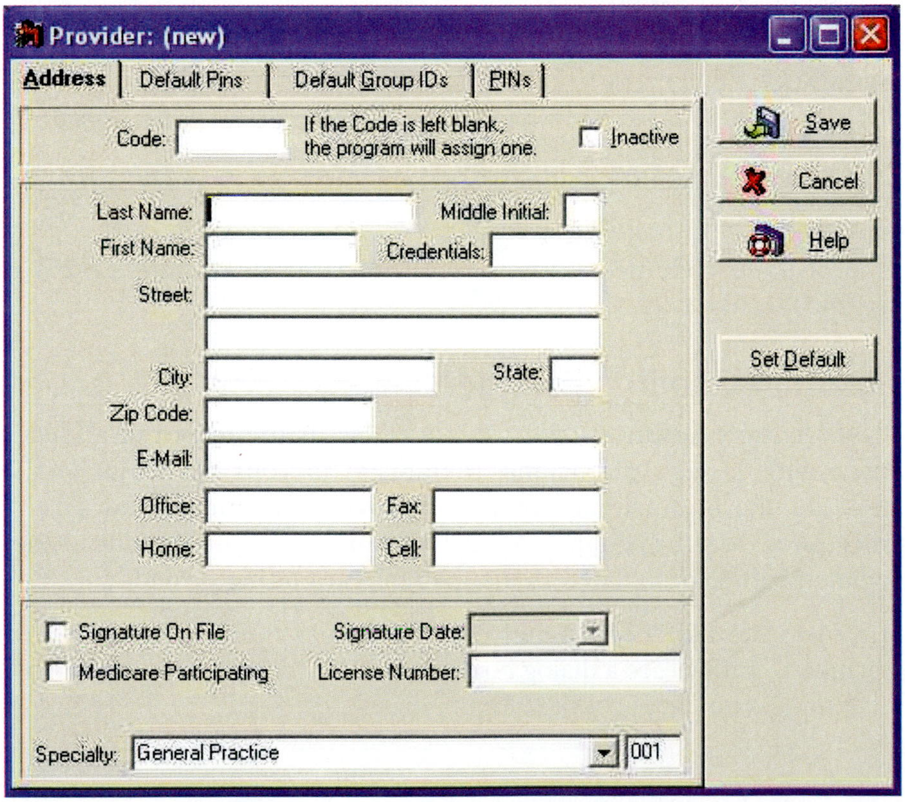

FIGURE 11-16
Provider: (new) dialog box.

3. You will see that there are four tabs across the upper portion of the screen. We will begin with the first—the Address tab. Allow the computer to assign a code for this provider by clicking in the first blank field, next to the words Last Name. Key in the appropriate data.

Last Name:	Healer	Middle Initial:	C
First Name:	James	Credentials:	MD
Street:	123 Main Street		
City:	Anytown	State:	FL
Zip Code:	32711		
E-mail:	jhealer@famdoc.com		
Office:	(407) 555-1234	Fax:	407-555-4321
Home:	(407) 555-9876	Cell:	407-555-0987

CMS-1500
Box 31

☑ Signature On File   Signature Date: 12/30/2003
☑ Medicare Participating   License Number: 1234567890
Specialty: Family Practice

For your classwork, you will need to complete only this one screen in the Provider section. However, before leaving this dialog box, take a moment to look at the Default Pins, the Default Group IDs, and the PINs tabs and the information they each require.

Now take a minute and *CHECK, DOUBLE-CHECK and TRIPLE-CHECK* what you have entered into the computer in comparison with what you see in this portion of the chapter. Capitals, lowercase letters, numbers, punctuation, and spaces are all important. It must match *exactly*. When you are certain that everything is correct, then

Click on the Save button.

[Save]

Notice that Dr. Healer's name is now on the list. Click on the Close button in the lower right-hand corner of this dialog box.

Entering Referring Providers

The list of referring providers is the record of all health care providers (e.g., physicians, therapists) that recommend, send, or refer patients to your facility for evaluation and/or treatment. These are the professionals that will need to get a report from your office as to what your provider (the attending physician) thinks, recommends, and/or does regarding this patient. Generally, you will find that there will be a select group of referring providers that you work with most often. However, every now and then, you may find a patient being referred by a provider that has not sent anyone to your office before.

1. Go to the LISTS Menu and click on Referring Providers from the drop-down menu. You will see a dialog box entitled Referring Provider List (Figure 11-17).

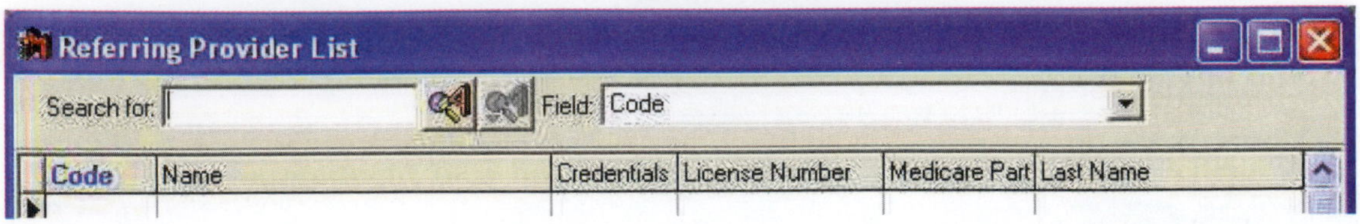

FIGURE 11-17
Referring Provider List box.

2. At the bottom of this dialog box, click on the button that says New.

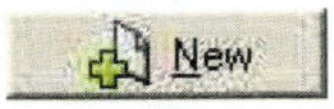

You will see a second dialog box, entitled Referring Provider: (new) (Figure 11-18).

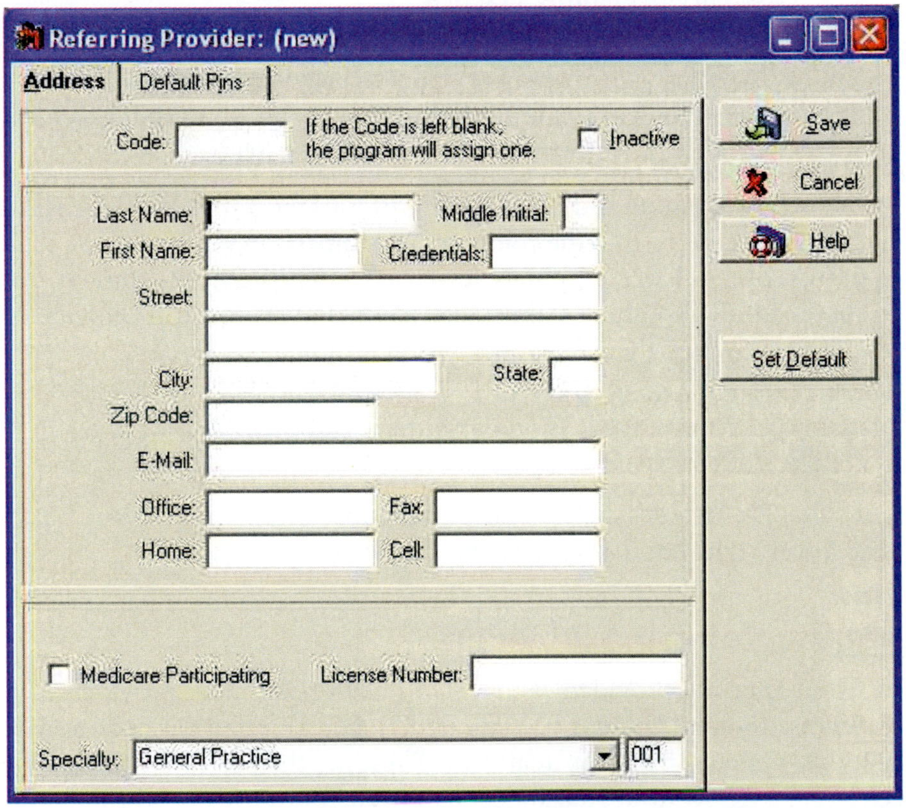

FIGURE 11-18
Referring Provider: (new) dialog box.

3. You will see that there are two tabs across the upper portion of the screen. We will begin with the first—the Address tab.

Allow the computer to assign a code for this referring provider by clicking in the first blank field, next to Last Name. If the patient brings a referral form, you will have all the data you need. If not, most health care facilities have a directory with information on other members of the health care community in the area. This is where you might find the information on the referring provider, Dr. Mark C. Welby. Key in the appropriate data.

Last Name:	Welby	Middle Initial:	C
First Name:	Mark	Credentials:	MD
Street:	432 Elm Avenue		CMS-1500 Box 17
City:	Drama	State:	FL
Zip Code:	32710		
E-mail:	mwelby@dramadoc.com		
Office:	(407) 555-8877	Fax:	(407) 555-9966
Home:	(407) 555-6565	Cell:	(407) 555-1112
☑ Medicare Participating		License Number:	7766554
Specialty:	General Practice		CMS-1500 Box 17a

For your classwork, you will need to complete only this one screen in the Referring Provider section. However, before leaving this dialog box, take a moment to look at the Default Pins tab and the information it requires.

Now take a minute and *CHECK, DOUBLE-CHECK, and TRIPLE-CHECK* what you have entered into the computer in comparison with what you see here. Capitals, lowercase letters, numbers, punctuation, and spaces are all important. It must match *exactly*. When you are certain that everything is correct, then

Click on the Save button.

[Save button]

Notice that Dr. Welby is listed in the Referring Provider List. Click on the Close button in the lower right-hand corner of this dialog box.

You now have the same insurance carrier, an employer, diagnosis codes, procedure codes, a provider, and a referring provider as this book. Also, as you continue with the exercises, you will know how to enter additional information, such as another diagnosis code, should you need to. Just refer back to these pages if you need a reminder.

As we discussed earlier, almost all health insurance claim forms are created on a computer and sent electronically. In order for the computer to have the data to fill out the form, someone (that's right—YOU!) has to input everything, accurately. You provide these elements of information—the ingredients, and the computer will finish the recipe and complete the health claim form. Then, another computer will review the information on the form and either approve the claim for payment or reject it and send it back to you. You just have to copy the data from the documentation you have and key it into the correct places in the computer.

Figure 11-21 is the patient registration form and Figure 11-25 is the superbill for Harvey Practice. You worked with his file in Chapters 5 and 7 when you coded his family history of colon cancer and his diagnostic colonoscopy. Because you already did the coding for this patient, you will accept the superbill for having the best, most accurate codes marked for the services provided. You will begin with the data on the patient registration form (Figure 11-21), so you can enter Mr. Practice as a new patient at this health care facility.

Entering a New Patient

Every person seen by any one of your facility's providers must be entered into the computer as a new patient when he or she comes in for the first time. This is also true for any person agreeing to be a guarantor for another person, *even if the guarantor will never become a patient* of this facility. Any guarantor that fits this definition must be entered in the new patient list as well.

1. Go to the LISTS Menu and click on Patients/Guarantors and Cases from the drop-down menu. You will see a dialog box entitled Patient List (Figure 11-19).

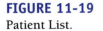

Patient List

Chart Nu...	Name	Date of Birth	Soc Sec Num
DOEMA000	Doe, Marvin D	7/6/1963	777-09-1247
LOYPA000	Loyal, Patience Z	12/12/1940	445-09-0988
MCGHA000	McGraw, Harold H	9/12/1933	123-45-6789
PRAMA000	Practice, Maxwell P	1/7/1948	225-66-9981
STUSA000	Student, Sarah S	6/1/1978	987-02-4739
SWEMA000	Sweet, Mary Lou	5/21/1973	554-98-2638

List of cases for: Sweet, Mary Lou

Number	Case Description
3	Wrist Pain

Edit Patient | New Patient | Delete Patient | Print Grid | Close

FIGURE 11-19
Patient List.

2. At the bottom of this dialog box, click on the button that says New Patient.

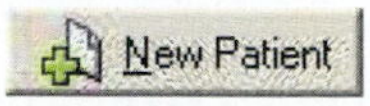

    ⊞ New Patient

    You will see a second dialog box, entitled Patient/Guarantor: (new) (Figure 11-20).

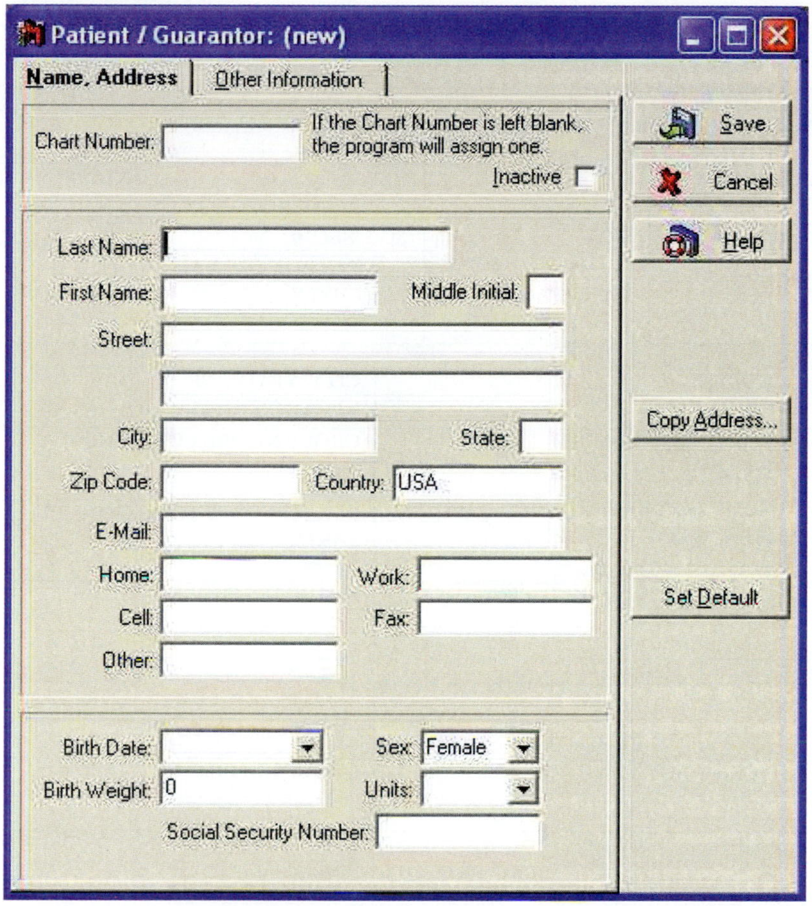

FIGURE 11-20
Patient/Guarantor: (new).

3. You will see that there are two tabs across the upper portion of the screen. We will begin with the first—the Name, Address tab.

    Allow the computer to assign a code for this patient by clicking in the first blank field, next to the words Last Name. Key in the appropriate data from Harvey Practice's patient registration form (Figure 11-21). Go line by line, pressing your Tab key or your Enter key to move from field to field. Take your time and type carefully. Remember, *accuracy is most important.* If there is a piece of data that the computer asks for that is not shown on the registration form, such as an e-mail address or a cell phone number, you may leave it blank.

    Enter Mr. Practice's name, address, phone number, birth date, and sex.

    ┌──────────────┐
    │ CMS-1500   │
    │ Boxes 2, 3, 5│
    └──────────────┘

On this screen, you will also enter the patient's work and cell phone numbers (if available) and his Social Security number. This information is for use in your office, should you need to contact the patient or send an account to a collection agency.

PATIENT REGISTRATION FORM

RESPONSIBLE PARTY			DATE *March 3, 2006*	
LAST NAME *Practice*	FIRST NAME *Harvey*	MI *N*	SOCIAL SECURITY # *533-96-6654*	DATE OF BIRTH *Dec. 12, 1987*
ADDRESS *841 Rabbit Way*	CITY *Cityville*	STATE *FL*	ZIP CODE *32901*	SEX *M* — MARITAL STATUS *Single*
HOME PHONE *407-555-7317*	WORK PHONE *407-555-9110*		REFERRED BY: *Mark C. Welby, M. D.*	

EMPLOYER INFORMATION		WORK STATUS:	FULL-TIME PART-TIME (STUDENT)
COMPANY NAME	ADDRESS		CITY, STATE, ZIP

DEPENDENT INFORMATION

DEPENDENT'S NAME		DEPENDENT'S NAME		DEPENDENT'S NAME	
RELATIONSHIP	DATE OF BIRTH	RELATIONSHIP	DATE OF BIRTH	RELATIONSHIP	DATE OF BIRTH
SOC. SEC. #	SEX	SOC. SEC. #	SEX	SOC. SEC. #	SEX
EMPLOYER	WORK PHONE	EMPLOYER	WORK PHONE	EMPLOYER	WORK PHONE

INSURANCE INFORMATION–PRIMARY POLICY

COMPANY NAME *McGraw Insurance Co.*	ADDRESS *P. O. Box 5544*	CITY, STATE, ZIP *Wilson, OH 45533*
PHONE NUMBER *800-555-6654*	ID OR POLICY NUMBER *533966654*	GROUP NUMBER OR NAME *TS9023*
INSURED'S NAME (IF DIFFERENT) *Roger Practice*	SOCIAL SECURITY # *243-33-1924*	RELATIONSHIP TO RESPONSIBLE PARTY *Father*
INSURED'S ADDRESS (IF DIFFERENT)	INSURED'S CITY, STATE, ZIP	INSURED'S PHONE NUMBER

INSURANCE INFORMATION–SECONDARY POLICY

COMPANY NAME	ADDRESS	CITY, STATE, ZIP
PHONE NUMBER	ID OR POLICY NUMBER	GROUP NUMBER OR NAME
INSURED'S NAME (IF DIFFERENT)	SOCIAL SECURITY #	RELATIONSHIP TO RESPONSIBLE PARTY
INSURED'S ADDRESS (IF DIFFERENT)	INSURED'S CITY, STATE, ZIP	INSURED'S PHONE NUMBER

OTHER INFORMATION

ALLERGIES	REASON FOR TODAY'S VISIT *Colon checkup*
PATIENT'S SIGNATURE *Harvey Practice*	DATE *3/3/06*

FOR OFFICE USE ONLY		
CO-PAY $ _15.00_	CO-INSURANCE $ _____	DEDUCTIBLE $ _____
CHECK ☒ # _5533_	CASH ☐ CHARGE ☐ PAID IN FULL ☐	
ASSIGNED PROVIDER _J. Healer, MD_		

FIGURE 11-21
Harvey Practice's patient registration form.

4. When you have completed this screen, click on the Other Information tab (Figure 11-22) and continue entering the appropriate data. The first line on this screen asks you to tell the computer whether this person is a Patient or a Guarantor.

Type: | Patient ▼ |

In NDCMedisoft Advanced, the only time you will choose Guarantor from this drop-down menu is if, as stated earlier in this chapter, the person is only the Guarantor for another individual and they themselves will never be a patient of this facility. This is not necessarily true in other software programs.

The Assigned Provider can be found at the bottom of this patient registration form. Each office will have a different way to note which physician in the office has been assigned to this new patient. You will be able to learn that quickly in your new job.

Patient ID #2, Patient Indicator, Flag, and Healthcare ID might be used for an internal coding system. For our purposes, we will leave these blank.

Accept the default Patient Billing Code.

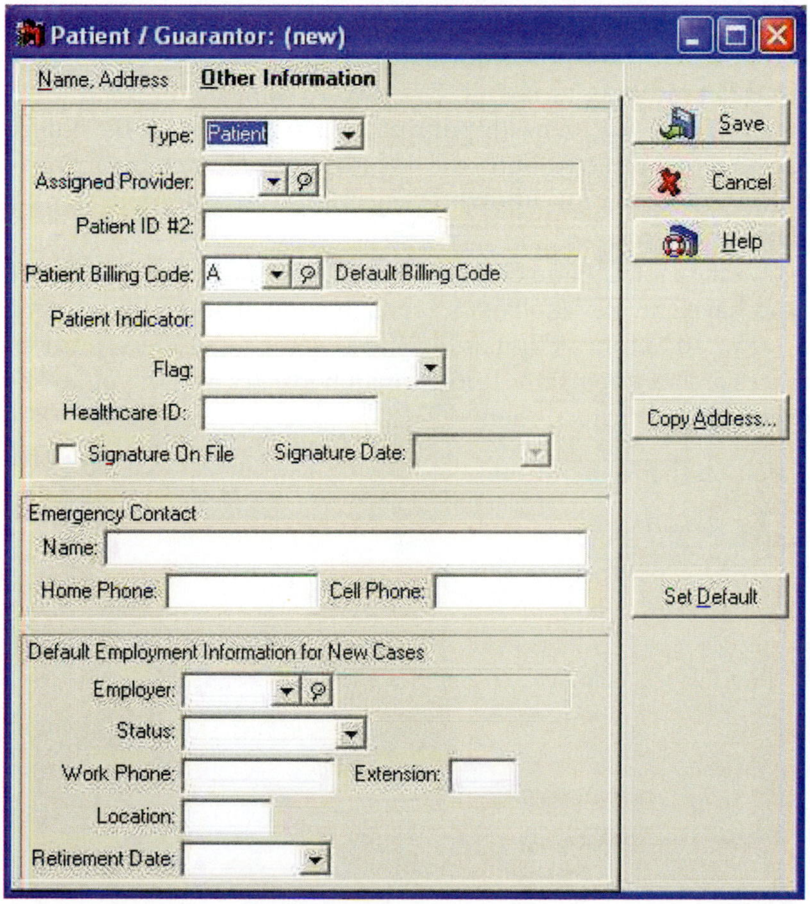

FIGURE 11-22
Patient/Guarantor—Other Information screen.

5. Check the new patient paperwork and make certain that the patient has signed the form and dated it. Then check off the box next to Signature on File and enter the date the patient signed the form.

CMS-1500
Box 12

☑ Signature On File   Signature Date: 03/03/06

You will find Mr. Practice's signature toward the bottom of the registration form, with the date alongside it. This signature gives your office permission to release the patient's private health care information to the insurance carrier, so you can be paid. Without it, your claim will be rejected—even if everything else is correct. This tells the insurance company that you have the patient's original signature giving you permission to release his or her confidential protected health information (PHI) to the company for purposes of payment.

The next section will hold the Emergency Contact information for this patient, along with his or her Employment Information. NDCMedisoft Advanced will automatically place the information you enter here into the appropriate fields as needed.

Check every box on the screen and compare it with everything on the registration form (from top to bottom) to make certain that you are not skipping anything. Chances are good that the form at your office will look different. However, the information will be same as everywhere else, just in a different order or layout. Get used to hunting for the information you need. There are very important items that must be completed, because they go directly onto the health insurance claim form (CMS-1500) and are reason for automatic rejection if they are left blank or are completed incorrectly.

Now take a minute and *CHECK, DOUBLE-CHECK, and TRIPLE-CHECK* what you have entered into *both* screens in comparison with what you see on the registration form. Capitals, lowercase letters, numbers, punctuation, and spaces are all important. It must match *exactly.* When you are certain that everything is correct, then

Click on the Save button.

Entering a New Case

You should now be back in the Patient List dialog box (Figure 11-23). On the left-hand side, you will see our new patient, Harvey Practice, now listed with a chart number (assigned automatically by NDCMedisoft). Mr. Practice's name should be highlighted.

On the right side of the same dialog box, you will see a section titled

List of cases for: Practice, Harvey N

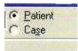

FIGURE 11-23
Patient List dialog box showing Patient and Case radio buttons.

Directly above this section, on the top right side, you will see two radio buttons:

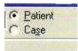

You now have to open a **case** for the patient in order to input data regarding the specific reason that caused the patient to come to see the provider for this encounter. You will only open a new case for each new condition or concern—that is, each new chief complaint or diagnosis (or group of diagnoses).

Key Term

Case: In NDCMedisoft Advanced, a case is a file that will be created each time the patient sees the provider for a new chief complaint or diagnosis.

1. OK, Let's proceed with opening a new case for Harvey Practice. Go up to the radio buttons on the top right and click on the button next to the word Case.

   ○ Patient
   ⊙ Case

   You will notice that the buttons across the bottom of the dialog box have now changed. Before, they were named

       Edit Patient   New Patient   Delete Patient

   Now they have changed to

       Edit Case   New Case   Delete Case

2. Click on the New Case button.

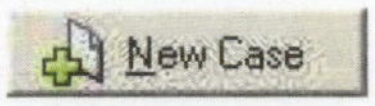

Now a new dialog box has opened, entitled Case: PRAHA000 Practice, Harvey [new] (Figure 11-24).

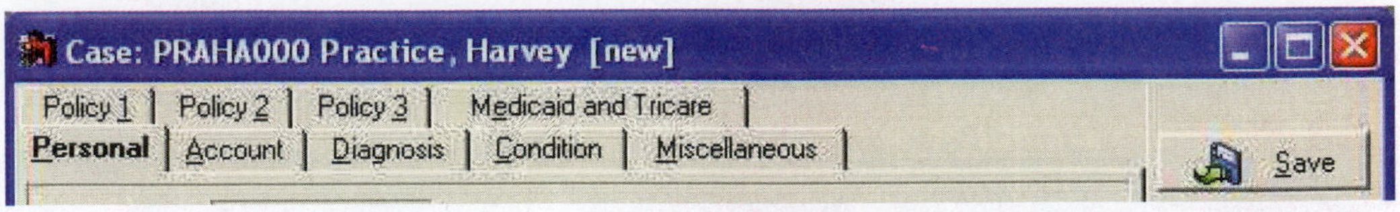

FIGURE 11-24
New Case dialog box.

3. You will see that there are nine tabs across the upper portion of the screen. We will begin with the first—the Personal tab. Using the information on the patient registration form and the superbill, key in the appropriate data.

As you complete each screen, double-check your work before you click on the next tab. If you click on the Save button while moving between tabs, NDCMedisoft will take you back to the Patient List dialog box. Don't worry; simply click on the Case Description shown in the List of cases for: and then click the Edit Case button at the bottom left side of the dialog box. This will reopen the case dialog box, and you will be able to continue to input data from where you were last.

4. All the data you need to complete all nine tab screens can be found on the patient registration form (Figure 11-21) and the superbill (Figure 11-25). You will not need to fill in every line because some may not apply. However, make certain to look at *every* field on *every* tab before determining that you do not need to provide an answer to something.

Remember that, if the correct answer is not available to you in a drop-down menu, you will have to go to the LISTS Menu, go to the particular type (such as a provider, referring provider, or diagnosis code), and enter the new information so it will show in that drop-down menu. Let's go through all nine tabs together.

Family Doctors Associates
123 Main Street • Anytown, FL 32711
(407) 555-1200

Date: *March 3, 2006*   Attending Physician: *J. Healer, MD*

Patient Name: *Harvey Practice*

CPT DESCRIPTION	CPT DESCRIPTION	CPT DESCRIPTION
OFFICE/HOSPITAL	**PATHOLOGY/LAB/RADIOLOGY**	**PROCEDURES/TESTS**
☒ 99201 OFFICE-NEW; FOCUSED	☐ 73100 X-RAY WRIST TWO VIEWS	☐ 12011 SIMPLE SUTURE, FACE
☐ 99202 OFFICE-NEW; EXPANDED	☐ 73590 X-RAY TIBIA/FIBULA, TWO	☐ 29125 SPLINT-SHORT ARM
☐ 99203 OFFICE-NEW; DETAILED	☐ 73600 X-RAY ANKLE TWO VIEWS	☐ 29355 WALKER CAST-LONG LEG
☐ 99204 OFFICE-NEW; COMPREHEN	☐ 76085 MAMMOGRAM-COMP DET	☐ 29540 STRAPPING-ANKLE
☐ 99205 OFFICE-NEW; COMPREHEN	☐ 76092 MAMMOGRAM SCREENING	☒ 45378 COLONOSCOPY-DIAGNOSTIC
☐ 99211 OFFICE-ESTB; MINIMAL	☐ 80050 BLOOD TEST-GEN HEALTH	☐ 45385 COLONOSCOPY-POLYP REM.
☐ 99212 OFFICE-ESTB; FOCUSED	☐ 80061 BLOOD TEST-LIPID PANEL	☐ 50390 ASPIRATION, RENAL CYST
☐ 99213 OFFICE-ESTB; EXPANDED	☐ 82947 BLOOD TEST-GLUCOSE	☐ 90703 TETANUS INJECTION
☐ 99214 OFFICE-ESTB; DETAILED	☐ 83718 BLOOD TEST-HDL	☐ 92081 VISUAL FIELD EXAM
☐ 99215 OFFICE-ESTB; COMPREHEN	☐ 85025 BLOOD TEST-CBC	☐ 93000 ECG, 12 LEADS, W/RPT
☐ 99281 EMER DEPT; FOCUSED	☐ 86403 STREP TEST, QUICK	☐ 93015 TREADMILL STRESS TEST
☐ 90844 COUNSELING—50 MIN.	☐ 87430 ENZY IMMUNOASSAY-STREP	☐ 99173 VISUAL ACUITY SCREEN

ICD DESCRIPTION	ICD DESCRIPTION	ICD DESCRIPTION
☐ 034.0 STREP THROAT	☐ 522 LOW RED BLOOD COUNT	☐ V01.5 RABIES EXPOSURE
☐ 042 HUMAN IMMUNO VIRUS	☐ 538.8 STOMACH PAIN	☒ V16.0 FAMILY HISTORY-COLON
☐ 250.51 DIABETES W/ VISION	☐ 643 HYPEREMESIS	☐ V16.3 FAMILY HISTORY-BREAST
☐ 250.80 DIABETES, TYPE II	☐ 707.14 ULCER OF HEEL/MID FOOT	☐ V20.2 WELL CHILD
☐ 307.51 BULIMIA NON-ORGANIC	☐ 788.30 ENURESIS	☐ V22.0 PREGNANCY-FIRST NORM
☐ 354.0 CARPAL TUNNEL SYNDROME	☐ 815.00 FRACTURE, HAND	☐ V22.1 PREGNANCY-NORMAL
☐ 362.01 RETINOPATHY (DIABETIC)	☐ 823.20 FRACTURE, TIBIA	☐ E816.2 MOTORCYCLE ACCT
☐ 401.9 HYPERTENSION, UNSPEC	☐ 831.00 DISLOCATION, SHOULDER	☐ E826.1 FALL FROM BICYCLE
☐ 482.30 PNEUMONIA	☐ 845.00 SPRAINED ANKLE	☐ E849.0 PLACE OF OCCUR-HOME
☐ 490 BRONCHITIS, UNSPECIFIED	☐ 880.03 OPEN WOUND UPPER ARM	☐ E881.0 FALL FROM LADDER
☐ 493.92 ASTHMA, UNSPECIFIED	☐ 912.0 ABRASION, SHOULDER	☐ E906.0 DOG BITE

FOLLOW UP

PRN _____

WEEKS _____*6*_____

NXT APPT. _____*✓*_____

TIME _____*3 p. m.*_____

FIGURE 11-25
Superbill for Harvey Practice.

Personal tab: (Figure 11-26) All information can be found on the patient registration form. On this screen, Description is the patient's chief complaint, or the reason he or she has come to this health care provider for this visit. Remember, the guarantor is the person who guarantees payment to the health care office, who will pay the bill if the insurance does not. Enter the patient's Marital Status and Student Status from the drop-down menu. The employment information has been entered by NDCMedisoft Advanced because you entered it into the New Patient dialog box.

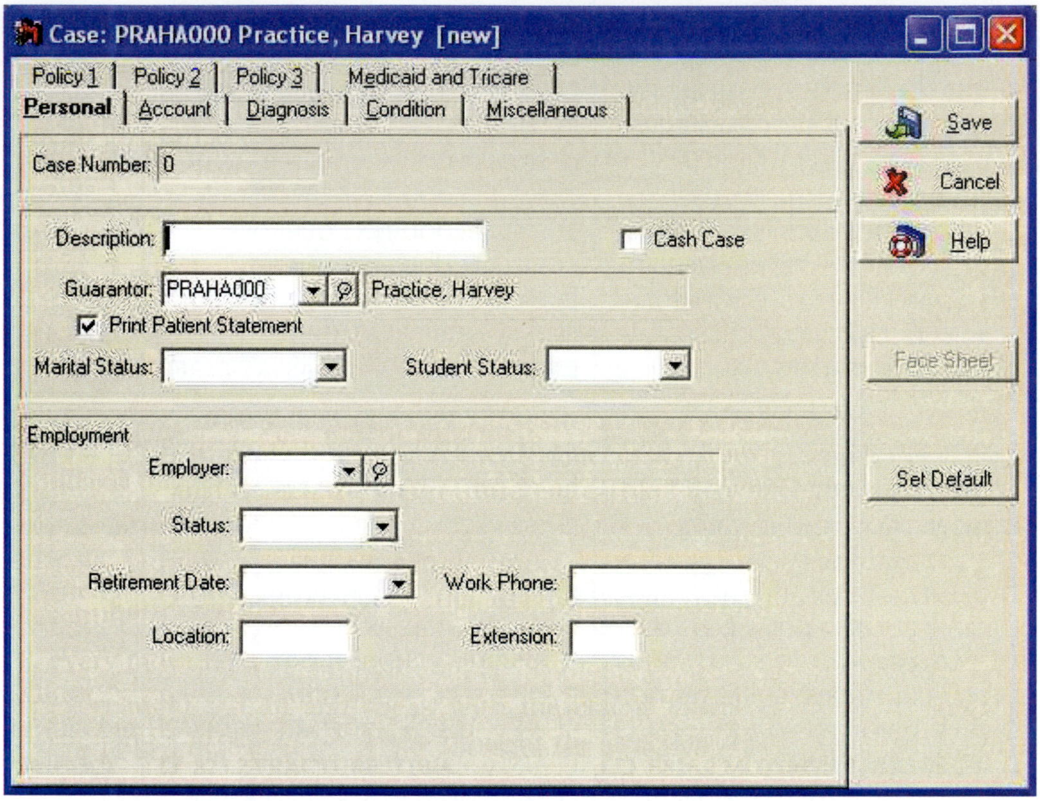

CMS-1500
Box 8

FIGURE 11-26
Case dialog
box—Personal screen.

> **IMPORTANT NOTE**
>
> On the Personal tab, there is a line for the input of a retirement date (toward the bottom of the screen). If the patient is employed full-time, there will not be a retirement date, so you will need to leave this blank.

CMS-1500
Boxes 33
and 17

Account tab: (Figure 11-27) All information can be found on the patient registration form. Both the Assigned Provider and the Referring Provider are shown on that form. Accept default Case Billing Code A and Price Code A. There is no authorization information for this referral, because the physician is in the network. However, if this were an HMO referral, for example, you would enter the dates, number of visits, and authorization number copied from the referral authorization form in this section of the screen.

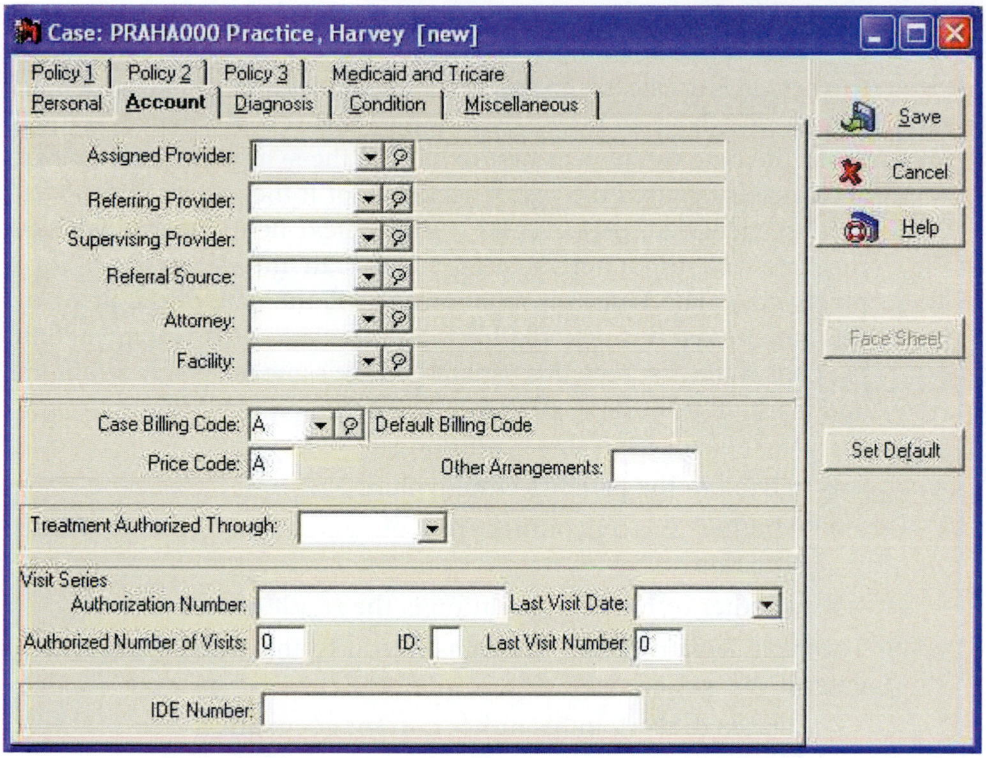

FIGURE 11-27
Case dialog
box–Account screen.

Diagnosis tab: (Figure 11-28) The diagnosis code for this patient can be found on the superbill, and the patient's allergies can be found on the patient registration form. At least one diagnosis code *must* be entered. We will discuss the EDI notes (same as EMC) and the EDI Report information later in this chapter.

CMS-1500
Box 21

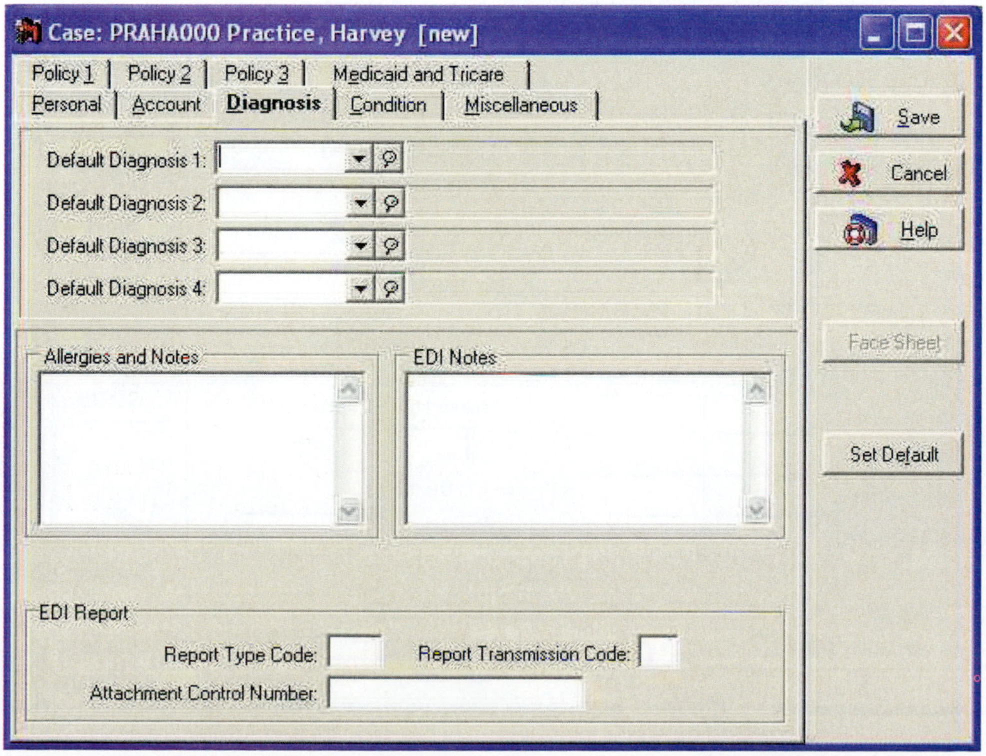

FIGURE 11-28
Case dialog
box—Diagnosis screen.

CMS-1500
Box 14

Condition tab: (Figure 11-29) Mr. Practice's visit has nothing to do with either an illness or an injury. Therefore, none of the data requested on this screen is applicable to this particular encounter. However, when a patient does have an illness or an injury, this screen is where you will input the date the patient first exhibited the symptoms, the date the accident that caused the injury occurred, or if the patient is pregnant, her last menstrual period (LMP). In the next field, indicate whether the date you input refers to an illness, an injury, or LMP (for a pregnancy). The First Consultation Date is the date of the first time this patient saw this provider for this condition. Next you must input

CMS-1500
Box 15

the date of the first time this patient had the same or similar symptoms and mark off if the date reflects that information.

CMS-1500
Box 10

Next check off if this condition is:

→ related to the patient's employment

whether this encounter was an emergency (life or death) situation

→ whether or not this condition is the result of an accident

The next section of this screen asks you to input the From and To dates if this patient was:

unable to work in his or her current occupation

CMS-1500
Boxes 16
and 18

→ hospitalized as a result of having this condition

totally or partially disabled

This information is usually found in the patient's chart. None of these items are true for Mr. Practice so leave these fields blank.

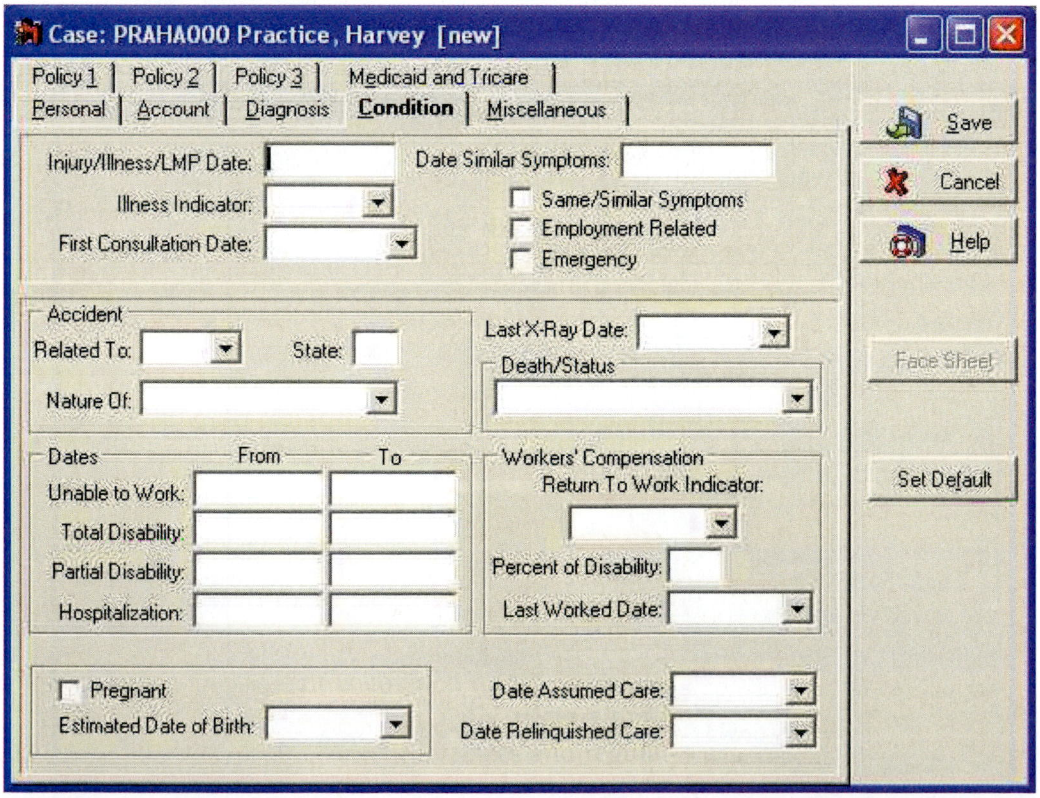

FIGURE 11-29
Case dialog
box—Condition screen.

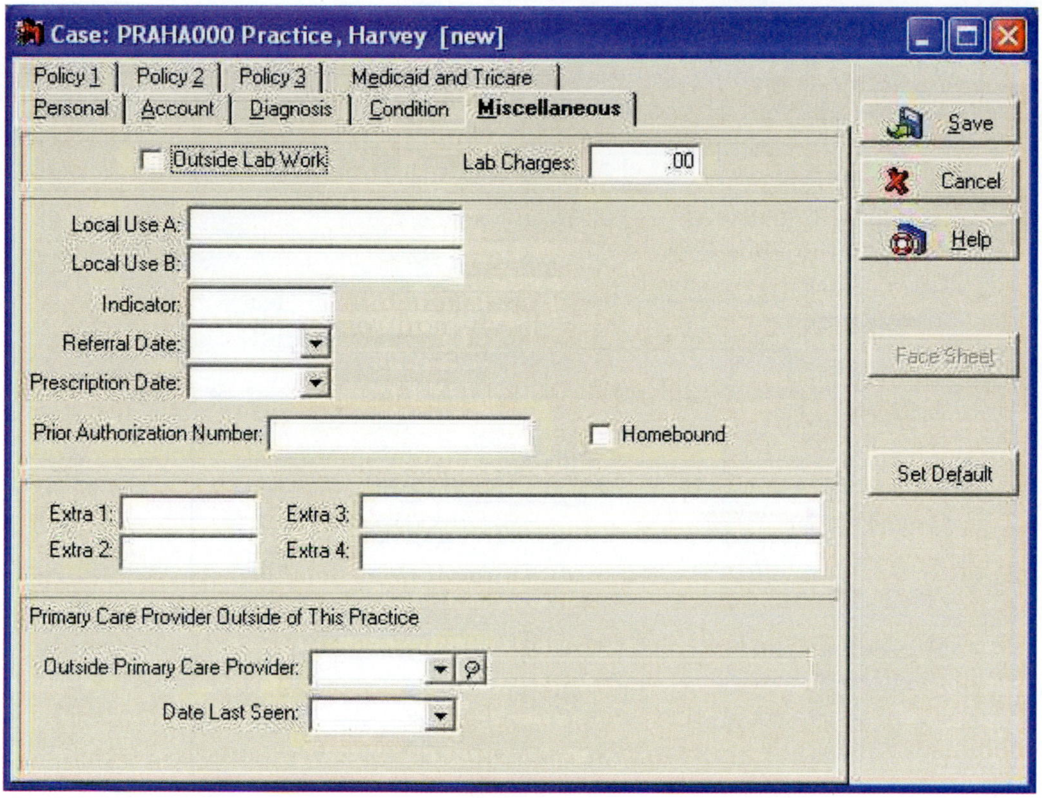

FIGURE 11-30
Case dialog
box—Miscellaneous
screen.

Miscellaneous tab: (Figure 11-30) This tab is for information regarding lab work. This patient has not had any lab work, so there is no applicable information for this screen.

> CMS-1500
> Box 20

Policy 1 tab: (Figure 11-31) This is for the information regarding the patient's primary insurance policy. All information can be found on the patient registration form and patient's insurance ID card. At least one insurance policy must be entered, unless the patient is designated as a Cash Case on the Personal tab. Remember that, in some cases, the policyholder is not the patient. Look on the patient registration form to make certain. Then indicate what the relationship is between the patient and the policyholder. Remember to check off the box for Assignment of Benefits/Accept Assignment, so that your office can get paid. Information on the patient's deductible, co-payment, and co-insurance is also entered on this screen. You will get most of this information from the patient's insurance card and when you called for coverage and eligibility verification.

> CMS-1500
> Boxes 1a, 4,
> 6, 7, and 11

> CMS-1500
> Box 27

Policy 2 tab: (Figure 11-32) This is for the information regarding the patient's secondary insurance policy. All information can be found on the patient registration form. (Mr. Practice does not have secondary insurance coverage.) If this screen is left blank, then NO in Box 11d on the insurance form will be checked off by NDCMedisoft. If information is entered in this screen, then YES in Box 11d will be checked, and the information entered here will be placed in Boxes 9a–d.

> CMS-1500
> Boxes 11d
> and 9a–d

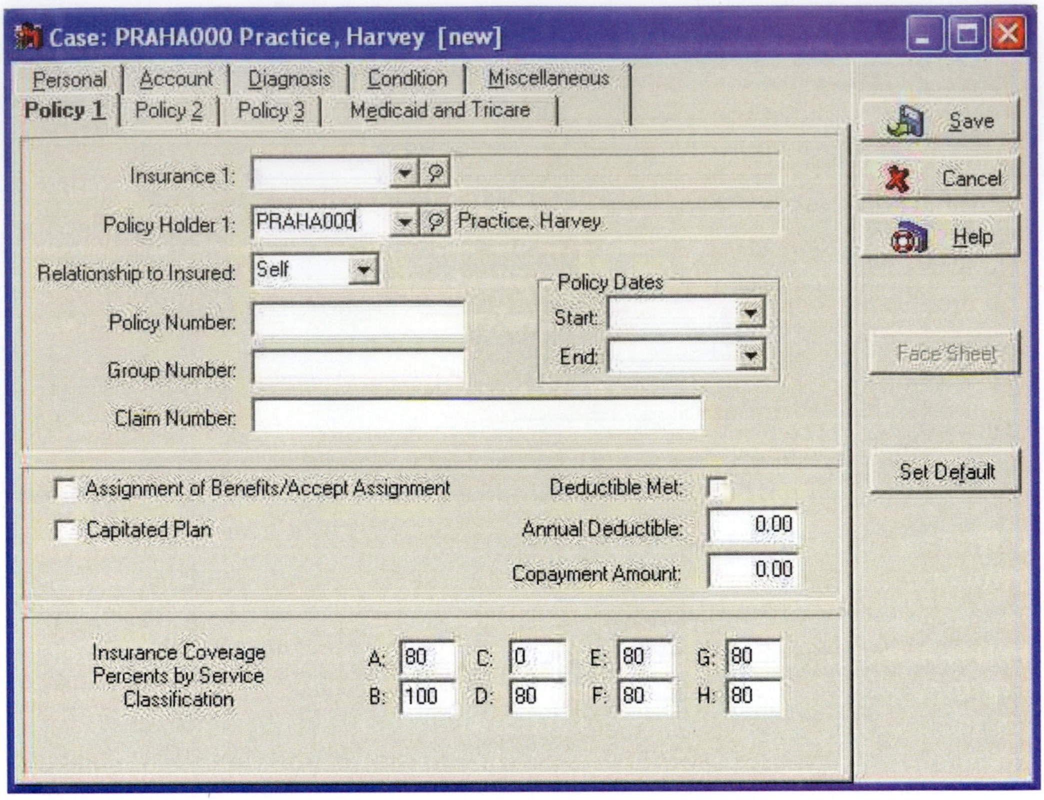

FIGURE 11-31
Case dialog
box—Policy 1 screen.

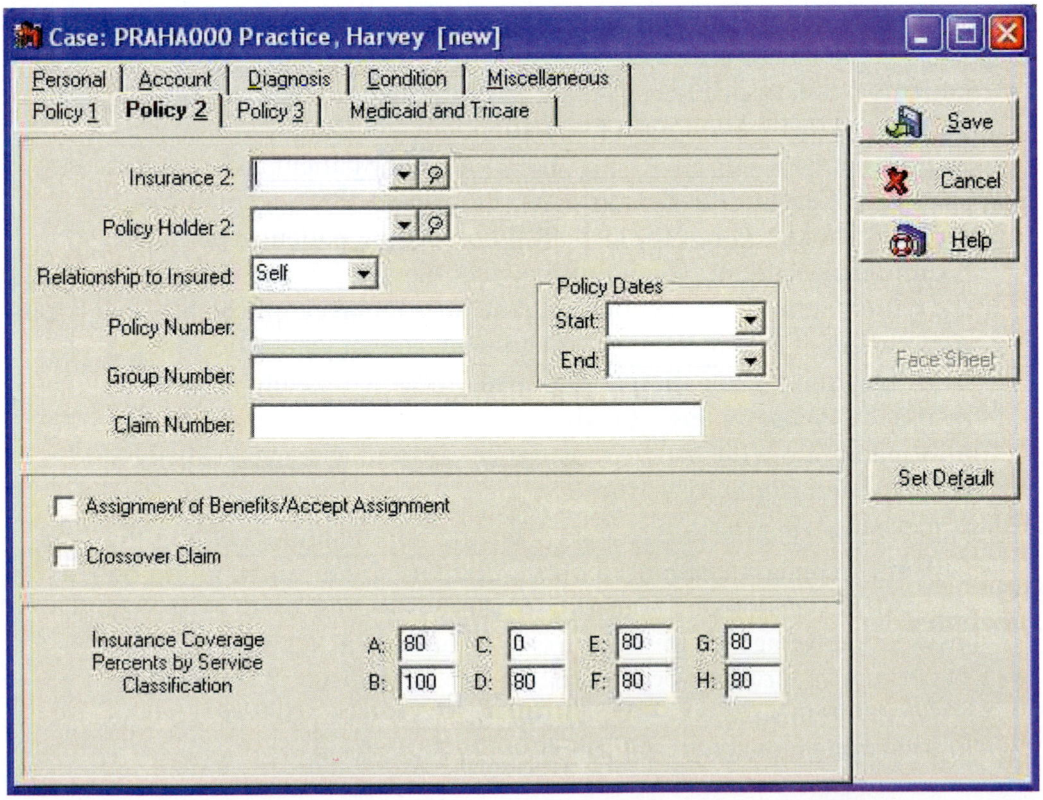

FIGURE 11-32
Case dialog
box—Policy 2 screen.

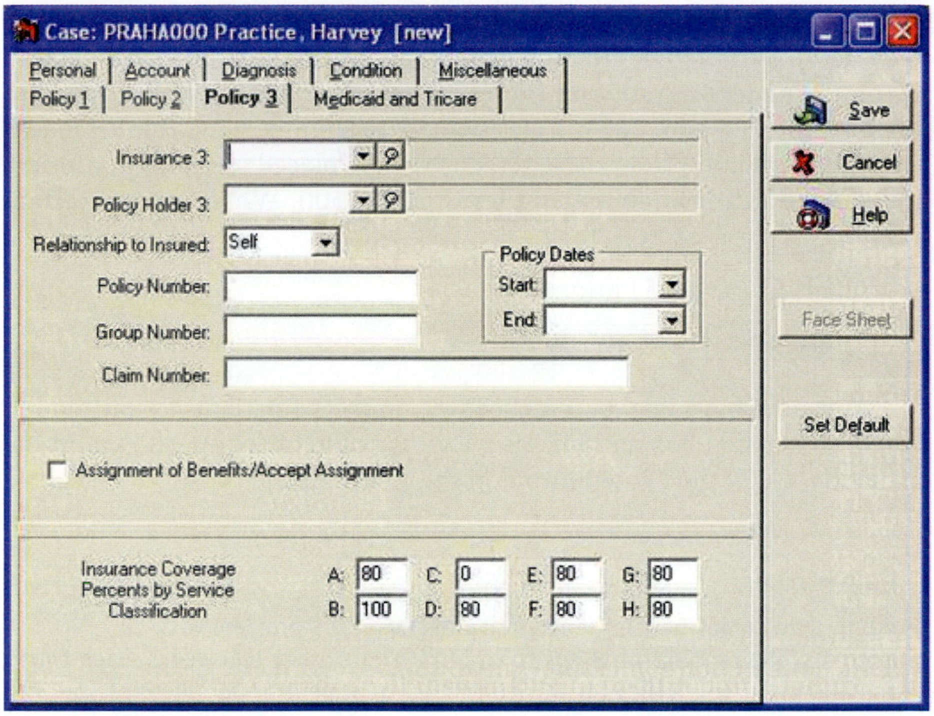

FIGURE 11-33
Case dialog
box—Policy 3 screen.

Policy 3 tab: (Figure 11-33) This is for the information regarding the patient's tertiary insurance policy. All information can be found on the patient registration form. (Harvey Practice does not have a third policy.)

Medicaid and TriCare tab: (Figure 11-34) This is for information on patients covered by either Medicaid or TriCare/CHAMPUS. Mr. Practice is not on either plan, so this screen will be left blank in his file. However, if one of your future patients is covered by either type of policy, you must enter the appropriate information on this screen. Medicaid information will be entered onto the insurance claim form. TriCare and CHAMPUS use a different form, not CMS-1500.

CMS-1500
Boxes 22
and 23

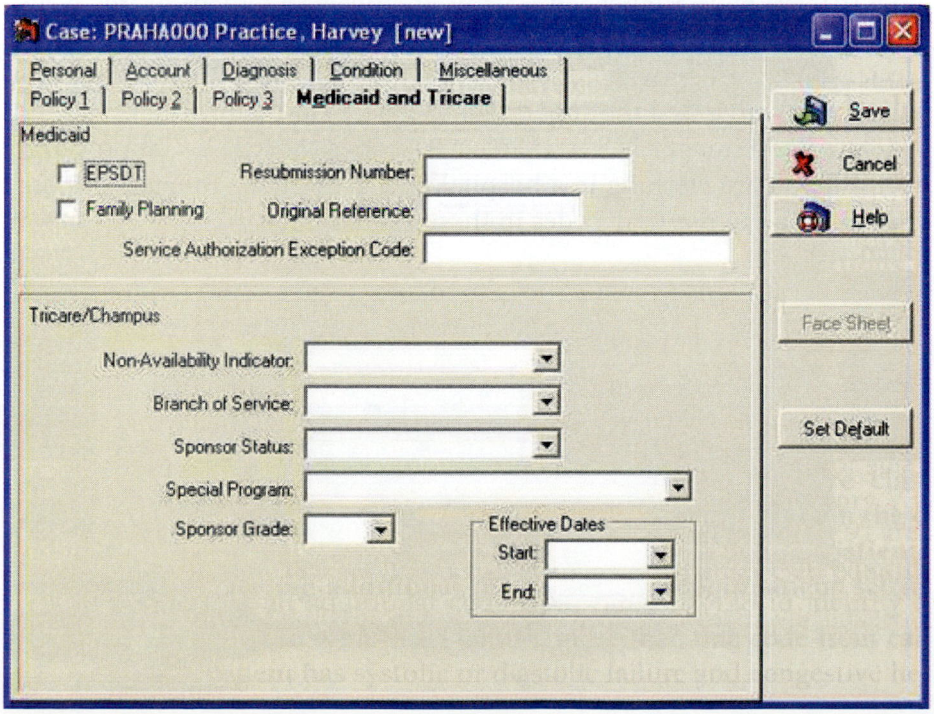

FIGURE 11-34
Case dialog
box—Medicaid and
TriCare screen.

Now take a minute and *CHECK, DOUBLE-CHECK, and TRIPLE-CHECK* what you have entered into *all nine* screens in comparison with what you see on the patient registration form and the superbill. Capitals, lowercase letters, numbers, punctuation, and spaces are all important. It must match *exactly.* Information from these screens will be placed in their appropriate boxes on health insurance claim form CMS-1500. When you are certain that everything is correct, then

Click on the Save button.

You now have Harvey Practice's name in the patient list on the left side of this dialog box and his case, for his colon checkup, shown on the right side. Click the Close button on the lower right.

Examples

Robin Byrd comes to see the physician because of a problem with her allergies. The physician has her come in for shots every two weeks. Each time she is seen in your office for this continued treatment of her allergies you will *not* open a new case. You will enter new transactions (procedure codes) for each visit and create a new claim form but they will all be connected to this one case with the same diagnosis.

Mr. Smith has been a patient here for many years. Last month, he came in for his annual physical. Earlier this week, he came in with a suspected case of the flu. Because this visit is for a different reason (flu) than the last visit (annual physical), you will need to open a new case. Mr. Smith's file will then have two cases—one for physical and one for flu.

Entering Procedures and Patient Co-Payments

Now that we have established Harvey Practice as a patient of this health care facility in the computer, the next step is to key in the procedures and services that were provided for his colon checkup visit. By this time, you have already reviewed the superbill and have read the provider's notes in order to determine the best available CPT codes (or ICD-9-CM procedure codes, if you are working in a hospital that uses them. To make it easier, you are going to use CPT codes in these exercises).

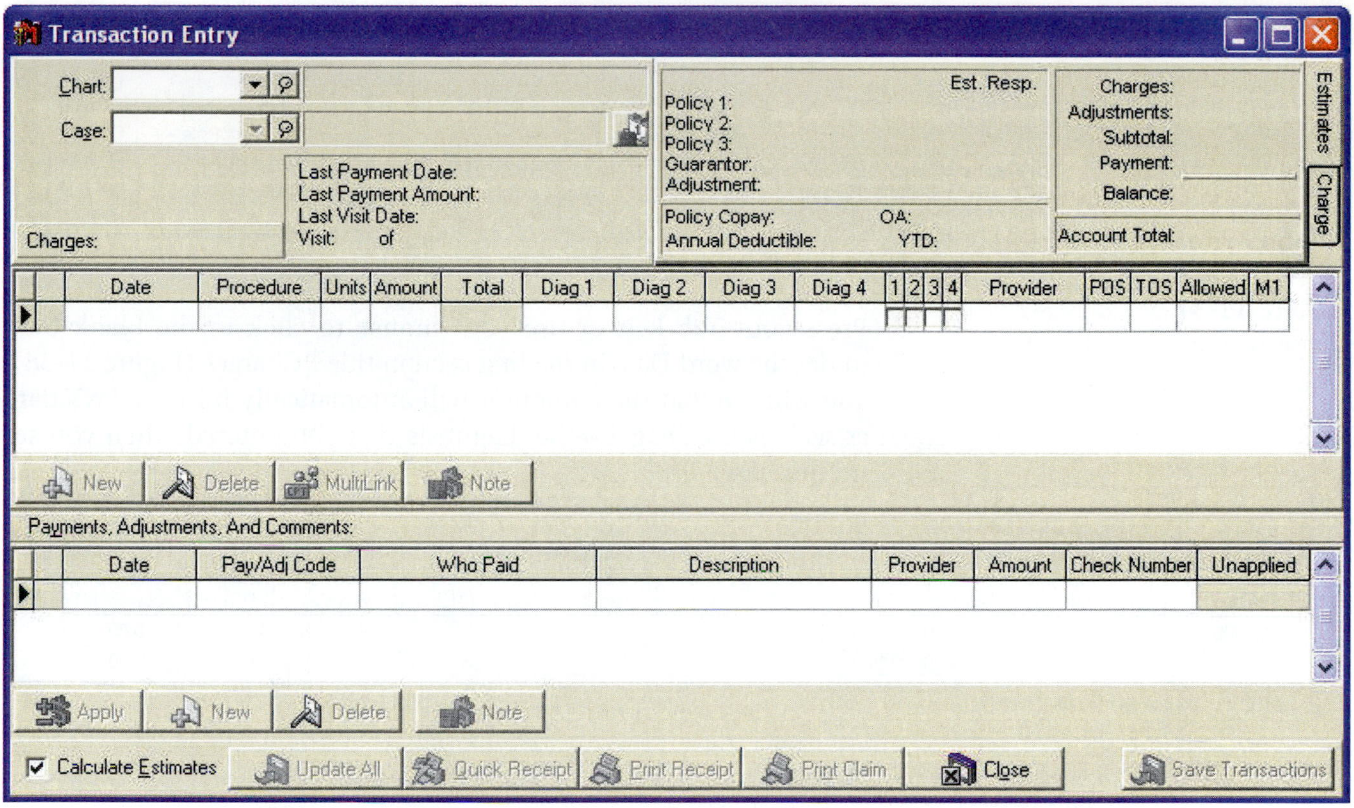

FIGURE 11-35
Transaction Entry screen.

1. Go to the ACTIVITIES Menu and click on Enter Transactions from the drop-down menu. You will see a dialog box entitled Transaction Entry (Figure 11-35). At the upper left side of this dialog box, you will see the chart field with a drop-down menu (Figure 11-36).

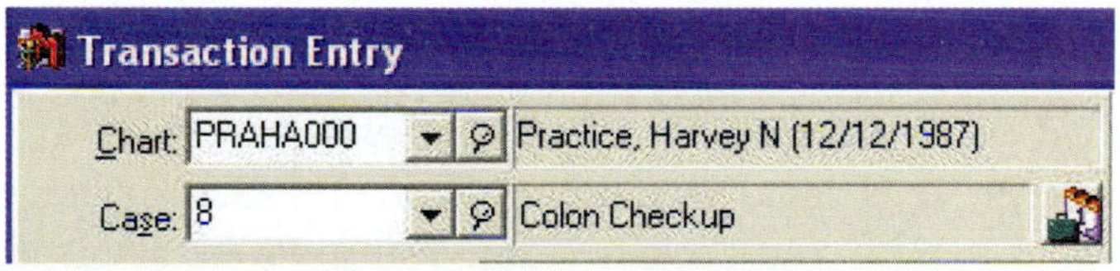

FIGURE 11-36
Chart drop-down menu showing Harvey Practice.

IMPORTANT NOTE

Your case number may be different than what is shown in Figure 11-36. These numbers are assigned, in order, by the computer as each case is entered. Therefore, if more people have been working on your computer, this number may be higher. It doesn't matter.

2. Click on the down arrow and choose the name of the patient for whom you want to enter information. Find Harvey Practice's name and click on it. Or type in the first few letters of the patient's last name into the field. You will notice that NDCMedisoft will fill in information across the screen for you. Toward the right side you should see the insurance policies, guarantor's name, and co-payment amount listed for this patient (Figure 11-37). NDCMedisoft took this information from the screens when you set up this case for this individual. This is a good example of how the computer uses information you enter once and places it wherever you need it.

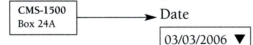

FIGURE 11-37
Transaction Entry screen.

3. Press your Tab key, or use your mouse to click in the blank field under the word Date in the first section titled Charges (Figure 11-38). You will see that the computer will automatically fill in today's date as well as the Diag 1—the diagnosis that you entered when you set up this case.

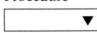

FIGURE 11-38
Transaction Entry—Charges.

4. Key in the date shown on the patient's superbill. When you are working, you will not always be able to enter today's patients today. Therefore, you must get in the habit of paying close attention to this date. The date shown in this computer file *must* match the date the procedures and services were actually provided. This data will not only be used to create an insurance claim form; it is legal documentation of exactly what happened between a patient and the provider. You must be accurate. You can choose from the drop-down calendar or key in MMDDCCYY. The wrong date could be considered fraud.

CMS-1500
Box 24A → Date

03/03/2006 ▼

5. Press your Tab key one time and your cursor will be moved into the blank field below the word Procedure.

Procedure

▼

Key in the first procedure code from Mr. Practice's superbill, or click on the down arrow and choose it from the list of CPT codes. Always begin with the E/M code.

CMS-1500
Box 24D → Procedure

99201 ▼

Press your Tab key and the computer will automatically complete the boxes that follow on that line, including the amount being charged for this procedure (Figure 11-39).

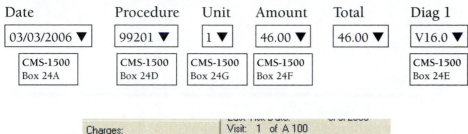

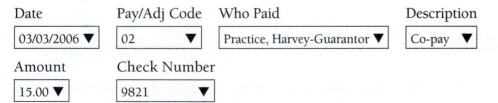

FIGURE 11-39
Transaction Entry—Charges screen.

6. Enter the next CPT code that you find on Mr. Practice's superbill. (You will find a button at the bottom of this section that says New. Click on this, and a new line above will appear, so that you can enter additional procedures.) Remember, if the code you need is not available to you from the drop-down menu, you will need to go to the LISTS Menu, choose Procedure Codes, and enter the codes you need. Then, return here, to the Transaction Entry dialog box, and finish entering the patient's information.

7. If you look at the bottom of the patient registration form, you will see that Mr. Practice paid his $15.00 insurance co-payment by check. This will need to be entered into the computer, as well, so you can keep an accurate record of his account. In the bottom half of this Transaction Entry screen, you will see the second section, titled Payments, Adjustments, And Comments.

8. Using your mouse, click in the blank field under the word Date. Make certain the date matches the date on the check; then press your Tab key.

9. Finish entering the information regarding Mr. Practice's co-payment (Figure 11-40). If you do not find a payment code in that field's drop-down box, go to the LISTS Menu and enter it in the same screen as you did the procedure codes. Just remember to indicate the code type as a payment code.

		Date	Pay/Adj Code	Who Paid	Description	Provider	Amount	Check Number
▶		3/3/2006	02	Practice, Harvey -Guarantor	Co-pay	JCH	-15.00	5533

Payments, Adjustments, And Comments:

[Apply] [New] [Delete] [Note]

☑ Calculate Estimates   [Update All] [Quick Receipt] [Print Receipt] [Print Claim] [Close] [Save]

FIGURE 11-40

Transaction Entry—co-payment entry.

10. Click on the Apply button in the lower left of this section of the screen. You will see a dialog box entitled Apply.

In the upper right corner of this screen, notice the box that says Unapplied-15.00 (Figure 11-41). This indicates that you have received $15.00 but you have not yet credited this payment to a specific charge. Unless the manager in your health care facility instructs you differently, the co-payment is always applied to the E/M code charge. Therefore, go ahead and enter $15.00 into the box under the heading This Payment, on the line with the charge for code 99201—the CPT code for the office visit.

FIGURE 11-41

Apply Payment to Charges.

Apply Payment to Charges

Payment From: G
For: Practice, Harvey

Unapplied
-15.00

	Date From	Document	Procedure	Charge	Balance	Payor Total	This Payment
	3/3/2006	0410240000	99201	46.00	46.00	0.00	0.00
	3/3/2006	0410240000	45378	145.00	145.00	0.00	0.00

There are 2 charge entries.   [Apply To Oldest] [Close] [Help]

11. Click on the Close button on the bottom right on this dialog box. You are now back in the Transaction Entry dialog box.

Now take a minute and *CHECK, DOUBLE-CHECK, and TRIPLE-CHECK* what you have entered into *all* fields in comparison with what you see on the patient's documentation. Capitals, lowercase letters, numbers, punctuation, and spaces are all important. It must match *exactly*. Information from these screens will be placed in the appropriate boxes on health insurance claim form CMS-1500. When you are certain that everything is correct, then

Click on the Save Transactions button.

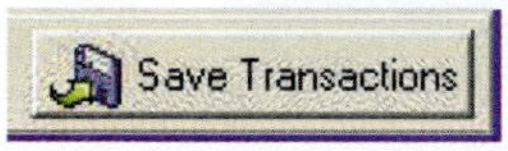

[Save Transactions]

Printing a Receipt

1. Click on the Print Receipt button in the center, along the bottom of the Transaction Entry dialog box.

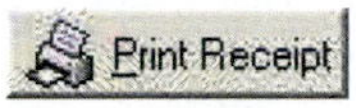

[Print Receipt]

You are going to use this printout to double-check your work. In your office, you will print this out when a patient would like a copy of all the charges and payments related to this visit for his or her records.

2. Click once on Walkout Receipt (All Transactions) to highlight it and click on OK (Figure 11-42).

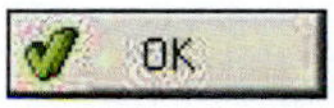

[OK]

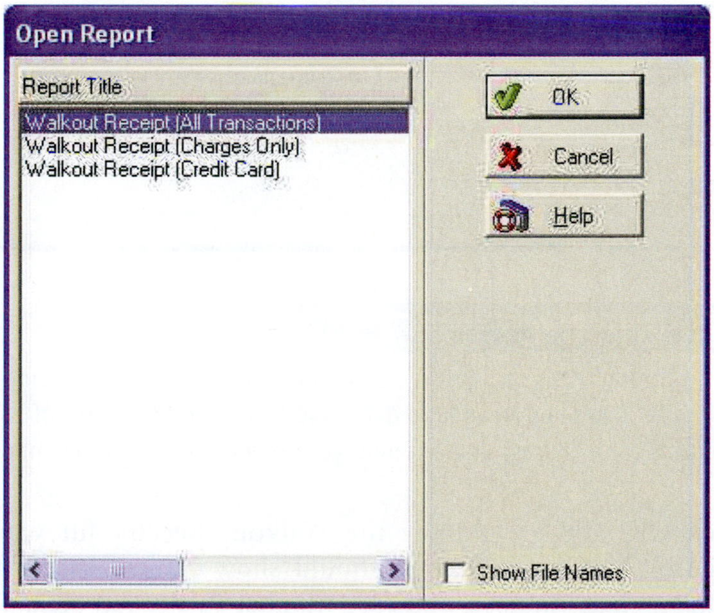

FIGURE 11-42
Open Report dialog box.

3. You should always check the report on the screen first (Figure 11-43). Then you can make certain it is the correct report for the correct patient with the correct information, rather than waiting until the printout shows you made an error.

Click on Start.

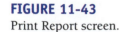

FIGURE 11-43
Print Report screen.

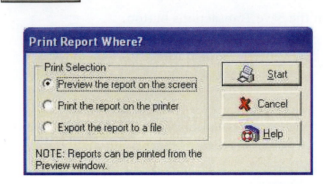

4. Make certain the dates you enter match the dates of the transactions you want to show on your receipt (Figure 11-44). Make certain you take your time and check the dates.

Date From Range: 03/03/2006 ▼   to   03/03/2006 ▼

FIGURE 11-44
Data Selection Questions box.

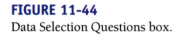

IMPORTANT NOTE

If you go through this too quickly, and you click OK without noticing that the computer has filled in today's date, and that is *not* the date of the transactions (procedures) you entered, your receipt will have nothing on it.

---

5. Click OK. You should see the Walkout Receipt fill your screen (Figure 11-45). The receipt should show Harvey Practice's name, address, chart number, and case number in the top area. The main section should indicate the date each procedure was performed, the description, the CPT code for each procedure, the related diagnosis (ICD-9-CM) code, and the amount charged for each procedure. You should also see Mr. Practice's co-payment of $15.00. Either on the screen, or from the printout, match every piece of data to the patient registration form and the superbill for Mr. Practice's visit.

Family Doctors Associates
123 Main Street • Anytown, FL 32711
(407) 555-1200

Page 1

Patient:	Harvey N. Practice 841 Rabbit Way Cityville, FL 32901

Chart #: PRAHA000
Case #: 8

Instructions:
Complete the patient information portion of your insurance claim form. Attach this bill, signed and dated, and all other bills pertaining to the claim. If you have a deductible policy, hold your claim forms until you have met your deductible. Mail directly to your insurance carrier.

Date	Description	Procedure	Modify	Dx 1	Dx 2	Dx 3	Dx 4	Units	Charge
3/3/2006	Office visit-focused	99201		V16.0				1	46.00
3/3/2006	Colonoscopy-diag	45378		V16.0				1	145.00
3/3/2006	Patient Payment Check	02						1	-15.00

Provider Information

Provider Name: James C. Healer, MD
License: 1234567890
Insurance PIN:
NoxPIN: 3452331123

Total Charges:	$191.00
Total Payments:	-$15.00
Total Adjustments:	$0.00
Total Due This Week:	$176.00
Total Account Balance:	$176.00

Assigned Release: I hereby authorize payment of medical benefits to the physician for the services described above. I also authorize the release of any information necessary to process this claim.

Patient Signature: _____   Date: _____

FIGURE 11-45
Walkout Receipt for Harvey Practice.

6. When you are ready, click on the Print button at the top of the screen (it is a drawing of a printer). If you need to make any corrections, do so before printing. When you are finished, click on the Close button on the bottom right of the Transaction Entry dialog box. Your receipt should look like Figure 11-45. If you notice any errors in what you have entered, go to the original screen where you entered that information by clicking Edit. Then just rekey in the data correctly and resave that screen. (More on correcting errors in Appendix D: NDCMedisoft Advance Issues & Answers.)

Creating a Health Insurance Claim Form

Now that all the information on Mr. Practice's visit has been entered and proofed for accuracy, you need to create the health insurance claim form (CMS-1500). This will be sent electronically from your health care facility, most of the time. However, for your classwork, you will be printing the claims on paper, so that you can review them more carefully.

1. Go to the ACTIVITIES Menu and choose Claim Management. You will see a dialog box (Figure 11-46).

FIGURE 11-46
Claim Management screen.

Claim Management
Search: [   ]   Sort By: Claim Number ▼   List Only...   Change Status   ◄ ◄ ► ► ► ↻

	Claim Number	Chart Num	Carrier 1	Status 1	Media 1	Batch 1	Bill Date 1	EDI Receiver 1	Carrier
►									

2. Click on the Create Claims button on the bottom of the dialog box, toward the left.

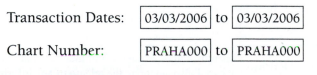

You will get another dialog box, titled Create Claims (Figure 11-47).

3. The first section of this dialog box requires you to enter a range of transaction dates and chart numbers. Here, you will be creating the claim form for Mr. Practice's most recent visit only, so the range will be only the date on his superbill and his chart number. Enter the information:

Transaction Dates: 03/03/2006 to 03/03/2006

Chart Number: PRAHA000 to PRAHA000

IMPORTANT NOTE

You must complete both parts of the range, even though the information is the same.

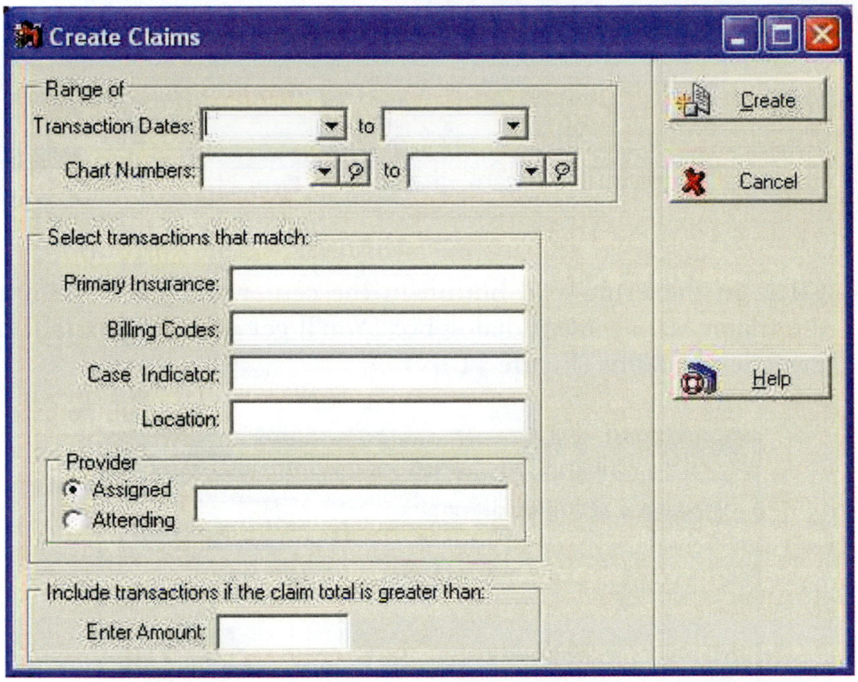

FIGURE 11-47
Create Claims dialog box.

4. For creating this claim, you do not need to complete any other fields in this dialog box, so click the Create button on the upper right section. However, when you are working, if you are going to create several claims at once (to be efficient and save time), you might create all the claims for one insurance carrier. Then, you would also complete the primary insurance field, for example.

IMPORTANT NOTE

If you get a dialog box that says

> Information

no new claims were created. If you expected some to be created, check the following items:

> Go back and check all your information. Chances are good that the dates you entered in your Create Claims Transaction Dates don't match the dates of the actual procedures entered in your Transaction Entry dialog box.

---

5. If everything is correct, you should now see your claim listed in the Claim Management dialog box (Figure 11-48). You will see the claim number assigned by the computer, along with the chart number for the patient (PRAHA000) and the Carrier 1 code (MCG00) assigned to the insurance carrier. You should also see the column titled Media 1 with Paper shown. This indicates that the claim created will be printed rather than sent electronically. Click once on this line that lists the claim you want to print out.

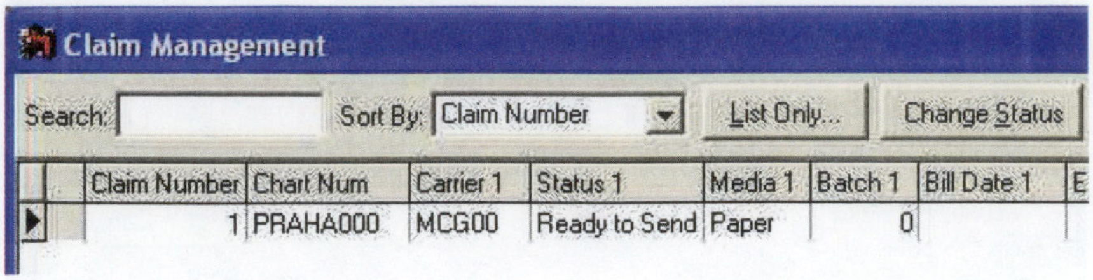

FIGURE 11-48
Claim Management screen.

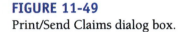

6. Click on the Print/Send button in the center along the bottom of the Claim Management dialog box. You'll get a dialog box that says Print/Send Claims (Figure 11-49).

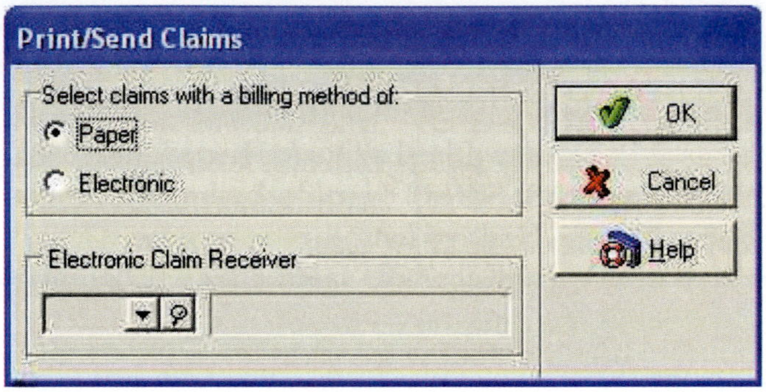

FIGURE 11-49
Print/Send Claims dialog box.

7. Click on the OK button on the right side of the dialog box. You'll get a dialog box that says Open Report (Figure 11-50). Choose the form depending on what type of printer you are using. If you pick any option with "W/Form" next to it the actual CMS-1500 form will print with your patient's information, rather than just the information alone. It is much easier to understand it all when you can see all the data you have entered, placed into the actual CMS-1500 form.

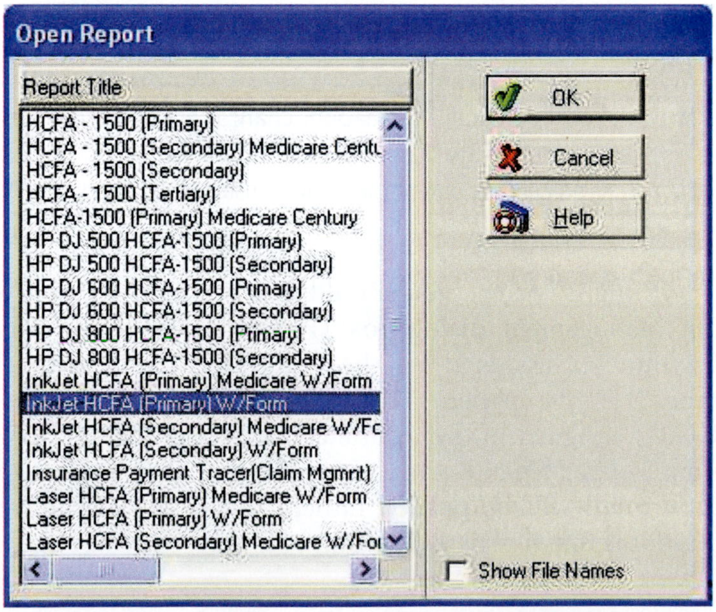

FIGURE 11-50
Open Report screen.

IMPORTANT NOTE

The HCFA-1500 form is now called the CMS-1500. However, it often takes time for all the computer applications and organizations to catch up. The form itself has not changed, so don't worry about which name is used.

8. Click on the OK button on the right side of the dialog box. It's not time for the form yet. Another dialog box with more questions appears (Figure 11-51).

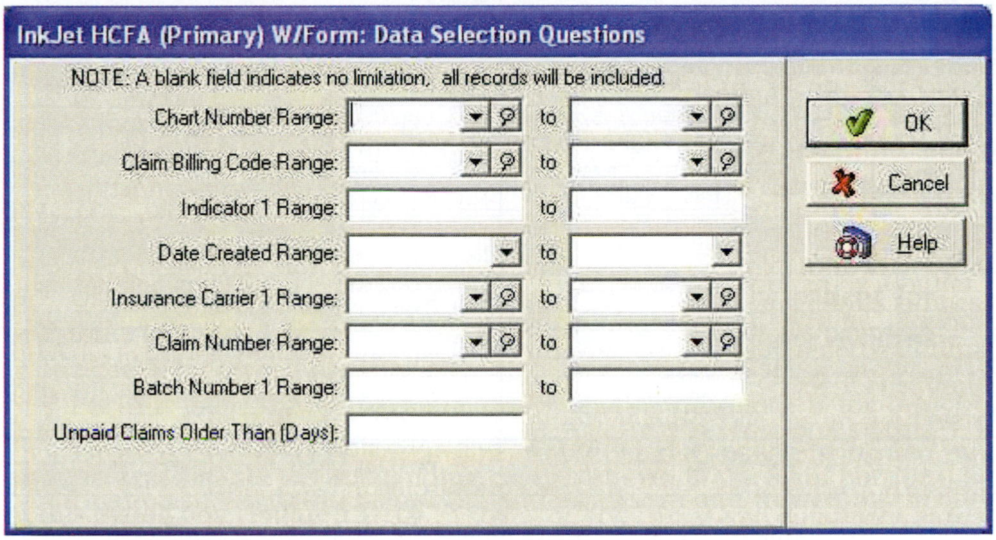

FIGURE 11-51
Data Selection screen.

9. You must enter information on both sides of Chart Number Range. For our purposes, this is the only field in this dialog box that you will fill in. Click on the OK button.

   Finally, your claim form should appear on the screen. It is a good idea to scroll down and look through all the information on the screen to see if you notice anything incorrect. If so, close this screen, delete this existing claim form, go back and make the appropriate corrections, and create a new claim form for this patient.

IMPORTANT NOTE

NDCMedisoft Advanced does not automatically update an existing claim form with changes made after the claim form has been created. Therefore, you must delete the old claim form and create a new one to show the changes that were made.

10. When you are ready, go ahead and print the form by clicking on the Print button along the top of the dialog box, near the center. Your printout should look like the form you see in Figure 11-52.

    Good job!

PLEASE
DO NOT
STAPLE
IN THIS
AREA

MCGRAW INSURANCE CO.
P.O. BOX 5544
WILSON, OH 45533

P

| | PICA | | | | | | HEALTH INSURANCE CLAIM FORM | | PICA | |

HEALTH INSURANCE CLAIM FORM

| 1. MEDICARE (Medicare #) | MEDICAID (Medicaid #) | CHAMPUS (Sponsor's SSN) | CHAMPVA (VA File #) | GROUP HEALTH PLAN [X] (SSN OR ID) | FECA BLK LUNG (SSN) | OTHER (ID) | 1a. INSURED'S I.D. NUMBER (FOR PROGRAM IN ITEM 1) 533966654 |

| 2. PATIENT'S NAME (Last Name, First Name, Middle Initial) PRACTICE, HARVEY N | 3. PATIENT'S BIRTH DATE MM 12 DD 12 YY 87 SEX M [X] F [ ] | 4. INSURED'S NAME (Last Name, First Name, Middle Initial) PRACTICE, ROGER P |

2nd Fold

| 5. PATIENT'S ADDRESS (No., Street) 841 RABBIT WAY | 6. PATIENT RELATIONSHIP TO INSURED Self [ ] Spouse [ ] Child [X] Other [ ] | 7. INSURED'S ADDRESS (No., Street) 327 MAIN STREET |

| CITY CITYVILLE | STATE FL | 8. PATIENT STATUS Single [X] Married [ ] Other [ ] | CITY OURTOWN | STATE FL |

| ZIP CODE 32901 | TELEPHONE (Include Area Code) (407) 555 7317 | Employed [ ] Full-Time Student [X] Part-Time Student [ ] | ZIP CODE 32706 | TELEPHONE (INCLUDE AREA CODE) (407) 555 6985 |

| 9. OTHER INSURED'S NAME (Last Name, First Name, Middle Initial) | 10. IS PATIENT'S CONDITION RELATED TO: | 11. INSURED'S POLICY GROUP OR FECA NUMBER TS9023 |

| a. OTHER INSURED'S POLICY OR GROUP NUMBER | a. EMPLOYMENT? (CURRENT OR PREVIOUS) YES [ ] NO [X] | a. INSURED'S DATE OF BIRTH MM 01 DD 07 YY 48 SEX M [X] F [ ] |

| b. OTHER INSURED'S DATE OF BIRTH MM DD YY SEX M [ ] F [ ] | b. AUTO ACCIDENT? PLACE (State) YES [ ] NO [X] | b. EMPLOYER'S NAME OR SCHOOL NAME PRIME INCORPORATED |

| c. EMPLOYER'S NAME OR SCHOOL NAME | c. OTHER ACCIDENT? YES [ ] NO [X] | c. INSURANCE PLAN NAME OR PROGRAM NAME MCGRAW HMO |

| d. INSURANCE PLAN NAME OR PROGRAM NAME | 10d. RESERVED FOR LOCAL USE | d. IS THERE ANOTHER HEALTH BENEFIT PLAN? YES [ ] NO [X] **if yes**, return to and complete item 9 a-d. |

READ BACK OF FORM BEFORE COMPLETING AND SIGNING THIS FORM.

| 12. PATIENT'S OR AUTHORIZED PERSON'S SIGNATURE. I authorize the release of any medical or other information necessary to process this claim. I also request payment of government benefits either to myself or to the party who accepts assignment below. SIGNED SIGNATURE ON FILE DATE 03/03/06 | 13. INSURED'S OR AUTHORIZED PERSON'S SIGNATURE. I authorize payment of medical benefits to the undersigned physician or supplier for services described below. SIGNED SIGNATURE ON FILE |

1st Fold

| 14. DATE OF CURRENT: ILLNESS (First symptom) OR INJURY (Accident) OR PREGNANCY(LMP) MM DD YY | 15. IF PATIENT HAS HAD SAME OR SIMILAR ILLNESS GIVE FIRST DATE MM DD YY | 16. DATES PATIENT UNABLE TO WORK IN CURRENT OCCUPATION FROM MM DD YY TO MM DD YY |

| 17. NAME OF REFERRING PHYSICIAN OR OTHER SOURCE MARK C. WELBY MD | 17a. I.D. NUMBER OF REFERRING PHYSICIAN 7766554 | 18. HOSPITALIZATION DATES RELATED TO CURRENT SERVICES FROM MM DD YY TO MM DD YY |

| 19. RESERVED FOR LOCAL USE | 20. OUTSIDE LAB? YES [ ] NO [X] $ CHARGES |

| 21. DIAGNOSIS OR NATURE OF ILLNESS OR INJURY (RELATE ITEMS 1,2,3 OR 4 TO ITEM 24E BY LINE) 1. V16.0   3. 2.   4. | 22. MEDICAID RESUBMISSION CODE ORIGINAL REF. NO. |
| | 23. PRIOR AUTHORIZATION NUMBER |

24. A DATE(S) OF SERVICE						B Place of Service	C Type of Service	D PROCEDURES, SERVICES, OR SUPPLIES (Explain Unusual Circumstances) CPT/HCPCS | MODIFIER	E DIAGNOSIS CODE	F $ CHARGES	G DAYS OR UNITS	H EPSDT Family Plan	I EMG	J COB	K RESERVED FOR LOCAL USE
From MM	DD	YY	To MM	DD	YY										
03	03	06	03	03	06	11		99201 |	1	46.00	1				HEALER
03	03	06	03	03	06	11		45378 |	1	145.00	1				HEALER

| 25. FEDERAL TAX I.D. NUMBER 3452331123 SSN [ ] EIN [X] | 26. PATIENT'S ACCOUNT NO. PRAHA000 10 | 27. ACCEPT ASSIGNMENT? (For govt. claims, see back) [X] YES [ ] NO | 28. TOTAL CHARGE $ 191.00 | 29. AMOUNT PAID $ | 30. BALANCE DUE $ 191.00 |

| 31. SIGNATURE OF PHYSICIAN OR SUPPLIER INCLUDING DEGREES OR CREDENTIALS (I certify that the statements on the reverse apply to this bill and are made a part thereof.) SIGNATURE ON FILE SIGNED DATE 12/30/03 | 32. NAME AND ADDRESS OF FACILITY WHERE SERVICES WERE RENDERED (If other than home or office) | 33. PHYSICIAN'S, SUPPLIER'S BILLING NAME, ADDRESS, ZIP CODE & PHONE# JAMES C. HEALER MD 123 MAIN STREET ANYTOWN, FL 32711 PIN# 6654321 GRP# |

FIGURE 11-52

CMS-1500 claim form for Harvey Practice.

SENDING CLAIMS ELECTRONICALLY

Most insurance carriers prefer claims to be submitted electronically rather than on paper via the regular mail. It is faster and more efficient for everyone concerned. Electronic claims are processed and paid more quickly, as we discussed earlier. In addition, electronic claims do not require paper, toner, postage, and time, thereby costing less to create and submit.

Electronic Data Interchange (EDI) is the electronic roadway used for businesses to exchange important documents. This is similar to the electronic pathway that e-mail travels when you send a letter. This type of electronic system is also used to communicate between an ATM (automatic teller machine), for example, and the bank's main computers when you want to withdraw some money. EDI, using HIPAA electronic transmission standards, is what is used to send your completed claim form to the insurance carrier, or to a health care clearinghouse.

Health care clearinghouses are used to assist health care providers in filing electronic claims. Basically, you send the claim form created in your computer program (such as NDCMedisoft Advanced, Intergy, or Medical Manager) electronically to the clearinghouse. Its computers then check the claim for missing information and legitimate diagnosis and procedure codes. They can also review the claim form for specific elements that may be required by particular insurance carriers. Then the clearinghouse will either return the claim to you with a report telling you of any problems, so you can correct the claim, or they will forward your correct claim electronically to the appropriate carrier for payment. Having this service will cost your health care facility extra money. There might be a sign-up fee, a monthly fee, and a per claim fee. Not all health care facilities use the services of an electronic claims processor. But whether they do or not, you still need to enter every piece of data correctly. In addition, if a claim comes back for correction, that will cost your office time and money. Clearinghouses do not provide the insurance coder and biller with a reason to do a sloppy job. They just help make the entire process more effective.

Your computer needs some information to send your claims electronically. Let's go through the process of setting this up.

1. Go to the LISTS Menu and choose EDI RECEIVERS. You will see the EDI Receiver List dialog box (Figure 11-53).

Key Terms

Electronic Data Interchange (EDI): The electronic system used to send health insurance claim forms, and other sensitive information, from one business to another in a protected manner.

Health Care Clearinghouses: A company that offers electronic processing services for health care claims.

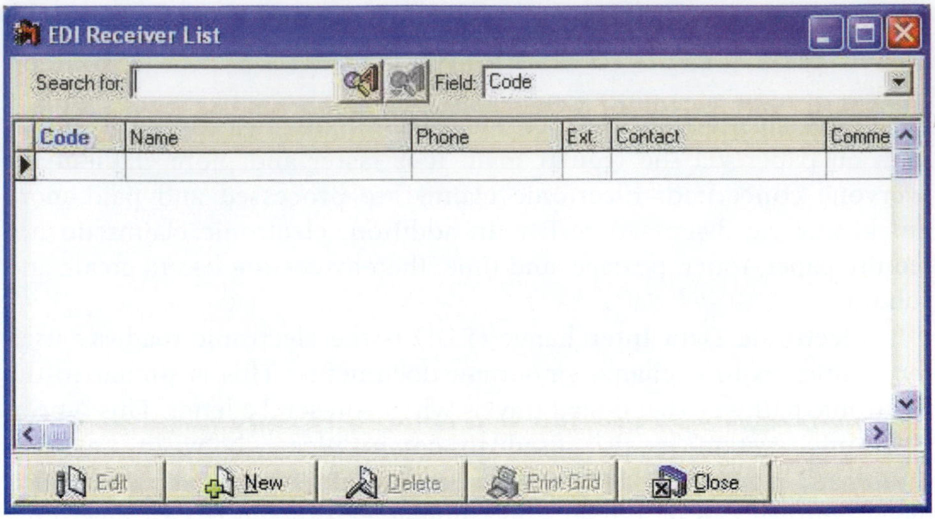

FIGURE 11-53
EDI Receiver List screen.

2. Click on the [New] button. A new dialog box opens (Figure 11-54). The clearinghouse with which your office is contracted will supply this information to you. Because we do not have a contract for our learning here, the idea is for you to understand about electronic claims and have you complete the information for the experience.

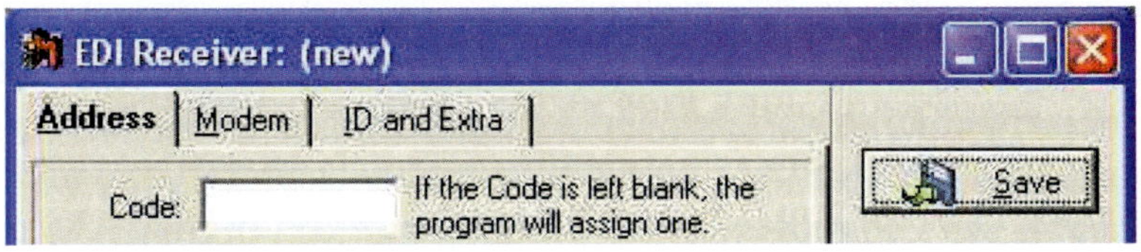

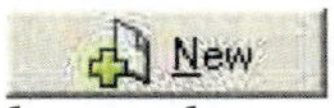

FIGURE 11-54
EDI Receiver: (new) screen.

3. Permit NDCMedisoft to assign the code for this receiver and use your mouse to click into the first field, Name. Key in the appropriate data (Figure 11-55).

Name:	NDC Health	
Street:	5222 E. Baseline Road	
	Suite 101	
City:	Gilbert	State: AZ
Zip Code:	85234	
Phone 1:	800-333-4747	
Phone 2:	800-334-4006	
Fax:	(Leave blank)	
Contact:	(Leave blank)	
Comment:	(Leave blank)	

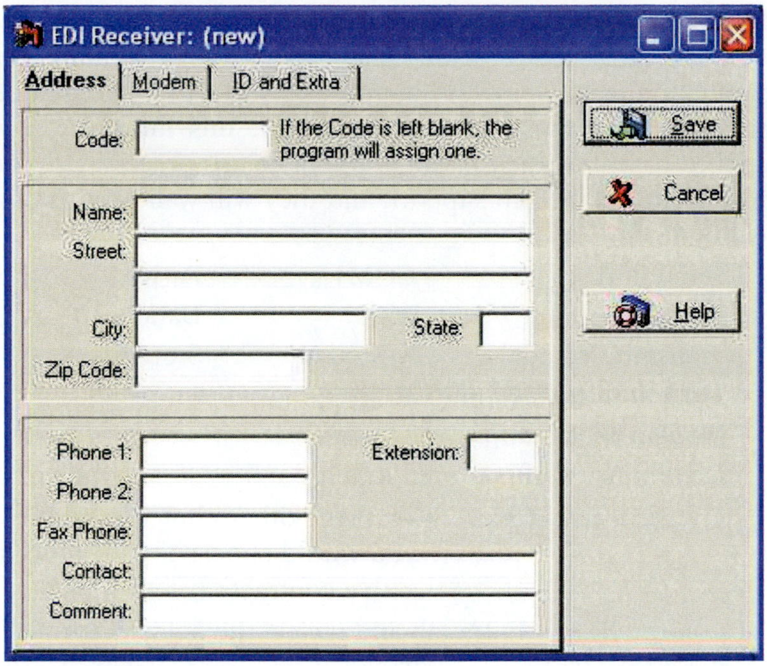

FIGURE 11-55
EDI Receiver Address screen.

4. Click on the Modem tab and look at the fields for data the computer will need (Figure 11-56).

Data Phone: This is the phone number used for transmittal.
Dialing Prefix: Some offices require the dialing of 9 for an outside line.
Dialing Suffix: Some offices require a code to be entered to track long distance calls.

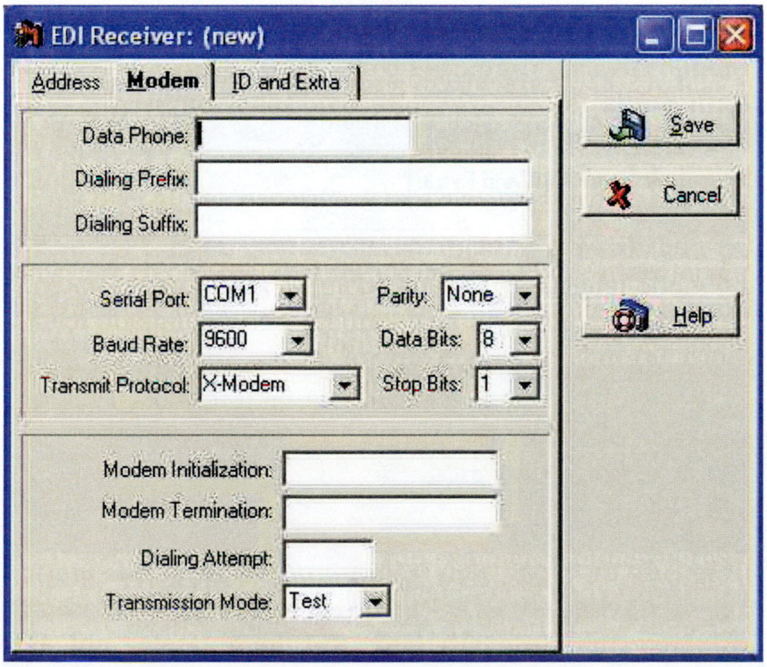

FIGURE 11-56
EDI Receiver Modem screen.

Most of you will find the rest of the information requested gobbledy-gook. In most cases, your office's technology administrator or information technology (IT) support person will take care of setting this up. If you must do it, don't worry; this information will be supplied to you by the clearinghouse or claims processor. If you need to, you can call its tech support, and they will walk you through this field-by-field.

Serial Port:	COM1	Parity:	None
Baud Rate:	9600	Data Bits:	8
Transmit Protocol:	X-Modem	Stop Bits:	1
Modem Initialization:	8		
Modem Termination:	(Leave blank)		
Dialing Attempt:	(Leave blank)		
Transmission Mode:	Test (the other choice is Active, which you would choose if your office had an active contract)		

5. Click on the ID and Extra tab and review the fields (Figure 11-57).

Submitter ID 1:	This is for a number that identifies the organization submitting the claim, so that the computer can recognize the account.
Submitter ID 2:	This is a second or an alternate ID number.
Submitter Password 1:	This is the password that would accompany the Submitter ID 1 number.
Submitter Password 2:	This is the password that would accompany the Submitter ID 2 number.
Program File:	This identifies the code for the software application.

FIGURE 11-57
EDI Receiver ID and Extra screen.

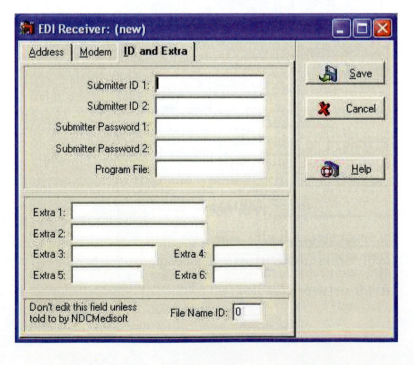

Now take a minute and *CHECK, DOUBLE-CHECK, and TRIPLE-CHECK* what you have entered into the first screen in comparison with what you see in this book. Capitals, lowercase letters, numbers, punctuation, and spaces are all important. It must match *exactly*. Information from these screens will tell the computer how to send health insurance claim form CMS-1500 electronically and make certain it gets to the correct place. When you are certain that everything is correct, then

Click on the Save button.

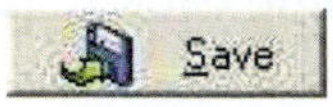

You will see that NDC Health is now shown on the EDI Receiver List. Click the Close button on the lower right hand side of the dialog box.

For insurance carriers that accept electronic claims, you must make certain that the correct information is entered accurately into the computer for each carrier. This is done in the carrier's listing in your computer. Let's take a look.

1. Go to the LISTS Menu and choose Insurance Carrier.
2. Click once on the listing for McGraw Insurance Co. and click the Edit button. Let's review this listing, which we put in earlier, and look at the fields that would change for electronic submission of claims, rather than paper.

   Address tab: Nothing changes on this screen.

   Options tab: (Figure 11-58) The one field that would change on this tab is at the very bottom of the screen. If you were converting from paper claims to electronic claims with this carrier, you would change Default Billing Method from Paper to Electronic.

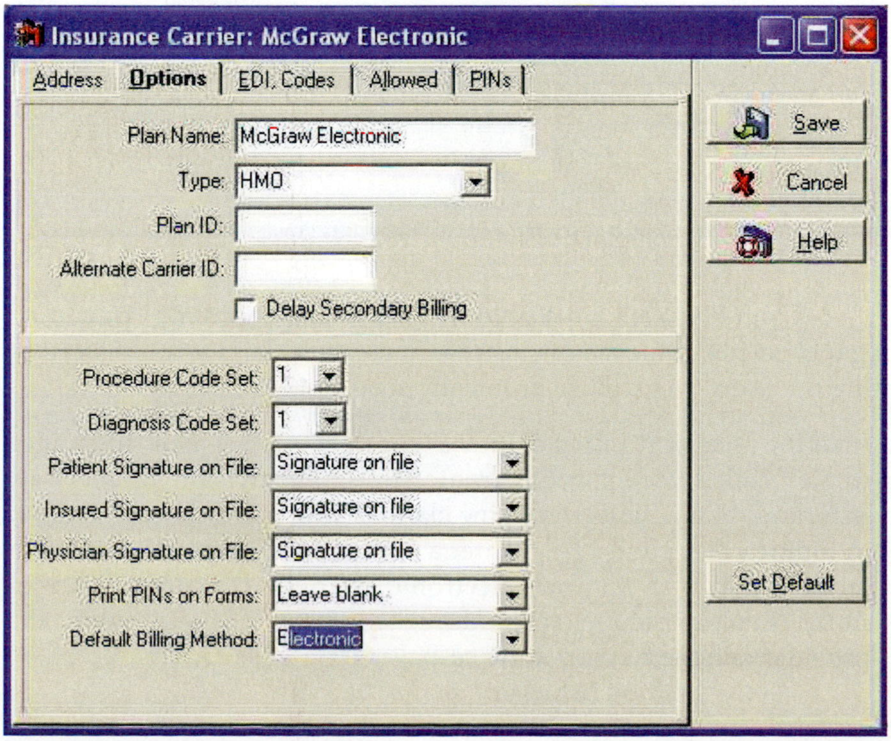

FIGURE 11-58
Insurance Carrier Options screen.

EDI, Codes tab: With a carrier accepting paper claims, this screen would be left blank (Figure 11-59). However, if you were going to file electronic claims, this screen would need to be completed with information given to you by the insurance carrier. The first field, EDI Receiver, would be chosen from those you have entered in your EDI Receiver list, as you did with NDC Health. If the receiver were not already in the system, you would need to go to the LISTS Menu and enter the receiver in the EDI Receiver List first, then come back here and choose it from the drop-down menu.

Because we do not have a current contract with an EDI Receiver, we will not change any of the above fields. However, now that you have seen it and gone through it, this review should help you actually do it in the office if you need to.

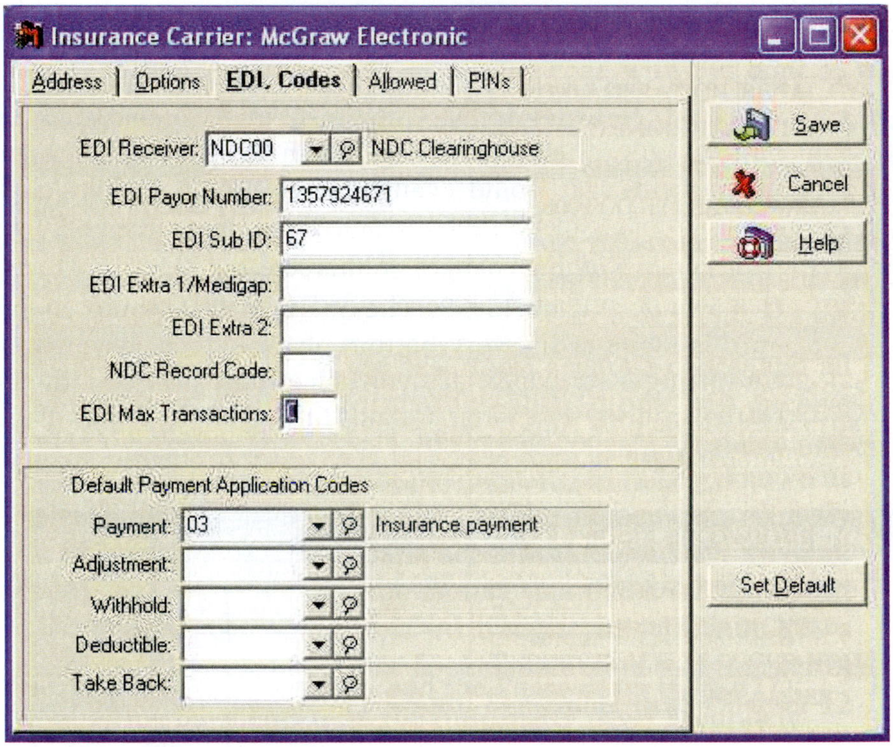

FIGURE 11-59
EDI Codes Screen.

The Claim Management screen will also change were we converting from paper to electronic claims. After you create a claim form, instead of printing the form, you will electronically send it. Let's go through it.

1. Imagine that you entered into a contract with a new insurance carrier called McGraw Electronic. It is the division of McGraw Insurance that accepts electronic claims. Now, using the information in Figures 11-60 and 11-61, enter a new patient, Bridgette Sweet and create a case with McGraw Electronic as Policy 1 insurance carrier. Enter the transaction (procedure) code for her visit with the provider and the receipt of the co-pay.

PATIENT REGISTRATION FORM

RESPONSIBLE PARTY			DATE *October 12, 2006*	
LAST NAME *Sweet*	FIRST NAME *Bridgette*	MI	SOCIAL SECURITY # *157-37-4290*	DATE OF BIRTH *July 16, 1974*

ADDRESS *397 Electronic Avenue*	CITY *Cityville*	STATE *FL*	ZIP CODE *32901*	SEX *F*	MARITAL STATUS *Single*

HOME PHONE *407-555-1507*	WORK PHONE *407-555-4451*	REFERRED BY:

EMPLOYER INFORMATION	WORK STATUS: (FULL-TIME) PART-TIME STUDENT

COMPANY NAME *Prime Incorporated*	ADDRESS *5580 Rehearsal Lane*	CITY, STATE, ZIP *Our Town, FL 32704*

DEPENDENT INFORMATION

DEPENDENT'S NAME	DEPENDENT'S NAME	DEPENDENT'S NAME
RELATIONSHIP / DATE OF BIRTH	RELATIONSHIP / DATE OF BIRTH	RELATIONSHIP / DATE OF BIRTH
SOC. SEC. # / SEX	SOC. SEC. # / SEX	SOC. SEC. # / SEX
EMPLOYER / WORK PHONE	EMPLOYER / WORK PHONE	EMPLOYER / WORK PHONE

INSURANCE INFORMATION–PRIMARY POLICY

COMPANY NAME *McGraw Electronic*	ADDRESS *P.O. Box 5544*	CITY, STATE, ZIP *Wilson, OH 45533*
PHONE NUMBER *800-555-6654*	ID OR POLICY NUMBER *157374290A*	GROUP NUMBER OR NAME *PT1023*
INSURED'S NAME (IF DIFFERENT)	SOCIAL SECURITY #	RELATIONSHIP TO RESPONSIBLE PARTY
INSURED'S ADDRESS (IF DIFFERENT)	INSURED'S CITY, STATE, ZIP	INSURED'S PHONE NUMBER

INSURANCE INFORMATION–SECONDARY POLICY

COMPANY NAME	ADDRESS	CITY, STATE, ZIP
PHONE NUMBER	ID OR POLICY NUMBER	GROUP NUMBER OR NAME
INSURED'S NAME (IF DIFFERENT)	SOCIAL SECURITY #	RELATIONSHIP TO RESPONSIBLE PARTY
INSURED'S ADDRESS (IF DIFFERENT)	INSURED'S CITY, STATE, ZIP	INSURED'S PHONE NUMBER

OTHER INFORMATION

ALLERGIES	REASON FOR TODAY'S VISIT *Scraped shoulder*
PATIENT'S SIGNATURE *Bridgette Sweet*	DATE *10/12/06*

FOR OFFICE USE ONLY

CO-PAY $ *15.00*	CO-INSURANCE $	DEDUCTIBLE $

CHECK ☒ # *4571*   CASH ☐   CHARGE ☐   PAID IN FULL ☐

ASSIGNED PROVIDER *J. Healer, MD*

FIGURE 11-60
Bridgette Sweet's new patient registration form.

Family Doctors Associates
123 Main Street • Anytown, FL 32711
(407) 555-1200

Date: *October 12, 2006*   Attending Physician: *J. Healer, MD*

Patient Name: *Bridgette Sweet*

CPT DESCRIPTION	CPT DESCRIPTION	CPT DESCRIPTION
OFFICE/HOSPITAL	**PATHOLOGY/LAB/RADIOLOGY**	**PROCEDURES/TESTS**
☐ 99201 OFFICE-NEW; FOCUSED	☐ 73100 X-RAY WRIST TWO VIEWS	☐ 12011 SIMPLE SUTURE, FACE
☒ 99202 OFFICE-NEW; EXPANDED	☐ 73590 X-RAY TIBIA/FIBULA, TWO	☐ 29125 SPLINT-SHORT ARM
☐ 99203 OFFICE-NEW; DETAILED	☐ 73600 X-RAY ANKLE TWO VIEWS	☐ 29355 WALKER CAST-LONG LEG
☐ 99204 OFFICE-NEW; COMPREHEN	☐ 76085 MAMMOGRAM-COMP DET	☐ 29540 STRAPPING-ANKLE
☐ 99205 OFFICE-NEW; COMPREHEN	☐ 76092 MAMMOGRAM SCREENING	☐ 45378 COLONOSCOPY-DIAGNOSTIC
☐ 99211 OFFICE-ESTB; MINIMAL	☐ 80050 BLOOD TEST-GEN HEALTH	☐ 45385 COLONOSCOPY-POLYP REM.
☐ 99212 OFFICE-ESTB; FOCUSED	☐ 80061 BLOOD TEST-LIPID PANEL	☐ 50390 ASPIRATION, RENAL CYST
☐ 99213 OFFICE-ESTB; EXPANDED	☐ 82947 BLOOD TEST-GLUCOSE	☐ 90703 TETANUS INJECTION
☐ 99214 OFFICE-ESTB; DETAILED	☐ 83718 BLOOD TEST-HDL	☐ 92081 VISUAL FIELD EXAM
☐ 99215 OFFICE-ESTB; COMPREHEN	☐ 85025 BLOOD TEST-CBC	☐ 93000 ECG, 12 LEADS, W/RPT
☐ 99281 EMER DEPT; FOCUSED	☐ 86403 STREP TEST, QUICK	☐ 93015 TREADMILL STRESS TEST
☐ 90844 COUNSELING—50 MIN.	☐ 87430 ENZY IMMUNOASSAY-STREP	☐ 99173 VISUAL ACUITY SCREEN

ICD DESCRIPTION	ICD DESCRIPTION	ICD DESCRIPTION
☐ 034.0 STREP THROAT	☐ 522 LOW RED BLOOD COUNT	☐ V01.5 RABIES EXPOSURE
☐ 042 HUMAN IMMUNO VIRUS	☐ 538.8 STOMACH PAIN	☐ V16.0 FAMILY HISTORY-COLON
☐ 250.51 DIABETES W/VISION	☐ 643 HYPEREMESIS	☐ V16.3 FAMILY HISTORY-BREAST
☐ 250.80 DIABETES, TYPE II	☐ 707.14 ULCER OF HEEL/MID FOOT	☐ V20.2 WELL CHILD
☐ 307.51 BULIMIA NON-ORGANIC	☐ 788.30 ENURESIS	☐ V22.0 PREGNANCY-FIRST NORM
☐ 354.0 CARPAL TUNNEL SYNDROME	☐ 815.00 FRACTURE, HAND	☐ V22.1 PREGNANCY-NORMAL
☐ 362.01 RETINOPATHY (DIABETIC)	☐ 823.20 FRACTURE, TIBIA	☐ E816.2 MOTORCYCLE ACCT
☐ 401.9 HYPERTENSION, UNSPEC	☐ 831.00 DISLOCATION, SHOULDER	☐ E826.1 FALL FROM BICYCLE
☐ 482.30 PNEUMONIA	☐ 845.00 SPRAINED ANKLE	☐ E849.0 PLACE OF OCCUR-HOME
☐ 490 BRONCHITIS, UNSPECIFIED	☐ 880.03 OPEN WOUND UPPER ARM	☐ E881.0 FALL FROM LADDER
☐ 493.92 ASTHMA, UNSPECIFIED	☒ 912.0 ABRASION, SHOULDER	☐ E906.0 DOG BITE

FOLLOW UP

PRN _____

WEEKS _____

NXT APPT. _____

TIME _____

FIGURE 11-61
The superbill for Bridgette Sweet's encounter with Dr. Healer.

2. Go to the ACTIVITIES Menu, choose Claim Management, and create the claim form for Ms. Sweet. Everything is the same as you did earlier in this chapter. The new claim is now shown in the Claim Management dialog box (Figure 11-62). You will see the claim number assigned by the computer, along with the chart number for the patient (SWEBR000) and the Carrier 1 code (MCG01) assigned to the new insurance carrier. Take a look at the column titled Media 1 with EDI shown. This indicates that the claim created will be sent electronically. You can compare this with the claim shown above it in Figure 11-62. See how that claim's Media 1 listing shows us that that claim form will be printed on paper. Click once on Bridgette Sweet's claim.

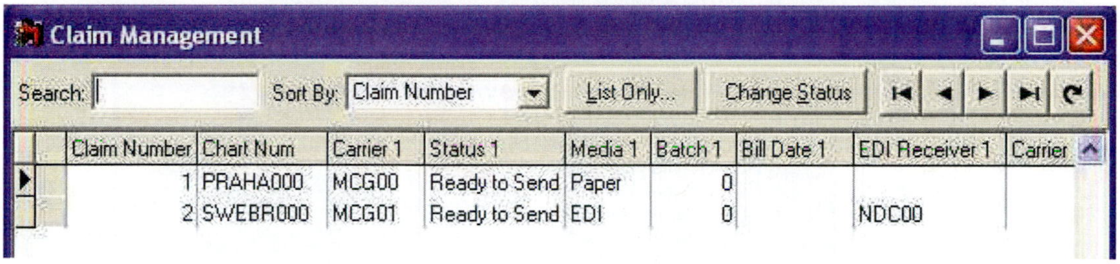

FIGURE 11-62
Claim Management screen.

3. Click on the Print/Send button in the center along the bottom of the Claim Management dialog box. You will get a dialog box titled Print/Send Claims (Figure 11-63). Make certain that the Electronic radio button is chosen and that the correct EDI Receiver is selected from the drop-down menu.

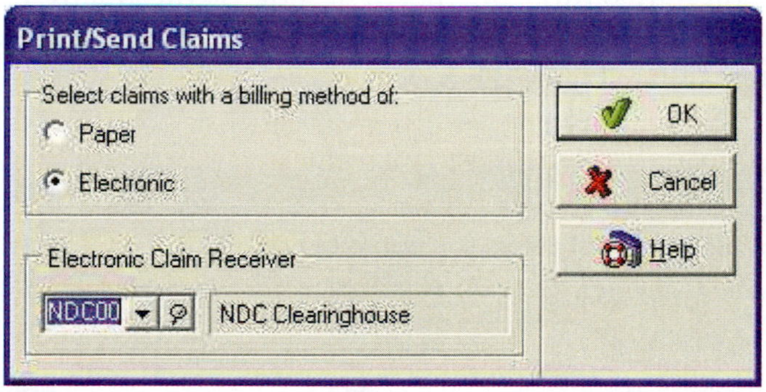

FIGURE 11-63
Print/Send Claims screen.

Note: If your Print/Send claims dialog box does not look exactly like Figure 11-63, check the following two items before continuing:
   a. Double-check that Bridgette Sweet's insurance carrier is identified as McGraw Electronic and not McGraw Insurance.
   b. Go to the LISTS Menu and select Insurance Carriers. Select McGraw Electronic, click Edit and open the listing. On the Options Tab screen, the Default Billing Method should show Electronic. Then, on the EDI Codes Tab screen, the EDI receiver should show NDC Clearinghouse. Check pages 269–270 of this text for more instructions.
   c. If you had to amend either of the above, you will need to delete the claim form you created for Bridgette Sweet and create a new one. The software will not update an existing claim.

4. Click the OK button on the right side of the dialog box. You will get a dialog box that says Open Report (Figure 11-64).

FIGURE 11-64
Open Report screen.

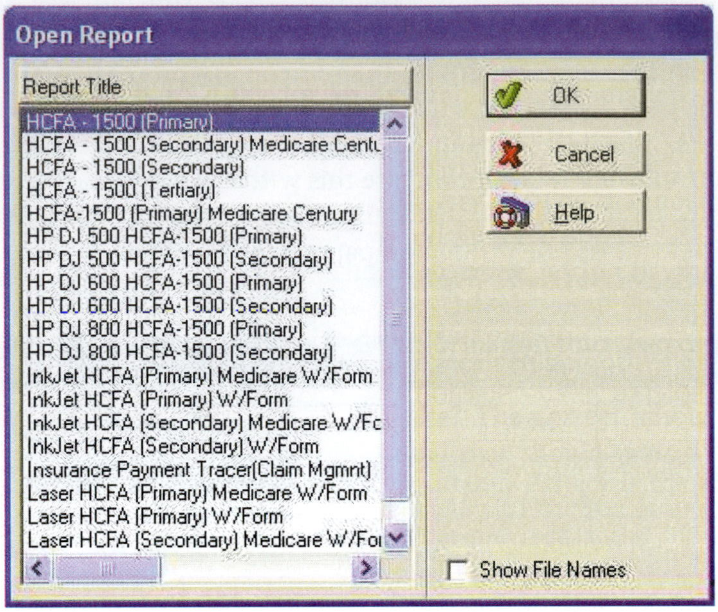

5. Choose the form, depending on the type of insurance carrier you are transmitting to—Medicare or other; Primary, Secondary, or Tertiary payer. (Remember, the HCFA-1500 form is now called the CMS-1500.)
6. Click the OK button on the right side of the dialog box. It's not time for the form yet. There is another dialog box with more questions first (Figure 11-65).

FIGURE 11-65
Data Selection screen.

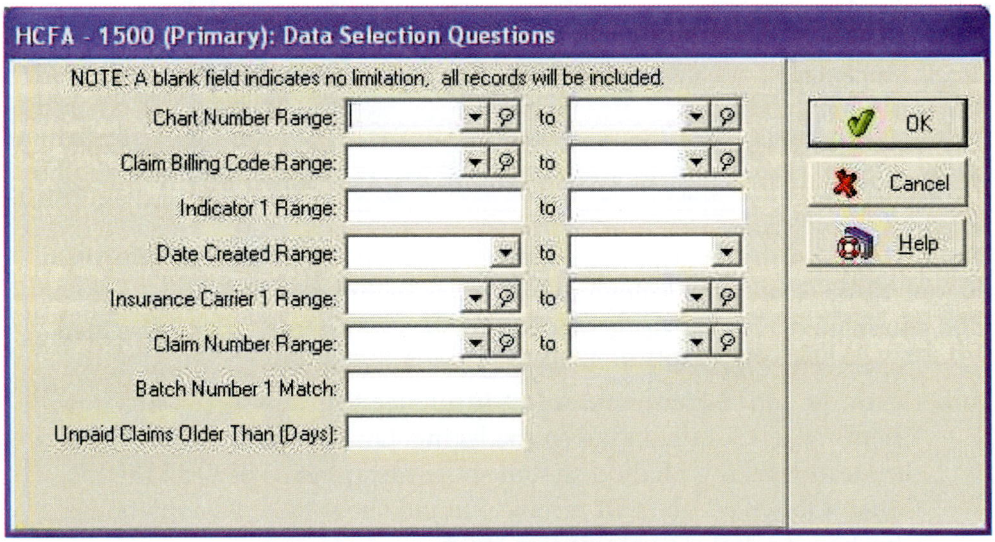

7. Enter the information next to the Chart Number Range for Bridgette Sweet's Claim SWEBR000 to SWEBR000.

8. Click on the OK button.

Finally, your claim form should appear on the screen. It is a good idea to scroll down and look through all the information on the screen to see if you notice anything that is incorrect. If so, close this screen, go back and correct any errors that you noticed, delete this claim form, and create a new claim form. Remember, NDCMedisoft Advanced does not automatically update existing claim forms with new or changed information. Therefore, you must delete the claim with the wrong information and create a new one once the data has been fixed.

9. When the claim form is correct, you then click on the Print/Send button to send this claim form electronically to either the clearinghouse or the insurance carrier.

Now you are familiar with the way to send a claim form electronically.

837 HEALTH CARE PROFESSIONAL CLAIM

In Chapter 2, you learned about HIPAA's Privacy Rule. Another portion of HIPAA created transaction sets as standards for electronically sending claim and encounter data. The 837 Professional is one of the transaction sets used to submit provider data to a third party payer and is the electronic version of the paper CMS-1500 claim form. Data used to create a CMS-1500 form correlates to the 837 Professional form when submitting electronically. The UB-92 claim form converts to its electronic version, the 837 Institutional.

CHAPTER SUMMARY

While converting the provider's diagnoses and procedures into their proper codes is very important, so is the creation of the claim form. After all, if the information is not entered correctly into the computer, all of your coding work is a waste of time. There are many different brands of patient accounting software programs. We used NDCMedisoft Advanced in this book. Now that you have completed this chapter, you understand more than how to key information into a computer program—you understand all the reasons why that information is important to the claims and reimbursement process. The coding (finding the best codes) and the billing (entering of the data into the patient accounting software application) go hand in hand.

Chapter Review

On the following pages, you will find patient registration forms and superbills for five of the patients you worked with in Chapter 9:

1. Marvin Doe
2. Patience Loyal
3. Mary Lou Sweet
4. Tex T. Books
5. Sarah Student

Use their information to rehearse what you have learned about entering information into NDCMedisoft Advanced and creating claim forms. Print out the claim forms for each of these patients.

IMPORTANT NOTE

Watch the dates carefully.

Don't forget to check, double-check, and triple-check what you have entered into every field of every screen in comparison with what you see on the patient registration forms and superbills. Capitals, lowercase letters, numbers, punctuation, and spaces are all important. It must match exactly.

1. Marvin Doe patient registration form

RESPONSIBLE PARTY			DATE *February 27, 2006*		
LAST NAME *Doe*	FIRST NAME *Marvin*	MI	SOCIAL SECURITY # *944-73-8929*		DATE OF BIRTH *July 6, 1964*
ADDRESS *342 Fifth Avenue*	CITY *Cityville*	STATE *FL*	ZIP CODE *32901*	SEX *M*	MARITAL STATUS *Married*
HOME PHONE *407-555-9903*	WORK PHONE *407-555-4451*		REFERRED BY: *Mark C. Welby, M. D.*		

EMPLOYER INFORMATION		WORK STATUS:	(FULL-TIME) PART-TIME STUDENT	
COMPANY NAME *Prime Incorporated*	ADDRESS *5580 Rehearsal Lane*		CITY, STATE, ZIP *Our Town, FL 32704*	

DEPENDENT INFORMATION					
DEPENDENT'S NAME *Mitzi*		DEPENDENT'S NAME		DEPENDENT'S NAME	
RELATIONSHIP *Wife*	DATE OF BIRTH *May 6, 1965*	RELATIONSHIP	DATE OF BIRTH	RELATIONSHIP	DATE OF BIRTH
SOC. SEC. # *251-55-1912*	SEX *F*	SOC. SEC. #	SEX	SOC. SEC. #	SEX
EMPLOYER *Jones & Co.*	WORK PHONE *407-555-1000*	EMPLOYER	WORK PHONE	EMPLOYER	WORK PHONE

INSURANCE INFORMATION–PRIMARY POLICY		
COMPANY NAME *McGraw Insurance Co.*	ADDRESS *P. O. Box 5544*	CITY, STATE, ZIP *Wilson, OH 45533*
PHONE NUMBER *800-555-6654*	ID OR POLICY NUMBER *944738929A*	GROUP NUMBER OR NAME *PT1023*
INSURED'S NAME (IF DIFFERENT)	SOCIAL SECURITY #	RELATIONSHIP TO RESPONSIBLE PARTY
INSURED'S ADDRESS (IF DIFFERENT)	INSURED'S CITY, STATE, ZIP	INSURED'S PHONE NUMBER

INSURANCE INFORMATION–SECONDARY POLICY		
COMPANY NAME	ADDRESS	CITY, STATE, ZIP
PHONE NUMBER	ID OR POLICY NUMBER	GROUP NUMBER OR NAME
INSURED'S NAME (IF DIFFERENT)	SOCIAL SECURITY #	RELATIONSHIP TO RESPONSIBLE PARTY
INSURED'S ADDRESS (IF DIFFERENT)	INSURED'S CITY, STATE, ZIP	INSURED'S PHONE NUMBER

OTHER INFORMATION	
ALLERGIES	REASON FOR TODAY'S VISIT *diabetic checkup*
PATIENT'S SIGNATURE *Marvin D. Doe*	DATE *2/27/06*

FOR OFFICE USE ONLY		
CO-PAY $ *15.00*	CO-INSURANCE $ _____	DEDUCTIBLE $ _____
CHECK ☒ # *9821* CASH ☐ CHARGE ☐ PAID IN FULL ☐		
ASSIGNED PROVIDER *J. Healer, MD*		

2. Marvin Doe superbill

Family Doctors Associates
123 Main Street • Anytown, FL 32711
(407) 555-1200

Date: *February 27, 2006*   Attending Physician: *J. Healer, MD*

Patient Name: *Marvin Doe*

CPT DESCRIPTION	CPT DESCRIPTION	CPT DESCRIPTION
OFFICE/HOSPITAL	**PATHOLOGY/LAB/RADIOLOGY**	**PROCEDURES/TESTS**
☐ 99201 OFFICE-NEW; FOCUSED	☐ 73100 X-RAY WRIST TWO VIEWS	☐ 12011 SIMPLE SUTURE, FACE
☐ 99202 OFFICE-NEW; EXPANDED	☐ 73590 X-RAY TIBIA/FIBULA, TWO	☐ 29125 SPLINT-SHORT ARM
☐ 99203 OFFICE-NEW; DETAILED	☐ 73600 X-RAY ANKLE TWO VIEWS	☐ 29355 WALKER CAST-LONG LEG
☐ 99204 OFFICE-NEW; COMPREHEN	☐ 76085 MAMMOGRAM-COMP DET	☐ 29540 STRAPPING-ANKLE
☐ 99205 OFFICE-NEW; COMPREHEN	☐ 76092 MAMMOGRAM SCREENING	☐ 45378 COLONOSCOPY-DIAGNOSTIC
☐ 99211 OFFICE-ESTB; MINIMAL	☐ 80050 BLOOD TEST-GEN HEALTH	☐ 45385 COLONOSCOPY-POLYP REM.
☐ 99212 OFFICE-ESTB; FOCUSED	☐ 80061 BLOOD TEST-LIPID PANEL	☐ 50390 ASPIRATION, RENAL CYST
☐ 99213 OFFICE-ESTB; EXPANDED	☒ 82947 BLOOD TEST-GLUCOSE	☐ 90703 TETANUS INJECTION
☐ 99214 OFFICE-ESTB; DETAILED	☐ 83718 BLOOD TEST-HDL	☒ 92081 VISUAL FIELD EXAM
☒ 99215 OFFICE-ESTB; COMPREHEN	☐ 85025 BLOOD TEST-CBC	☐ 93000 ECG, 12 LEADS, W/RPT
☐ 99281 EMER DEPT; FOCUSED	☐ 86403 STREP TEST, QUICK	☐ 93015 TREADMILL STRESS TEST
☐ 90844 COUNSELING—50 MIN.	☐ 87430 ENZY IMMUNOASSAY-STREP	☒ 99173 VISUAL ACUITY SCREEN

ICD DESCRIPTION	ICD DESCRIPTION	ICD DESCRIPTION
☐ 034.0 STREP THROAT	☐ 522 LOW RED BLOOD COUNT	☐ V01.5 RABIES EXPOSURE
☐ 042 HUMAN IMMUNO VIRUS	☐ 538.8 STOMACH PAIN	☐ V16.0 FAMILY HISTORY-COLON
☒ 250.51 DIABETES W/VISION	☐ 643 HYPEREMESIS	☐ V16.3 FAMILY HISTORY-BREAST
☐ 250.80 DIABETES, TYPE II	☐ 707.14 ULCER OF HEEL/MID FOOT	☐ V20.2 WELL CHILD
☐ 307.51 BULIMIA NON-ORGANIC	☐ 788.30 ENURESIS	☐ V22.0 PREGNANCY-FIRST NORM
☐ 354.0 CARPAL TUNNEL SYNDROME	☐ 815.00 FRACTURE, HAND	☐ V22.1 PREGNANCY-NORMAL
☒ 362.01 RETINOPATHY (DIABETIC)	☐ 823.2 FRACTURE, TIBIA	☐ E816.2 MOTORCYCLE ACCT
☐ 401.9 HYPERTENSION, UNSPEC	☐ 831.00 DISLOCATION, SHOULDER	☐ E826.1 FALL FROM BICYCLE
☐ 482.30 PNEUMONIA	☐ 845.00 SPRAINED ANKLE	☐ E849.0 PLACE OF OCCUR-HOME
☐ 490 BRONCHITIS, UNSPECIFIED	☐ 880.03 OPEN WOUND UPPER ARM	☐ E881.0 FALL FROM LADDER
☐ 493.92 ASTHMA, UNSPECIFIED	☐ 912.0 ABRASION, SHOULDER	☐ E906.0 DOG BITE

FOLLOW UP

PRN _____

WEEKS _____7_____

NXT APPT. _____✓_____

TIME _____*10 a. m.*_____

3. Patience Loyal patient registration form

RESPONSIBLE PARTY			DATE *March 1, 2006*	
LAST NAME *Loyal*	FIRST NAME *Patience*	MI	SOCIAL SECURITY # 102-55-9865	DATE OF BIRTH *Feb. 5, 1942*
ADDRESS *541 Colonial Drive*	CITY *Cityville*	STATE *FL*	ZIP CODE 32901	SEX *F*	MARITAL STATUS *Widowed*
HOME PHONE 407-555-1437	WORK PHONE 407-555-4405		REFERRED BY: *Mark C. Welby, M. D.*	

EMPLOYER INFORMATION		WORK STATUS:	(FULL-TIME) PART-TIME STUDENT
COMPANY NAME *Thompson Services*	ADDRESS *123 Service Way*		CITY, STATE, ZIP *Our Town, FL 32704*

DEPENDENT INFORMATION

DEPENDENT'S NAME		DEPENDENT'S NAME		DEPENDENT'S NAME	
RELATIONSHIP	DATE OF BIRTH	RELATIONSHIP	DATE OF BIRTH	RELATIONSHIP	DATE OF BIRTH
SOC. SEC. #	SEX	SOC. SEC. #	SEX	SOC. SEC. #	SEX
EMPLOYER	WORK PHONE	EMPLOYER	WORK PHONE	EMPLOYER	WORK PHONE

INSURANCE INFORMATION–PRIMARY POLICY

COMPANY NAME *McGraw Insurance Co.*	ADDRESS *P. O. Box 5544*	CITY, STATE, ZIP *Wilson, OH 45533*
PHONE NUMBER *800-555-6654*	ID OR POLICY NUMBER *102559865A4*	GROUP NUMBER OR NAME *TS9023*
INSURED'S NAME (IF DIFFERENT)	SOCIAL SECURITY #	RELATIONSHIP TO RESPONSIBLE PARTY
INSURED'S ADDRESS (IF DIFFERENT)	INSURED'S CITY, STATE, ZIP	INSURED'S PHONE NUMBER

INSURANCE INFORMATION–SECONDARY POLICY

COMPANY NAME	ADDRESS	CITY, STATE, ZIP
PHONE NUMBER	ID OR POLICY NUMBER	GROUP NUMBER OR NAME
INSURED'S NAME (IF DIFFERENT)	SOCIAL SECURITY #	RELATIONSHIP TO RESPONSIBLE PARTY
INSURED'S ADDRESS (IF DIFFERENT)	INSURED'S CITY, STATE, ZIP	INSURED'S PHONE NUMBER

OTHER INFORMATION

ALLERGIES	REASON FOR TODAY'S VISIT *Dizzy spell*
PATIENT'S SIGNATURE *Patience Loyal*	DATE 3/1/06

FOR OFFICE USE ONLY		
CO-PAY $ *15.00*	CO-INSURANCE $ _____	DEDUCTIBLE $ _____
CHECK ☒ # *1279*	CASH ☐ CHARGE ☐ PAID IN FULL ☐	
ASSIGNED PROVIDER *J. Healer, MD*		

4. Patience Loyal superbill

Family Doctors Associates
123 Main Street • Anytown, FL 32711
(407) 555-1200

Date: *March 1, 2006*   Attending Physician: *J. Healer, MD*

Patient Name: *Patience Loyal*

CPT DESCRIPTION	CPT DESCRIPTION	CPT DESCRIPTION
OFFICE/HOSPITAL	**PATHOLOGY/LAB/RADIOLOGY**	**PROCEDURES/TESTS**
☐ 99201 OFFICE-NEW; FOCUSED	☐ 73100 X-RAY WRIST TWO VIEWS	☐ 12011 SIMPLE SUTURE, FACE
☐ 99202 OFFICE-NEW; EXPANDED	☐ 73590 X-RAY TIBIA/FIBULA, TWO	☐ 29125 SPLINT-SHORT ARM
☐ 99203 OFFICE-NEW; DETAILED	☐ 73600 X-RAY ANKLE TWO VIEWS	☐ 29355 WALKER CAST-LONG LEG
☐ 99204 OFFICE-NEW; COMPREHEN	☐ 76085 MAMMOGRAM-COMP DET	☐ 29540 STRAPPING-ANKLE
☐ 99205 OFFICE-NEW; COMPREHEN	☐ 76092 MAMMOGRAM SCREENING	☐ 45378 COLONOSCOPY-DIAGNOSTIC
☐ 99211 OFFICE-ESTB; MINIMAL	☒ 80050 BLOOD TEST-GEN HEALTH	☐ 45385 COLONOSCOPY-POLYP REM.
☐ 99212 OFFICE-ESTB; FOCUSED	☐ 80061 BLOOD TEST-LIPID PANEL	☐ 50390 ASPIRATION, RENAL CYST
☐ 99213 OFFICE-ESTB; EXPANDED	☐ 82947 BLOOD TEST-GLUCOSE	☐ 90703 TETANUS INJECTION
☒ 99214 OFFICE-ESTB; DETAILED	☒ 83718 BLOOD TEST-HDL	☐ 92081 VISUAL FIELD EXAM
☐ 99215 OFFICE-ESTB; COMPREHEN	☐ 85025 BLOOD TEST-CBC	☒ 93000 ECG, 12 LEADS, W/RPT
☐ 99281 EMER DEPT; FOCUSED	☐ 86403 STREP TEST, QUICK	☐ 93015 TREADMILL STRESS TEST
☐ 90844 COUNSELING—50 MIN.	☐ 87430 ENZY IMMUNOASSAY-STREP	☐ 99173 VISUAL ACUITY SCREEN

ICD DESCRIPTION	ICD DESCRIPTION	ICD DESCRIPTION
☐ 034.0 STREP THROAT	☐ 522 LOW RED BLOOD COUNT	☐ V01.5 RABIES EXPOSURE
☐ 042 HUMAN IMMUNO VIRUS	☐ 538.8 STOMACH PAIN	☐ V16.0 FAMILY HISTORY-COLON
☐ 250.51 DIABETES W/VISION	☐ 643 HYPEREMESIS	☐ V16.3 FAMILY HISTORY-BREAST
☐ 250.80 DIABETES, TYPE II	☐ 707.14 ULCER OF HEEL/MID FOOT	☐ V20.2 WELL CHILD
☐ 307.51 BULIMIA NON-ORGANIC	☒ 785.0 RAPID HEART BEAT	☐ V22.0 PREGNANCY-FIRST NORM
☐ 354.0 CARPAL TUNNEL SYNDROME	☐ 815.00 FRACTURE, HAND	☐ V22.1 PREGNANCY-NORMAL
☐ 362.01 RETINOPATHY (DIABETIC)	☐ 823.2 FRACTURE, TIBIA	☐ E816.2 MOTORCYCLE ACCT
☒ 401.9 HYPERTENSION, UNSPEC	☐ 831.00 DISLOCATION, SHOULDER	☐ E826.1 FALL FROM BICYCLE
☐ 482.30 PNEUMONIA	☐ 845.00 SPRAINED ANKLE	☐ E849.0 PLACE OF OCCUR-HOME
☐ 490 BRONCHITIS, UNSPECIFIED	☐ 880.03 OPEN WOUND UPPER ARM	☐ E881.0 FALL FROM LADDER
☐ 493.92 ASTHMA, UNSPECIFIED	☐ 912.0 ABRASION, SHOULDER	☐ E906.0 DOG BITE

FOLLOW UP

PRN _____

WEEKS _____2_____

NXT APPT. ___✓_____

TIME _____2:30 p.m._____

5. Mary Lou Sweet patient registration form

RESPONSIBLE PARTY			DATE *February 24, 2006*	
LAST NAME *Sweet*	FIRST NAME *Mary Lou*	MI	SOCIAL SECURITY # *564-99-8731*	DATE OF BIRTH *May 21, 1973*
ADDRESS *907 Carter Street*	CITY *Cityville*	STATE *FL*	ZIP CODE *32901*	SEX *F*	MARITAL STATUS *Single*
HOME PHONE *407-555-9211*	WORK PHONE *407-555-6655*		REFERRED BY:	

EMPLOYER INFORMATION		WORK STATUS:	(FULL-TIME) PART-TIME STUDENT	
COMPANY NAME *Russell Foods*	ADDRESS *470 Village Lane*		CITY, STATE, ZIP *Our Town, FL 32704*	

DEPENDENT INFORMATION

DEPENDENT'S NAME		DEPENDENT'S NAME		DEPENDENT'S NAME	
RELATIONSHIP	DATE OF BIRTH	RELATIONSHIP	DATE OF BIRTH	RELATIONSHIP	DATE OF BIRTH
SOC. SEC. #	SEX	SOC. SEC. #	SEX	SOC. SEC. #	SEX
EMPLOYER	WORK PHONE	EMPLOYER	WORK PHONE	EMPLOYER	WORK PHONE

INSURANCE INFORMATION–PRIMARY POLICY

COMPANY NAME *McGraw Insurance Co.*	ADDRESS *P. O. Box 5544*	CITY, STATE, ZIP *Wilson, OH 45533*
PHONE NUMBER *800-555-6654*	ID OR POLICY NUMBER *XY564998731*	GROUP NUMBER OR NAME *3201KJ*
INSURED'S NAME (IF DIFFERENT)	SOCIAL SECURITY #	RELATIONSHIP TO RESPONSIBLE PARTY
INSURED'S ADDRESS (IF DIFFERENT)	INSURED'S CITY, STATE, ZIP	INSURED'S PHONE NUMBER

INSURANCE INFORMATION–SECONDARY POLICY

COMPANY NAME	ADDRESS	CITY, STATE, ZIP
PHONE NUMBER	ID OR POLICY NUMBER	GROUP NUMBER OR NAME
INSURED'S NAME (IF DIFFERENT)	SOCIAL SECURITY #	RELATIONSHIP TO RESPONSIBLE PARTY
INSURED'S ADDRESS (IF DIFFERENT)	INSURED'S CITY, STATE, ZIP	INSURED'S PHONE NUMBER

OTHER INFORMATION

ALLERGIES	REASON FOR TODAY'S VISIT *Wrist pain*
PATIENT'S SIGNATURE *Mary Lou Sweet*	DATE *2/24/06*

FOR OFFICE USE ONLY		
CO-PAY $ *15.00*	CO-INSURANCE $ _____	DEDUCTIBLE $ _____
CHECK ☒ # *1515*	CASH ☐ CHARGE ☐ PAID IN FULL ☐	
ASSIGNED PROVIDER *J. Healer, MD*		

6. Mary Lou Sweet superbill

Family Doctors Associates
123 Main Street • Anytown, FL 32711
(407) 555-1200

Date: *February 24, 2006*   Attending Physician: *J. Healer, MD*

Patient Name: *Mary Lou Sweet*

CPT DESCRIPTION	CPT DESCRIPTION	CPT DESCRIPTION
OFFICE/HOSPITAL	**PATHOLOGY/LAB/RADIOLOGY**	**PROCEDURES/TESTS**
☐ 99201 OFFICE-NEW; FOCUSED	☒ 73100 X-RAY WRIST TWO VIEWS	☐ 12011 SIMPLE SUTURE, FACE
☒ 99202 OFFICE-NEW; EXPANDED	☐ 73590 X-RAY TIBIA/FIBULA, TWO	☒ 29125 SPLINT-SHORT ARM
☐ 99203 OFFICE-NEW; DETAILED	☐ 73600 X-RAY ANKLE TWO VIEWS	☐ 29355 WALKER CAST-LONG LEG
☐ 99204 OFFICE-NEW; COMPREHEN	☐ 76085 MAMMOGRAM-COMP DET	☐ 29540 STRAPPING-ANKLE
☐ 99205 OFFICE-NEW; COMPREHEN	☐ 76092 MAMMOGRAM SCREENING	☐ 45378 COLONOSCOPY-DIAGNOSTIC
☐ 99211 OFFICE-ESTB; MINIMAL	☐ 80050 BLOOD TEST-GEN HEALTH	☐ 45385 COLONOSCOPY-POLYP REM.
☐ 99212 OFFICE-ESTB; FOCUSED	☐ 80061 BLOOD TEST-LIPID PANEL	☐ 50390 ASPIRATION, RENAL CYST
☐ 99213 OFFICE-ESTB; EXPANDED	☐ 82947 BLOOD TEST-GLUCOSE	☐ 90703 TETANUS INJECTION
☐ 99214 OFFICE-ESTB; DETAILED	☐ 83718 BLOOD TEST-HDL	☐ 92081 VISUAL FIELD EXAM
☐ 99215 OFFICE-ESTB; COMPREHEN	☐ 85025 BLOOD TEST-CBC	☐ 93000 ECG, 12 LEADS, W/RPT
☐ 99281 EMER DEPT; FOCUSED	☐ 86403 STREP TEST, QUICK	☐ 93015 TREADMILL STRESS TEST
☐ 90844 COUNSELING—50 MIN.	☐ 87430 ENZY IMMUNOASSAY-STREP	☐ 99173 VISUAL ACUITY SCREEN

ICD DESCRIPTION	ICD DESCRIPTION	ICD DESCRIPTION
☐ 034.0 STREP THROAT	☐ 522 LOW RED BLOOD COUNT	☐ V01.5 RABIES EXPOSURE
☐ 042 HUMAN IMMUNO VIRUS	☐ 538.8 STOMACH PAIN	☐ V16.0 FAMILY HISTORY-COLON
☐ 250.51 DIABETES W/VISION	☐ 643 HYPEREMESIS	☐ V16.3 FAMILY HISTORY-BREAST
☐ 250.80 DIABETES, TYPE II	☐ 707.14 ULCER OF HEEL/MID FOOT	☐ V20.2 WELL CHILD
☐ 307.51 BULIMIA NON-ORGANIC	☐ 788.30 ENURESIS	☐ V22.0 PREGNANCY-FIRST NORM
☒ 354.0 CARPAL TUNNEL SYNDROME	☐ 815.00 FRACTURE, HAND	☐ V22.1 PREGNANCY-NORMAL
☐ 362.01 RETINOPATHY (DIABETIC)	☐ 823.20 FRACTURE, TIBIA	☐ E816.2 MOTORCYCLE ACCT
☐ 401.9 HYPERTENSION, UNSPEC	☐ 831.00 DISLOCATION, SHOULDER	☐ E826.1 FALL FROM BICYCLE
☐ 482.30 PNEUMONIA	☐ 845.00 SPRAINED ANKLE	☐ E849.0 PLACE OF OCCUR-HOME
☐ 490 BRONCHITIS, UNSPECIFIED	☐ 880.03 OPEN WOUND UPPER ARM	☐ E881.0 FALL FROM LADDER
☐ 493.92 ASTHMA, UNSPECIFIED	☐ 912.0 ABRASION, SHOULDER	☐ E906.0 DOG BITE

FOLLOW UP

PRN _____

WEEKS _____*6*_____

NXT APPT. _____*✓*_____

TIME _____*3 p. m.*_____

7. Tex T. Books patient registration form

RESPONSIBLE PARTY			DATE *April 25, 2006*	
LAST NAME *Books*	FIRST NAME *Tex*	MI *T*	SOCIAL SECURITY # *123-44-8897*	DATE OF BIRTH *Jan. 9, 1970*
ADDRESS *3201 Student Street*	CITY *Cityville*	STATE *FL*	ZIP CODE *32901*	SEX *M* · MARITAL STATUS *Married*

EMPLOYER INFORMATION — WORK STATUS: (FULL-TIME) PART-TIME STUDENT

COMPANY NAME *Coding Incorporated*	ADDRESS *21 Reimbursement Lane*	CITY, STATE, ZIP *Casselberry, FL 32707*

HOME PHONE *407-555-7715*   WORK PHONE *407-555-5858*   REFERRED BY:

DEPENDENT INFORMATION

DEPENDENT'S NAME | DEPENDENT'S NAME | DEPENDENT'S NAME
RELATIONSHIP / DATE OF BIRTH | SOC. SEC. # / SEX | EMPLOYER / WORK PHONE (all blank)

INSURANCE INFORMATION–PRIMARY POLICY

COMPANY NAME *McGraw Insurance Co.*	ADDRESS *P. O. Box 5544*	CITY, STATE, ZIP *Wilson, OH 45533*
PHONE NUMBER *800-555-6654*	ID OR POLICY NUMBER *123448897*	GROUP NUMBER OR NAME *CI4411*
INSURED'S NAME (IF DIFFERENT)	SOCIAL SECURITY #	RELATIONSHIP TO RESPONSIBLE PARTY
INSURED'S ADDRESS (IF DIFFERENT)	INSURED'S CITY, STATE, ZIP	INSURED'S PHONE NUMBER

INSURANCE INFORMATION–SECONDARY POLICY (all blank)

OTHER INFORMATION

ALLERGIES *Eggs*   REASON FOR TODAY'S VISIT *Employment health exam*

PATIENT'S SIGNATURE *Tex T. Books*   DATE *4/25/06*

FOR OFFICE USE ONLY

CO-PAY $ *15.00*   CO-INSURANCE $ ____   DEDUCTIBLE $ ____

CHECK ☒ # *9821*   CASH ☐   CHARGE ☐   PAID IN FULL ☐

ASSIGNED PROVIDER *J. Healer, MD*

8. Tex T. Books superbill

Family Doctors Associates
123 Main Street • Anytown, FL 32711
(407) 555-1200

Date: *May 20, 2006*   Attending Physician: *J. Healer, MD*

Patient Name: *Tex T. Books*

CPT DESCRIPTION	CPT DESCRIPTION	CPT DESCRIPTION
OFFICE/HOSPITAL	**PATHOLOGY/LAB/RADIOLOGY**	**PROCEDURES/TESTS**
☐ 99201 OFFICE-NEW; FOCUSED	☐ 73100 X-RAY WRIST TWO VIEWS	☐ 12011 SIMPLE SUTURE, FACE
☐ 99202 OFFICE-NEW; EXPANDED	☒ 73590 X-RAY TIBIA/FIBULA, TWO	☐ 29125 SPLINT-SHORT ARM
☐ 99203 OFFICE-NEW; DETAILED	☐ 73600 X-RAY ANKLE TWO VIEWS	☒ 29355 WALKER CAST-LONG LEG
☐ 99204 OFFICE-NEW; COMPREHEN	☐ 76085 MAMMOGRAM-COMP DET	☐ 29540 STRAPPING-ANKLE
☐ 99205 OFFICE-NEW; COMPREHEN	☐ 76092 MAMMOGRAM SCREENING	☐ 45378 COLONOSCOPY-DIAGNOSTIC
☐ 99211 OFFICE-ESTB; MINIMAL	☐ 80050 BLOOD TEST-GEN HEALTH	☐ 45385 COLONOSCOPY-POLYP REM.
☐ 99212 OFFICE-ESTB; FOCUSED	☐ 80061 BLOOD TEST-LIPID PANEL	☐ 50390 ASPIRATION, RENAL CYST
☐ 99213 OFFICE-ESTB; EXPANDED	☐ 82947 BLOOD TEST-GLUCOSE	☐ 90703 TETANUS INJECTION
☐ 99214 OFFICE-ESTB; DETAILED	☐ 83718 BLOOD TEST-HDL	☐ 92081 VISUAL FIELD EXAM
☐ 99215 OFFICE-ESTB; COMPREHEN	☐ 85025 BLOOD TEST-CBC	☐ 93000 ECG, 12 LEADS, W/RPT
☐ 99281 EMER DEPT; FOCUSED	☐ 86403 STREP TEST, QUICK	☐ 93015 TREADMILL STRESS TEST
☐ 90844 COUNSELING—50 MIN.	☐ 87430 ENZY IMMUNOASSAY-STREP	☐ 99173 VISUAL ACUITY SCREEN

ICD DESCRIPTION	ICD DESCRIPTION	ICD DESCRIPTION
☐ 034.0 STREP THROAT	☐ 522 LOW RED BLOOD COUNT	☐ V01.5 RABIES EXPOSURE
☐ 042 HUMAN IMMUNO VIRUS	☐ 538.8 STOMACH PAIN	☐ V16.0 FAMILY HISTORY-COLON
☐ 250.51 DIABETES W/VISION	☐ 643 HYPEREMESIS	☐ V16.3 FAMILY HISTORY-BREAST
☐ 250.80 DIABETES, TYPE II	☐ 707.14 ULCER OF HEEL/MID FOOT	☐ V20.2 WELL CHILD
☐ 307.51 BULIMIA NON-ORGANIC	☐ 788.30 ENURESIS	☐ V22.0 PREGNANCY-FIRST NORM
☐ 354.0 CARPAL TUNNEL SYNDROME	☐ 815.00 FRACTURE, HAND	☐ V22.1 PREGNANCY-NORMAL
☐ 362.01 RETINOPATHY (DIABETIC)	☒ 823.20 FRACTURE, TIBIA	☐ E816.2 MOTORCYCLE ACCT
☐ 401.9 HYPERTENSION, UNSPEC	☐ 831.00 DISLOCATION, SHOULDER	☐ E826.1 FALL FROM BICYCLE
☐ 482.30 PNEUMONIA	☐ 845.00 SPRAINED ANKLE	☐ E849.0 PLACE OF OCCUR-HOME
☐ 490 BRONCHITIS, UNSPECIFIED	☐ 880.03 OPEN WOUND UPPER ARM	☐ E881.0 FALL FROM LADDER
☐ 493.92 ASTHMA, UNSPECIFIED	☐ 912.0 ABRASION, SHOULDER	☐ E906.0 DOG BITE

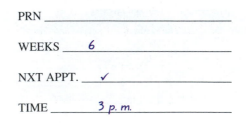

FOLLOW UP

PRN _____

WEEKS _____*6*_____

NXT APPT. _____✓_____

TIME _____*3 p.m.*_____

9. Sarah Student patient registration form

RESPONSIBLE PARTY			DATE *February 27, 2006*	
LAST NAME *Student*	FIRST NAME *Sarah*	MI	SOCIAL SECURITY # 387-49-5879	DATE OF BIRTH *June 1, 1978*
ADDRESS *8712 Career Path*	CITY *Cityville*	STATE *FL*	ZIP CODE 32901	SEX *F* / MARITAL STATUS *Single*
HOME PHONE 407-555-8843	WORK PHONE 407-555-4451		REFERRED BY: *Mark C. Welby, M. D.*	

EMPLOYER INFORMATION   WORK STATUS: (FULL-TIME)   PART-TIME   STUDENT

COMPANY NAME *Prime Incorporated*	ADDRESS *5580 Rehearsal Lane*	CITY, STATE, ZIP *Our Town, FL 32704*

DEPENDENT INFORMATION

DEPENDENT'S NAME		DEPENDENT'S NAME		DEPENDENT'S NAME	
RELATIONSHIP	DATE OF BIRTH	RELATIONSHIP	DATE OF BIRTH	RELATIONSHIP	DATE OF BIRTH
SOC. SEC. #	SEX	SOC. SEC. #	SEX	SOC. SEC. #	SEX
EMPLOYER	WORK PHONE	EMPLOYER	WORK PHONE	EMPLOYER	WORK PHONE

INSURANCE INFORMATION–PRIMARY POLICY

COMPANY NAME *McGraw Insurance Co.*	ADDRESS *P. O. Box 5544*	CITY, STATE, ZIP *Wilson, OH 45533*
PHONE NUMBER 800-555-6654	ID OR POLICY NUMBER 387495879A	GROUP NUMBER OR NAME PTI023
INSURED'S NAME (IF DIFFERENT)	SOCIAL SECURITY #	RELATIONSHIP TO RESPONSIBLE PARTY
INSURED'S ADDRESS (IF DIFFERENT)	INSURED'S CITY, STATE, ZIP	INSURED'S PHONE NUMBER

INSURANCE INFORMATION–SECONDARY POLICY

COMPANY NAME	ADDRESS	CITY, STATE, ZIP
PHONE NUMBER	ID OR POLICY NUMBER	GROUP NUMBER OR NAME
INSURED'S NAME (IF DIFFERENT)	SOCIAL SECURITY #	RELATIONSHIP TO RESPONSIBLE PARTY
INSURED'S ADDRESS (IF DIFFERENT)	INSURED'S CITY, STATE, ZIP	INSURED'S PHONE NUMBER

OTHER INFORMATION

ALLERGIES	REASON FOR TODAY'S VISIT *Severe leg pain, possible fracture*
PATIENT'S SIGNATURE *Sarah Student*	DATE 2/27/06

FOR OFFICE USE ONLY

CO-PAY $ *15.00*   CO-INSURANCE $ _____   DEDUCTIBLE $ _____

CHECK ☒ # *5719*   CASH ☐   CHARGE ☐   PAID IN FULL ☐

ASSIGNED PROVIDER _____ *J. Healer, MD*

10. Sarah Student superbill

Family Doctors Associates
123 Main Street • Anytown, FL 32711
(407) 555-1200

Date: *February 27, 2006*   Attending Physician: *J. Healer, MD*

Patient Name: *Sarah Student*

CPT DESCRIPTION	CPT DESCRIPTION	CPT DESCRIPTION
OFFICE/HOSPITAL	**PATHOLOGY/LAB/RADIOLOGY**	**PROCEDURES/TESTS**
☐ 99201 OFFICE-NEW; FOCUSED	☐ 73100 X-RAY WRIST TWO VIEWS	☐ 12011 SIMPLE SUTURE, FACE
☐ 99202 OFFICE-NEW; EXPANDED	☒ 73590 X-RAY TIBIA/FIBULA, TWO	☐ 29125 SPLINT-SHORT ARM
☐ 99203 OFFICE-NEW; DETAILED	☐ 73600 X-RAY ANKLE TWO VIEWS	☒ 29355 WALKER CAST-LONG LEG
☐ 99204 OFFICE-NEW; COMPREHEN	☐ 76085 MAMMOGRAM-COMP DET	☐ 29540 STRAPPING-ANKLE
☐ 99205 OFFICE-NEW; COMPREHEN	☐ 76092 MAMMOGRAM SCREENING	☐ 45378 COLONOSCOPY-DIAGNOSTIC
☐ 99211 OFFICE-ESTB; MINIMAL	☐ 80050 BLOOD TEST-GEN HEALTH	☐ 45385 COLONOSCOPY-POLYP REM.
☐ 99212 OFFICE-ESTB; FOCUSED	☐ 80061 BLOOD TEST-LIPID PANEL	☐ 50390 ASPIRATION, RENAL CYST
☐ 99213 OFFICE-ESTB; EXPANDED	☐ 82947 BLOOD TEST-GLUCOSE	☐ 90703 TETANUS INJECTION
☐ 99214 OFFICE-ESTB; DETAILED	☐ 83718 BLOOD TEST-HDL	☐ 92081 VISUAL FIELD EXAM
☐ 99215 OFFICE-ESTB; COMPREHEN	☐ 85025 BLOOD TEST-CBC	☐ 93000 ECG, 12 LEADS, W/RP
☒ 99281 EMER DEPT; FOCUSED	☐ 86403 STREP TEST, QUICK	☐ 93015 TREADMILL STRESS TEST
☐ 90844 COUNSELING—50 MIN.	☐ 87430 ENZY IMMUNOASSAY-STREP	☐ 99173 VISUAL ACUITY SCREEN

ICD DESCRIPTION	ICD DESCRIPTION	ICD DESCRIPTION
☐ 034.0 STREP THROAT	☐ 522 LOW RED BLOOD COUNT	☐ V01.5 RABIES EXPOSURE
☐ 042 HUMAN IMMUNO VIRUS	☐ 538.8 STOMACH PAIN	☐ V16.0 FAMILY HISTORY-COLON
☐ 250.51 DIABETES W/VISION	☐ 643 HYPEREMESIS	☐ V16.3 FAMILY HISTORY-BREAST
☐ 250.80 DIABETES, TYPE II	☐ 707.14 ULCER OF HEEL/MID FOOT	☐ V20.2 WELL CHILD
☐ 307.51 BULIMIA NON-ORGANIC	☐ 788.30 ENURESIS	☐ V22.0 PREGNANCY-FIRST NORM
☐ 354.0 CARPAL TUNNEL SYNDROME	☐ 815.00 FRACTURE, HAND	☐ V22.1 PREGNANCY-NORMAL
☐ 362.01 RETINOPATHY (DIABETIC)	☒ 823.20 FRACTURE, TIBIA	☐ E816.2 MOTORCYCLE ACCT
☐ 401.9 HYPERTENSION, UNSPEC	☐ 831.00 DISLOCATION, SHOULDER	☐ E826.1 FALL FROM BICYCLE
☐ 482.30 PNEUMONIA	☐ 845.00 SPRAINED ANKLE	☐ E849.0 PLACE OF OCCUR-HOME
☐ 490 BRONCHITIS, UNSPECIFIED	☐ 880.03 OPEN WOUND UPPER ARM	☐ E881.0 FALL FROM LADDER
☐ 493.92 ASTHMA, UNSPECIFIED	☒ 912.0 ABRASION, SHOULDER	☐ E906.0 DOG BITE

FOLLOW UP

PRN _____

WEEKS _____ *6* _____

NXT APPT. _____ *✓* _____

TIME _____ *3 p.m.* _____

Working with Insurance Companies

12

OBJECTIVES

- Understand the claims process.
- Understand how to work with a clearinghouse.
- Identify a system for organizing the claims process.
- Know what to do if a claim is lost.
- Identify the process to appeal a denied claim.

We all know that every organization needs to have money coming in so that it can stay in business. The physician provides a service to his or her patients and expects to be paid for those services. That money is what keeps the practice open and able to pay your salary. If enough people don't pay their bills, then the office must lay off people (and that could mean you!). Or you might not be able to get that next raise, even if you deserve it.

KEY TERMS

electronic media claim (EMC)

electronic remittance advice (ERA)

eligibility verification

explanation of benefits (EOB)

remittance advice (RA)

tracer

IMPORTANT NOTE

Remember that a health care practice is a business. The process of getting information and submitting claims to the insurance company is key to the survival of your health care office and all the people it employs.

By now, you understand how important all of this information is and that you have a personal stake in completing claim forms correctly. As you transfer information from patient registration forms and other documents, be certain to

- Double-check your work to make sure it is accurate.
- Confirm that the form is completely filled out, with no necessary information missing.
- Verify the spelling of every name and the accuracy of every number.

It all must be absolutely correct.

Key Term

Electronic media claim (EMC): A health care claim form that is transmitted electronically.

As you already know, most insurance companies, including Medicare, prefer claim forms to be submitted electronically. An **electronic media claim (EMC)** also called an electronic claim, is evaluated more quickly. Accepted claims are paid faster. Years ago, it was not unusual for physicians' offices to wait four to six months to receive payment from an insurance company. With electronic claims, this has been cut to two to three weeks.

The increase in the use of technology in this process also means that there is an excellent chance a computer will be reviewing your claim form. During the initial processing of the claim you have sent, the computer will only compare letter to letter and number to number, looking for an exact match to the letters and numbers in their files. Then, claims with errors such as invalid policy numbers or missing information will be rejected and returned to you.

Example

The computer cannot scan your claim form and say, "Oh, I can see this is a typo. They really meant to put a *W* instead of a *U*." No, all the computer knows is that the letter is supposed to be a *U* and it is not. And the claim will be rejected.

WORKING WITH CLEARINGHOUSES

As discussed in Chapter 11, clearinghouses are companies that offer electronic claims processing services. When working with a clearinghouse, you will send all your claims, electronically, to one location. The clearinghouse's computer will then check your claim for

1. Missing information
2. Valid diagnosis codes (ICD-9-CM) and procedure codes (CPT or ICD-9-CM)
3. Assurance that other specific requirements have been met

When the clearinghouse's computer finds that your claim is correct, it will forward that claim to the appropriate insurance carrier, also known as a payer.

If the clearinghouse finds any problem with the claim, it will return the claim to you, along with a report explaining the problem. It might be that something is missing, or perhaps the policy number is invalid. The clearinghouse will give you the opportunity to correct the mistake before the claim goes to the insurance carrier. However, this is not an excuse for you to be careless with your work. Clearinghouses will not do the work for you, or correct errors for you. They cannot tell you that a code is wrong or does not fit the requirement for medical necessity. They will not confirm that you used the best code available. These companies are there to back you up, not to do your work for you.

Also, these services are not free. Most often, your health care office will pay a monthly charge along with a per claim fee. This means that, every time you send a claim through the clearinghouse, it costs money.

> **IMPORTANT NOTE**
>
> Your office pays per claim, even if it is the same claim over and over again. Your office manager or physician will not be happy with you if your claims are constantly coming back to the office with errors.

Many physicians' offices do not work with clearinghouses. If your office does not, you will create the claim form, proof it for errors, and send it to the third-party payer directly. Such providers feel that they would rather put the money into your salary and benefits. After all, these tasks are what they are paying you to do.

ORGANIZING CLAIMS

One thing that is very important for the professional insurance biller to do is to keep track of all the claims sent out on behalf of his or her medical office. Even with the help of computers and clearinghouses, a claim can get lost. It happens on occasion with letters sent through the post office, and it can happen electronically as well. One little power surge, or a computer with a virus, and your claim can just disappear. The only way you may know about this is the absence of a response, such as a payment, a statement of rejection, or a denial. Therefore, you have to keep track of every claim form you send.

> **IMPORTANT NOTE**
>
> You are responsible for following up on every claim you send.

The following are two simple steps for staying organized.

1. Keep a log of every claim as you send it. If you are using a clearinghouse, you will receive a report, listing all the claims sent (complete with date and time sent) and to which payer they were forwarded. Place these notices in a file folder on your computer's desktop or print out these reports and place them in a three-ring binder or another type of file. If you are sending claims directly from your office, you should create a separate master index for logging in this information. If you prefer, you can keep a master index in a notebook on your desk and handwrite a notation for each claim you send, indicating the following:

   - Carrier name (the third-party payer to whom you sent the claim)
   - Patient name
   - Date of service
   - Date and time you sent the claim

2. Build into your schedule a specific day and time each week for following up claims. When you set an appointment with yourself, such as every Friday at 9 A.M., or Mondays after the morning staff meeting, you will reduce the number of times that your workday will prevent you from doing this. It is so easy to say, "Once a week I am going to follow up on the claims" and just never have the time for this very important task. Each week, or as often as required by the number of claims you send out, go over the list and separate the claims into three "piles":

Pile 1: claims that have been paid by the insurers

Pile 2: claims for which you have received rejection or denial notices

Pile 3: claims for which you have received no notices or payment

Pile 1: Claims That Have Been Paid by the Insurers

The HIPAA Health Care Payment and Remittance Advice is the electronic transmission of this payment, using HIPAA approved secure data sets. The transmission has two parts: the transaction and the document.

- The document is a **remittance advice (RA)** or an **electronic remittance advice (ERA)**. Some health care professionals also refer to this document as an **explanation of benefits or EOB**.
- The transaction is an electronic funds transfer (EFT) that sends the payment directly into your facility's bank account, like direct deposit.

The RA will provide all the details of this payment including

- the exact amount of monies your office is receiving,
- for which patient,
- for which procedures performed, and
- on which service dates.

Once you are certain that a claim has been approved and your office has received payment from the third-party payer, the first thing you should do is mark this claim as paid in your master index. Be very careful when doing this.

When you enter the deposits into the computer (and into the bank, if the funds were not electronically transferred), you must be very diligent. You might have two claims for the same patient for different dates or two patients with the same name or similar names. You do not want to mark the wrong claim paid and leave the wrong claim marked unpaid. This will cause a lot of confusion and aggravation in dealing with the insurance carrier. We will go over how to enter deposits into the computer and credit each patient's account, specifically in NDCMedisoft Advanced, in Chapter 13.

Key Terms

Remittance advice (RA): Notification identifying details about a payment from the third-party payer.

Electronic remittance advice (ERA): Remittance advice that is sent to the provider electronically.

Explanation of benefits (EOB): Another type of paper remittance advice, more typically sent to the policyholder. However, some in the industry use the term *EOB* interchangeably with *RA*.

Pile 2: Claims for Which You Have Received Denial Notices

We have reviewed the fact that you can avoid many denied claims by checking, double-checking, and triple-checking your work. Make certain that

1. Insurance coverage is confirmed
2. All the information (such as policyholder and policy number) is correct
3. The best, most appropriate codes are used
4. Medical necessity has been established by those codes
5. All the information has been correctly placed on the correct claim form

Despite doing everything correctly, some claims are denied and come back unpaid. However, this does not mean that you either have to go after the guarantor for the money or have your office go without the money it deserves. There are many reasons an insurance carrier, or payer, may deny a claim. Let's review some of the most common reasons for a claim to be denied and what you can do about it.

Denied Due to Office Personnel Error

If you discover that the claim has been denied by the insurance carrier due to an error made by you or someone in your office, this can be fixed. Simply find out what the error was and correct it.

Compare the policy number on the claim to the copy of the insurance card that you made when the patient was seen in your office for this encounter. It is important that you specifically check it against the copy taken at the encounter for which this claim form is billing the insurance company. The patient may have been in your office more recently with a new policy because his or her insurance changed between the most recent visit and the visit for which this claim was submitted.

IMPORTANT NOTE

Get into the habit of dating the copy you make of the insurance card each time the patient comes in to see the physician.

You might find that, when you keyed the number into the computer, you inadvertently switched two numbers. It can happen when you are in a busy, hectic, noisy office with many people talking to you at the same time.

If you find that the policy number matches the ID card, you will have to continue looking for the typo, going over the claim form one box at a time to check every piece of information that was entered. Once you find the error, all you have to do is correct it and resubmit the claim form.

IMPORTANT NOTE

Make certain that you mark a resubmission with the words "Corrected Claim," so there is no mistake that you are not double billing (which is against the law).

You should have caught the error when you double-checked your work, but . . . OK. It happens. You have wasted time (and if you are using a clearinghouse, you have wasted money as well), and you have delayed payment to your office, but follow the third-party payer's procedure for resubmitting corrected claims and the money will arrive.

Examples

The policy number or a CPT code is invalid (nonexistent) because it was entered improperly.

Anyone could look at the number 546998823 and accidentally key in 546998832.

Denied Due to Lack of Coverage

You look at the denial notice and it doesn't make sense. You have documentation in the file that, when you called for **eligibility verification**, the insurance carrier representative confirmed that the patient's coverage was valid and the policy carried no exclusions. The co-payment, co-insurance, and deductible were also confirmed. However, the claim was returned as denied, with the reason that the patient was not covered.

What may have happened is that, between your verification of the patient's coverage and the arrival of the claim at the insurance carrier's office, the policy was cancelled. When your claim arrived, the computer, or the person, simply looked at the file, saw that the policy was no longer in effect, and therefore denied the claim. If this is the case,

1. You will need to send a letter, not make a phone call, to the insurance carrier. In the letter, carefully state the date and time of the eligibility verification and the name of the insurance representative who told you the patient was covered for services by your office. (Make certain your office's procedure for eligibility verification includes the documentation of all of these details for just this reason.) Emphasize the date of the phone call as well as the date(s) of treatment or service and attach a fresh printout of the claim form.
2. Before you mail this letter, call the company and confirm the name, title, and address of the employee responsible for receiving your appeal request. If you send this information to the wrong person, it may get lost within the company, or at the very least it will delay your satisfaction of this issue.
3. Make certain you keep copies of everything, and follow up in a week or two if you have not heard from the insurer.

Key Term

Eligibility verification: The process of confirming with the insurance carrier that an individual is qualified for benefits which would pay for services provided by your health care professional on a particular day.

In other cases, claims have been denied because the individual's policy was cancelled prior to your treatment and the insurance representative did not have (or did not tell you) up-to-date information. Therefore, your office provided treatment based on misinformation. As a matter of policy, typically the insurance carrier will claim that its staff member's confirmation of coverage does not represent a guarantee that your office will be paid. Again, you do not want to take no for an answer.

IMPORTANT NOTE

Both federal and state courts have ordered insurance carriers to pay claims based on their statements of eligibility at the time treatment and services were provided. These courts have established that the insurance representative's confirmation of benefits serve as encouragement to the physician, or other provider, to offer that treatment or service.

When you think about it, if the insurance carrier had stated that the patient did not have coverage at the time you called for verification, your office may have chosen to not see the patient, to not take an X-ray, or to ask the patient to pay cash at that time. The fact that the insurance carrier told you, or a member of your office, that they would pay the claim encouraged your physician to treat the individual and reasonably expect to be paid for his or her work. Again, you must do the following:

1. Write a letter of appeal to the appropriate person at the insurance company, stating all the details of the verification conversation.
2. If your office does eligibility verification electronically, you should copy the printout of the electronic confirmation and attach it to the letter.
3. Always keep hard copy (paper) documentation or notes indicating to whom you spoke, what was said, and the date and time of the conversation.

If your appeal is denied again, your office may need to enlist the services of an attorney. The bottom line is that your office is entitled to this payment, but there are times you may need to fight for it.

Denied Due to Lack of Medical Necessity

Should your office receive a denial based on lack of medical necessity, there are some things you must do:

1. Go back and confirm the diagnosis (ICD-9-CM) and procedure (CPT or ICD-9-CM) codes that appear on the claim form are the best, most accurate codes.
   a. There is a possibility that there was a simple error in keying in the code (such as transposing two of the numbers or leaving off a digit). More than once, a health care office and a patient have gone through months of arguing with the insurance carrier for the coverage of a procedure, only to find that the entire problem was a simple typographical error.

b. Perhaps there was an error in coding. Go back and look at the physician's notes. Start from the beginning and recode the encounter. If there is another coder in your office, you might ask him or her to look at the notes and code the diagnosis and procedure(s). Then compare the other coder's determination of the best, most appropriate codes with yours. If you come up with different and/or additional codes this time, you might go ahead and resubmit the claim with the new codes. Or this review might confirm that the codes were correct on the original claim.

c. Review the linking of the procedure codes to diagnosis codes (CMS-1500 Box 24E). Confirm the links are correct.

2. Contact the insurance carrier and get a written copy of its definition of medical necessity. Often the list of criteria for medical necessity consists of any treatment or service that:

a. Is commonly performed by health care practitioners (considered accepted standard of care) for the treatment of the condition, illness, or injury as indicated by the diagnosis code(s) provided

b. Is provided at the most efficient level of care that ensures the patient's safety

c. Is not experimental

d. Is not elective

Using the criteria for medical necessity from the insurance carrier that denied the claim (different carriers may have different criteria), review the patient's health record to confirm that this individual and this particular encounter meet all of the requirements. Again,

- Double-check the diagnosis and procedure codes to make certain they all accurately represent what occurred during that visit.

- Call and speak with the claims examiner to identify exactly what he or she thought the problem was with the claim. This conversation may give you some insight into what you should be looking for as you review the patient's chart.

- Get support materials from your health care professionals, particularly the attending physician on this case. Copies of articles or pages from credible sources, such as The Merck Manual, the *New England Journal of Medicine,* or other qualified sources of research, will help support your claim.

- If this patient encounter was the result of another provider referring the individual to your physician for additional treatment, the referring physician might agree to write a letter supporting your office.

3. Write a letter to the third-party payer's appeals board, or to whomever the claims representative instructs you to send the documentation, outlining all of the information you have gathered to corroborate specifically why the denial should be overturned.

   a. Include copies of supporting documentation, such as pages from The Merck Manual or a letter from the referring provider.

   b. In addition, request that a qualified health care professional licensed in the area of treatment or service under discussion be the one to review your appeal. This may provide a more agreeable opinion as to the medical necessity of your claim and get it approved.

Example

Let's look at Patience Loyal's case, one of the patients from Chapter 9. It is easy to determine that there should be a diagnosis code for her essential hypertension. However, if you do not have a second code for her rapid heartbeat, the claim would be rejected. Without the code for rapid heartbeat, there is no medical justification provided on the claim form for performing an EKG.

Denied Due to Preexisting Condition

A denial on the grounds that the patient was treated for a preexisting excluded condition or illness reinforces the need for accurate confirmation of eligibility before the patient is seen and treated by the physician. If, in fact, your physician is about to treat a patient for a specific diagnosis, you must determine if the insurance carrier has excluded that condition, illness, or injury from coverage. This should be done during the eligibility verification. However, if you get to the point at which a submitted claim has been denied due to a preexisting condition that has been excluded, you still have several options to try to get your claim paid:

1. Start by reviewing the diagnosis code. There may be a difference in the diagnosis codes, now and for past treatment, making your claim valid.

2. Request a copy of the insurance carrier's definition of a preexisting condition. Once you clearly understand the requirements, you will be able to analyze better the details of this claim and its validity.

3. A review of the patient's past medical records may also assist you in appealing this denial. Examining specific diagnosis codes and physician's notes' diagnostic statements may find an opportunity to justify the insurance carrier's coverage of this claim.

When you have the information to support your claim, write an appeal letter outlining why the denial should be reversed.

Denied Due to Benefit Limitation on Treatment by an Assistant

Some medical offices have physician's assistants and nurse practitioners treat patients for routine examinations, vaccinations, and other medical services. However, some insurance carriers limit the types of treatments and services for which they will pay when provided by a health care worker who is not a licensed physician. There are a couple of approaches to appeal this type of denial.

1. Begin by authenticating the qualifications of the person who provided the service or treatment. You will also want to reinforce in your appeal that having this health care professional perform this procedure, under the supervision of the licensed physician, was the most cost-efficient way to provide the service to the patient.
2. Obtain a copy of the carrier's written policy regarding treatment to patients by assistants and search for language that specifically denies payment for services provided by a professional with the credentials of your staff member. If you do not find any such language, your appeal letter should include that the insurance carrier's policy does not specifically exclude services provided by this level of professional.

Subsequent Denials

There are additional steps that can be taken to appeal a second or third denial. Sometimes an insurance carrier will deny a claim, hoping that you will give up and it will not have to pay. However, most of the time, subsequent denials are just a matter of poor communication between the insurance carrier and the health care office. Remember, although it is an insurance carrier's responsibility and obligation to pay claims, it is also its responsibility and obligation to protect its assets from fraud. Primarily, it is this intention that creates the circumstance of a falsely denied claim. However, after you have exhausted all efforts within the insurance carrier's organization to get the carrier to see your side and pay the claim, you have additional options:

1. Many states have state boards and/or review panels for this type of situation. Experienced health care providers, with varying areas of specialization, sit on these review boards. Their duty is to go over all the details of the case; examine the patient's health record, the claim form, and all other documentation; and evaluate the insurance carrier's basis for denying the claim. They have the right, empowered by the state government, to override the insurance carrier's decision and force the carrier to pay the claim. Bringing an appeal to this type of review board is an option to both health care professionals and individuals alike.
2. If the patient is covered under an employer's self-insured health plan, the state board is usually not an option for appeal. However, the federal government oversees and regulates self-insured plans and can provide you with an appeals process. At the very least, these insurers are required to have an in-house appeal board that will hear your case.

Surprisingly, you have an excellent chance of winning an appeal when you handle it properly. Researchers have found very high success rates for providers who file appeals. Therefore, if a claim is denied, it is worth the time to look into the reasons for denial and possibly exercise the right to appeal.

Writing Letters of Appeal

When a claim has been denied and you have gathered all the documentation to support your position that the denial is incorrect, you need to write a formal letter of appeal. This letter should contain the following:

Recipient: Call the third-party payer and get the name, title, and address of the person to whom you should address this letter. Make certain you double-check the spelling of the person's name—don't assume. Even a name as straightforward as John can also be spelled Jon or Jahn. Just ask!

RE: In the space between the recipient's name and address, and the salutation, you need to include identification regarding the person to whom this letter refers. This should be indented to your 1 inch tab position. The details that should be shown in this area of the letter are

Patient Name:

Policyholder Name:

Policy Number:

Date(s) of Service:

Claim Number:

Total Amount of Claim: $

Salutation: Always begin the letter with a proper business salutation to the recipient by name. For example, Dear Mr. Smith: or Dear Ms. Jones (followed by a colon). Avoid generic salutations such as To Whom It May Concern unless the insurance carrier will not release the name of the person designated to receive appeal letters and has instructed you to address this letter to a department or title.

Paragraph 1: State briefly and directly why you are writing this letter. This is a summary or condensed version of the rest of the letter. Be factual not emotional. Be specific about when and/or how you were informed that the claim was denied and the reasons stated by the insurance carrier for the denial. This paragraph is to make certain that you and the reader of this letter are on the same page (pardon the pun!). It is difficult to capture and retain someone's attention to what you are saying if they don't know what you are talking about to begin with.

Examples

1. Our claims service representative, Raul Vega, told us that the above claim was denied due to a lack of medical necessity. This letter is an official notice that we wish to appeal this decision.
2. On November 3, 2005, our office received a notice stating that the above-mentioned claim was denied because of lack of coverage. This letter is to appeal this decision.

Paragraph 2: Itemize all the facts/evidence you have to support your position that you should be paid. Explain what documentation you have to encourage them to change their minds and approve/pay your claim. This list may contain highlights from the physician's notes outlining why the procedure was medically necessary. You might include statistics proving that this procedure is no longer considered experimental but is now widely accepted as the new standard of care. Attach copies (never originals) of documents that contain the information and refer to those attachments in this portion of the letter. In reality, this section of the letter may need to be longer than one paragraph. Write what you need to establish your rationale, but remember that this is not creative writing. Do not use flowery language or get long in your explanation. Be direct and to the point and include just the facts.

Examples

1. As you can see in the attached documentation, the X-rays confirmed that the patient had a compound fracture requiring immediate surgery.
2. On Thursday, September 4, 2005, at 1:35 P.M. eastern, I spoke with Emma Longwood in your Eligibility Verification department who confirmed that Mr. Smith was fully covered by your HMO plan for the following procedures. . . .

Paragraph 3: Use paragraph 3 (the last paragraph) to clearly define where this discussion should go next. Of course, you want them to just reconsider and pay the claim, however, you will need to keep this a bit more open-ended. Offer to provide any additional documentation the insurance carrier may feel necessary. Supply your contact information (office phone number, e-mail address, fax number) even if it is right there on the letterhead. Set an appointment generally (i.e., "I will call you next week") to follow up with this person. The purpose of this statement is to keep this appeal moving in a direction toward acceptance and payment. You do not want this letter to get buried on a busy desk. In addition, mark your calendar and call when you said you would. It is your responsibility to keep this issue on the top of the insurance carrier's priority list. You know that old saying, "The squeaky wheel gets the grease." This means that those that speak up get the attention. The more you are in their face, the sooner you will get this resolved.

Examples

1. If you need any more information, to bring this to a quick resolution, please contact me at . . .
2. I will call you at the end of the week to discuss this matter further. In the meantime, if you need to contact me, please do so at . . .

Closing and Signature: All business letters should contain a closing, as well as the signature and title of the person sending the correspondence. *Sincerely* or *Sincerely yours* (followed by a comma) are the most common closings. After leaving four lines blank to make room for your signature, key in your full name. Directly underneath your name, key in your title (e.g., Insurance Specialist). If you are going to attach copies of important documentation to this letter, you need to note this under your signature. Leave one empty line under your title, and key in Enclosure or Enclosures or Enc. This notation points the recipient to the additional pages included in the envelope.

Pile 3: Claims for Which You Have Received No Notices or Payment

If a reasonable time has passed after sending a claim and you have received no notices or payment, you will need to follow up with the insurance carrier. (The term *reasonable time* is specifically defined by each third-party payer.)

1. Call and speak with someone in customer service to determine which examiner or representative will be handling your claim. Try to confirm that he or she has received your claim by getting a date and time of receipt and ask which staff member received it. If you cannot get this information, or you get a vague statement, such as "Oh, I'm sure we have it somewhere. We are very busy. We'll get to it soon," you will need to take the next step.
2. Go back over all the paperwork that accompanied claims paid by this carrier in the same time frame, such as an explanation of benefits (EOB), an electronic remittance advice (ERA), and a remittance advice (RA). There may have been a mistake and the wrong claim was marked paid in your file (meaning that this claim has really already been paid) and it is another that is still outstanding.
3. Once you are certain the insurance company has not responded to this claim in any way, you may need to send a **tracer**, also known as a duplicate billing or second submission.

Key Term

Tracer: An official request for a third-party payer to search its system to find a missing health claim form. It is also a term used for a replacement health claim form resubmitted to replace one that was lost.

Most insurance carriers require you to wait a specific number of days or weeks after the original date of submission before you are permitted to send a tracer claim. Check with the carrier, as each may have a different waiting period. This second version of the same claim must be marked "Tracer." This is to make sure that the insurance carrier knows you are not attempting to bill a second time for the same services. Double billing is against the law; however, sending a bill a second time because you believe that the first claim has been lost is good business.

Make a note in your master index of the date and time that you refiled the claim. That way, you can follow up again if you need to.

CHAPTER SUMMARY

The procedures you develop and abide by for tracking the health insurance claim forms you submit is almost as important as the coding process itself. Some health care offices do not have a routine for handling situations, such as lost claims or denied claims. However, you must realize how important this is to the overall financial well-being of your facility.

When you are organized, and keep a tracking log of all the claims you submit, your work is easier and your success rate is higher. Appealing denied claims is a part of your career, and it is an important part of the entire medical billing and insurance claims process.

Chapter Review

For this chapter review, you will need to refer to the physician's notes and patient registration forms in Chapter 9. You may need to make up some of the details for your letter, such as dates and times of getting eligibility verification, or your instructor may supply you with those details. Read the following scenarios and decide what to do. Then state whether you would

1. *correct the claim and resubmit (include how and what you would correct)*

   and/or

2. *send a letter of appeal to the insurance carrier, asking it to reconsider the denial of the claim; write a sample of the letter you would send.*

   1. McGraw Insurance Company denied a claim from Family Doctors Associates on behalf of the treatment provided for Mary Lou Sweet's carpal tunnel syndrome due to an excluded preexisting condition. Ms. Sweet's left wrist had been treated by a previous physician, and coverage had been excluded from the present policy when it was issued.

   2. A claim to McGraw Insurance Company by Family Doctors Associates for treatment of Patience Loyal's hypertension was denied. The ECG was deemed not medically necessary. The diagnosis code on the claim form was 409.1 and the CPT code for the ECG was 93000.

   3. Family Doctors Associates' claim to McGraw Insurance Company on behalf of Sarah Student's fracture of the tibia was denied due to no coverage. Ms. Student had failed to pay her premium on time and her policy expired two weeks prior to her treatment by this health care facility.

   4. The claim to McGraw Insurance Company from Family Doctors Associates was denied for the treatment of Marvin Doe due to benefit limitation on treatment by an assistant. When Mr. Doe came to the physician's office for his diabetic checkup, the nurse practitioner in the office performed his visual field examination and visual acuity screening.

   5. McGraw Insurance Company denied payment on Family Doctors Associates' claim for treatment of Harvey Practice due to an invalid policy. The insurance company notice stated that it does not have a policy with that number belonging to that person.

13 Receiving Revenues

KEY TERMS

allowed amount

balance billing

electronic funds transfer (EFT)

payee

payer

remittance

OBJECTIVES

- Understand how electronic remittances work.
- Properly document revenues received.
- Properly credit a patient's account.

When everything is done precisely—the health insurance claim forms are submitted with: the best, most accurate codes; and all of the correct policy information, your office will receive payment for the services it has provided. Most often, an insurance carrier will send you payment electronically, known as an **electronic funds transfer (EFT)**. The money goes directly from the insurance carrier's bank account into your office's bank account. You will never see the money, just like a direct deposit program with your paycheck. Although you will not get a printed check, you will receive documentation of this transfer of money into your company's account. Remember from Chapter 12 that this documentation is called an electronic remittance advice, or ERA for short.

On occasion, you may receive a check in the mail. A remittance advice (RA), also called an explanation of benefits (EOB), will accompany this check. An RA or EOB is a notification detailing exactly what benefits are being paid for by the third-party payer with reference to specific claims.

IMPORTANT NOTE

In business, every dollar coming into the company's bank accounts must be identified as to

- Whom it came from
- Why the business received the money

It doesn't matter whether the company is a for-profit or not-for-profit organization, there are laws that require the tracking of all money. This is very important and, if you are responsible for the accounting in your office, you must take this very seriously.

Key Term

Electronic funds transfer (EFT): Money that is moved from one bank account to another bank account using a computer. No money or checks actually change hands.

REMITTANCE ADVICE REVIEW

You will find a sample RA in Figure 13-1. Different companies may use various versions of this form; however, they all contain the same basic information. Let's review the information typically found on this report.

1. *Name and address of the payer.* Across the top of the page, you will find the name and address of the **payer**—the company sending you the **remittance**, or payment.
2. *Name, address, ID# of payee.* The upper left side is the most common location for the name and address of the company or person to whom the payment is directed, the **payee**. On a rare occasion, you might receive a check or an electronic notification of monies sent to you in error, intended for another health care office. You must double-check this information and be certain that the money you deposit in the company account actually belongs to you. Should you find another health care provider's name and/or address on the form, you must call the insurance company immediately and get instructions for returning the funds or the check.
3. *RA or ERA number.* This is the document number. It is very important and will be needed in case there are any discussions with the insurance carrier about the payment. Usually, the payer will use this number to log or file the transaction.
4. *Claim number.* A distinct number assigned to a specific claim. More than one claim may be paid with one remittance.
5. *Patient's name.* This column is used to indicate to whom the procedure or service was provided, and will show the patient's last name, followed by his or her first name.

Key Terms

Payer: An individual or organization that sends payment to another individual or organization; also spelled payor.

Remittance: Payment for services provided.

Payee: An individual or organization that receives payment from another individual or organization.

IMPORTANT NOTE

If the policyholder/insured is a different person than the patient, this form shows the patient's name.

McGraw Insurance Company
P.O. Box 5544
Wilson, OH 45533
800-555-6654

To:
Family Doctors Associates
123 Main Street
Anytown, FL 32711
407-555-1200

Practice ID# 6654321   RA# 00055468

CLAIM # 426064005033

PATIENT NAME	DATES OF SERVICE FROM/TO	PROCEDURE CODE	AMOUNT CHARGED	ALLOWED AMOUNT	DEDUCTIBLE /CO-PAYMENT	AMOUNT PAID
Practice, Harvey	03/03/2006-03/03/2006	99201	$46.00	$ 40.00	$15.00	$ 25.00
Practice, Harvey	03/03/2006-03/03/2006	45378	$155.00	$ 145.00	0	$ 145.00
Total: Check # 55833						$ 170.00

Questions regarding this remittance should be directed to:

   McGraw Insurance Company

   P.O. Box 5544

   Wilson, OH 45533

 Customer Service: 800-555-6654

FIGURE 13-1
Example of a remittance advice.

6. *Dates of service.* Just as you indicated in Box 24A of the CMS-1500 insurance claim form for this visit, this column gives you a range of dates. If the procedure or service was given and completed on one day, the same date will appear on both sides of the range, as in "05/21/06 to 05/21/06."

7. *Procedure code.* This is the procedure code for which your office is receiving these funds.

8. *Amount charged.* This is the fee charged by the health care provider for the service. By law, the same fee must be charged to all individuals for the same service (treatment or procedure), regardless of whether the patient pays cash or which insurance plan is involved.

9. *Allowed amount.* The **allowed amount** is the maximum amount of money that a particular insurance company will pay for a specific procedure or service.

10. *Deductible/co-payment.* This column (not included on all RA or EOB forms) shows the amount the patient or policyholder is expected to pay to the health care provider. It is the provider's responsibility to collect this amount, and it is automatically subtracted from the allowed amount before payment is sent to the provider.

11. *Amount paid.* This figure is the exact amount of money included in this payment for this procedure code. It doesn't matter how much you asked for on the claim form; this is how much the payer is giving you. Keep in mind that the co-payments, deductible, and co-insurance percentages that are the responsibility of the patient, as well as any other discounts or adjustments, will be deducted by the insurance carrier from the original allowed charge.

> **IMPORTANT NOTE**
>
> If this payment amount is dramatically different from what your office charged, you might want to investigate. Perhaps the wrong code was indicated, or perhaps there is a dispute with the insurance carrier over the level of the procedure.

12. *Check number.* If it is a paper check, it will carry its own number. This check number is different than the remittance number.

13. *Total amount of the check or remittance.* This is the total amount that your office is receiving at this time. This is the amount that will be written on the deposit slip and the amount that will show on the bank statement.

These columns are very important, and you must check them very carefully, especially when you are entering the information about this payment into the patient accounting system. The danger is that you might mark the same procedure that was performed on a different date as paid, when, in fact, it hasn't been. You might say, why would it matter? We talked about this a little bit in Chapter 12. Let's look at this case study and see if there is a difference.

CASE STUDY

John Smith has been diagnosed with type I diabetes. In the past two weeks, he has seen his family doctor twice, once on February 23, 2006, and again on March 1, 2006, for an evaluation of his diabetes and a blood glucose test. As a result, two claim forms have been sent to his insurance company. The only difference between the two claim forms is the information in Box 24A—the date of service. The diagnosis code and the procedure codes are the same.

The RA comes in from the insurance carrier, noting payment for the March 1, 2006 E/M service and the blood glucose test. However, the person in the physician's office entering information into the computer applies the payment to the February 23, 2006, visit because it was the older charge. What difference does it make? The correct amount was credited to the correct patient and that's all that should matter, right? Hmm, let's see.

Later that week, the insurance billing professional in this same office does her weekly check of claims status. With the information shown in the computer, she marks the February 23 claim paid and the March 1 claim as still due. Doing her job properly, she calls the insurance carrier and asks about the March 1 claim. She is informed that that claim has been paid. An argument ensues, because she insists that her office has not received the money either electronically or by mail. The insurance representative insists that he has received confirmation that the office has received the money. They both end the call, thinking the other incompetent, and the matter remains unresolved.

What will it take to find the error?

_____

_____

What difference does it make if you mark the wrong claim paid? You decide. If you think that it wouldn't matter as much in an office where the person who enters the information also handles the follow-up with the insurance carriers—because that person would remember—you are too optimistic. What you should remember is that the average health care provider can easily see more than 50 patients a week. That can add up to 150 different claims filed with several different insurance companies over the course of just three weeks. You will be coding new patient encounters while creating claim forms for the encounters you have already coded and following up on payments, denials, and lost claims as well. Do you really think you will be able to remember a small detail about one patient's account, such as which date was paid for when? Even if you have a flawless, unshakeable, absolutely perfect memory, why would you want to use up precious brain cells remembering something you didn't need to if you had entered the information correctly to begin with?

> **IMPORTANT NOTE**
>
> A good professional leaves nothing to chance, and it is a gamble to depend on your memory, no matter how good it is.

Now that we have reviewed how very important it is to mark the correct claim and the correct codes for the correct date of service in the computer, do we need to review how important it is that you enter all of the information in the correct patient's chart? You must take time and care in entering it all. It is so easy to make a mistake, especially when you have two patients with the same or similar names. As you should be in this habit already, always *double-check and triple-check* your work.

Next, you are going to practice entering payments from the insurance company into the computer.

ENTERING INSURANCE PAYMENTS INTO NDCMEDISOFT ADVANCED, VERSION 9

You have just received an RA from McGraw Insurance Company (see Figure 13-1). The first thing you must do is to enter into the computer that the monies from this payer were received by the physician's office.

> **IMPORTANT NOTE**
>
> The process of entering payments received is the same whether you get a check in the mail with an RA or receive an ERA notifying you of an EFT.

Open NDCMedisoft Advanced, Version 9. Go to the ACTIVITIES Menu and choose Enter Deposits/Payments. This will bring up the Deposit List screen. (Figure 13-2). In the upper left-hand corner of this screen, you will see Deposit Date, and the field beside it will automatically show today's date. So that you can practice, and have your screens all look the same as this book, let's change this date to March 20, 2006.

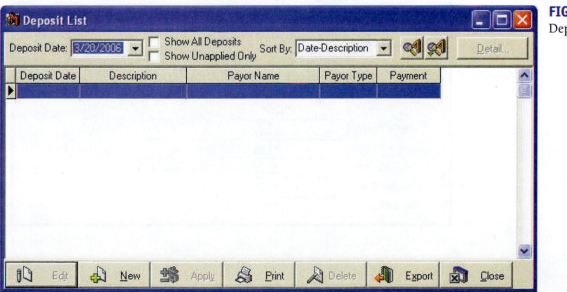

FIGURE 13-2
Deposit List screen.

IMPORTANT NOTE

If this date is in the future, you will see a dialog box that reads the following:

> You have entered a future date. Do you want to change it?
>
> Yes   No

Just click on No. It's not a problem. The computer knows what today's date is and wants to be certain that you did not enter a future date mistakenly.

Next to the Deposit Date field, you will see two check boxes that say Show All Deposits and Show Unapplied Only. These two boxes simply give you choices with regard to how much information you want to see in this dialog box. If you check the box in front of Show All Deposits, the section below will fill up with a listing of every deposit ever entered into the Deposit List. If you check in front of Show Unapplied Only, you will see only the deposits that have been entered but not applied to the specific patients. We will leave both unchecked.

To the right of the two check boxes, you will see the Sort By selection box (Figure 13-3). This gives you choices with regard to how you want to sort, or organize, the information in this dialog box.

Look down at the buttons across the bottom of this dialog box. The button that is second from the left says New (Figure 13-4).

Because you have a new deposit to make, click on the New button. Now you will see the Deposit: (new) dialog box (Figure 13-5). The deposit date will be the same one you indicated on the first screen, 3/20/2006.

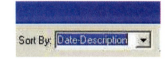

FIGURE 13-3
Sort By selection box.

FIGURE 13-4
New deposit button.

FIGURE 13-5
Deposit: (new) entry screen.

Using the RA in Figure 13-2, enter the information into the fields on this screen:

Payer Type: Insurance

This drop-down menu gives you three options to choose from: insurance; patient; and capitation. This field will indicate what category of payer sent the money. You received this payment from an insurance company, so you will choose Insurance.

Payment Method: Check

This field's drop-down menu gives you four choices: check, cash, credit card, and electronic. Here you must show what form the money was in. Our example payment is a check, so choose that option.

Check #: 55833

To the right of the Payment Method field is a field that will change, depending on what you choose for Payment Method. EFT Tracer will appear for an electronic payment, Check # will appear for a check, and nothing will appear for a cash payment. When Credit Card is chosen, a button will appear below that says Authorize. When you click on the Authorize button and complete the information in that dialog box, NDCMedisoft will assist you in contacting the credit card company to get this charge approved.

Description/Bank No: 00055468

In our make-believe office, we put the document number for the ERA or RA in this field. This way, you will be able to connect this computer entry with that piece of paper or electronic notification.

Payment Amount: $170.00

In this field, you must key in the *total* amount for the deposit, *not* the individual amounts per patient or per procedure code. You will use this entry to match against the bank statement that will show the *total* amount of the deposit.

Deposit Code: A

If the office you work in uses different deposit codes to identify types of funds received, such as capitation or insurance payments, you might change this code. For our exercises, accept the default code A.

Insurance: MCG00

Choose the name of the insurance company that sent you the money from the drop-down list.

Payment Code: 03

Choose insurance payment from the codes shown in the drop-down list. If it is not there, you may need to save and close this box and go to the LISTS Menu to Procedure/Payment/Adjustment Codes to enter 03 insurance payment.

Adjustment Code:

Withhold Code:

Deductible Code:

Take Back Code:

These next four fields are used to apply certain discounts automatically. If these fields need to be completed, you will be instructed to do so by the insurance company or your office manager. We will leave them blank.

Click on SAVE. You are now back in the Deposit List dialog box (Figure 13-6). You should see the information for this deposit now shown across the first line.

FIGURE 13-6
Deposit List dialog box return.

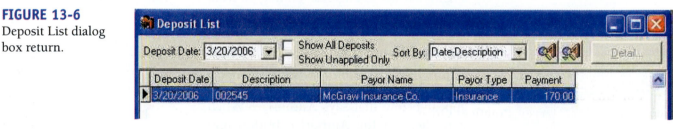

Next, you need to apply this insurance payment to each patient's account and mark the charges for these procedures as paid. At the bottom of this dialog box, click on the button third from the left, Apply. You will see a dialog box come up: Apply Payment/Adjustments to Charges (Figure 13-7).

FIGURE 13-7
Apply Payment/Adjustments to Charges dialog box.

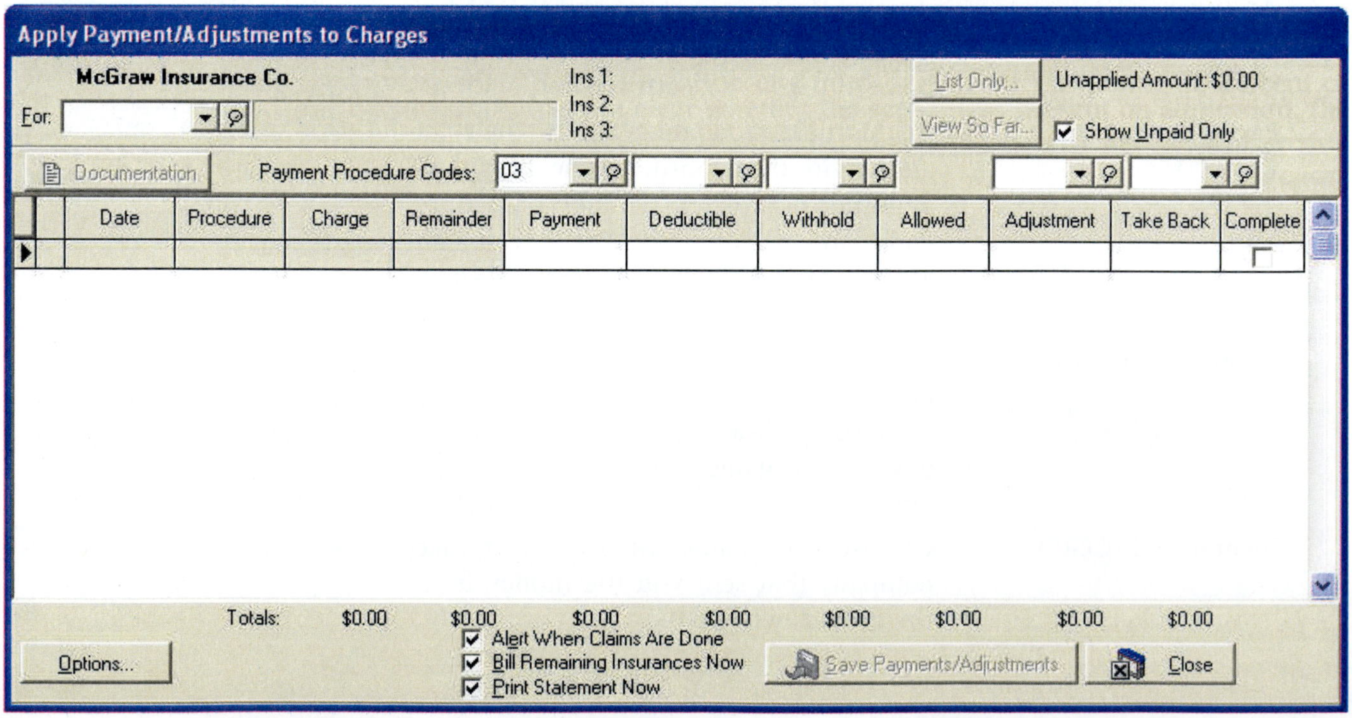

At the top left of the box, you should see the name of the insurance company, with a drop-down field right below it (Figure 13-8).

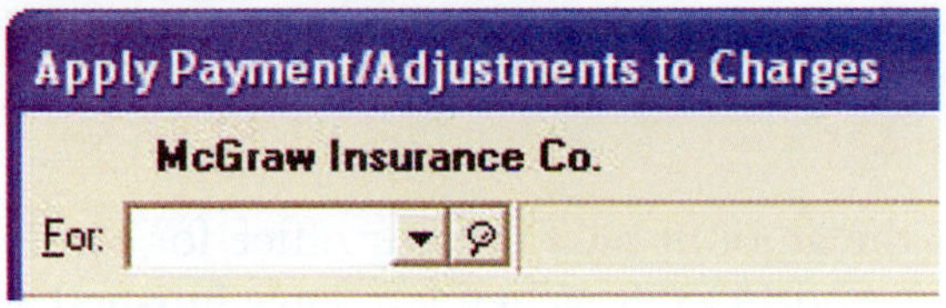

FIGURE 13-8
Apply Payment/Adjustments to Charges showing Insurance Carrier name.

In the upper right-hand corner of this dialog box, look at the field titled Unapplied Amount (Figure 13-9). This indicates how much of the money received from the insurance carrier has not yet been applied to a patient's account.

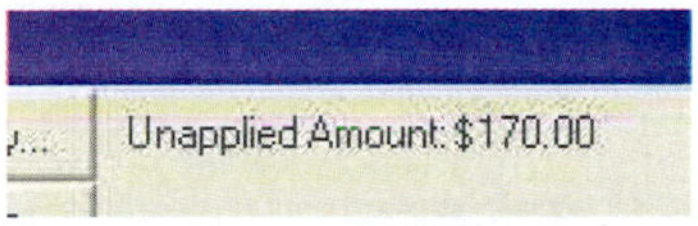

FIGURE 13-9
Unapplied Amount total.

Using the drop-down menu next to For: choose the patient for whom the insurance company sent you money. If the RA shows payment in one check for several patients, choose the name for the first one shown.

For this exercise, the payment from McGraw Insurance is for one patient only, Mr. Harvey Practice. Once you choose Mr. Practice's chart number, you will see his outstanding charges shown in the main portion of this dialog box (Figure 13-10).

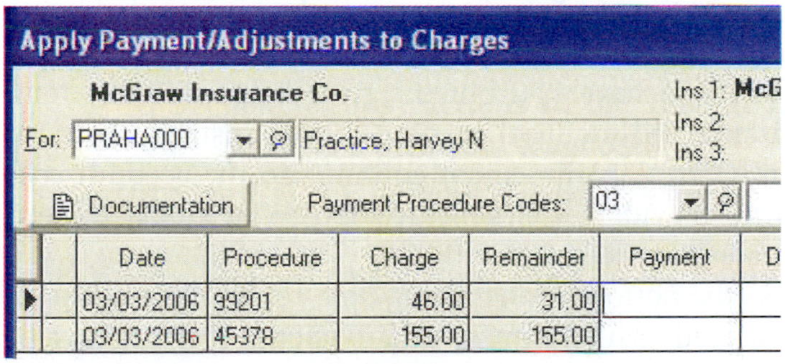

FIGURE 13-10
Outstanding charges for Harvey Practice.

The first line indicates that, on March 3, 2006, procedure code 99201 was provided to Mr. Harvey Practice. The physician's charge for this is $46.00. The remainder due for this charge is just $31.00. You may remember that Mr. Practice paid the office a $15.00 co-payment. When you entered that co-payment into the Transactions Entry screen, it was applied to (or designated to pay for a portion of the amount owed for) the procedure code 99201. The remainder is the same as balance due.

Click in the empty box on the first line below the word Payment and key in the amount shown on the RA as the Amount Paid for this procedure code on this date (Figure 13-11). You will notice that, once you key in $25.00 under Payment and hit the down arrow on your keyboard, the number in the remainder column changes to 6.00.

Memory Tip

Remainder is the amount that *REMAINS* to be paid.

PATIENT NAME	DATES OF SERVICE FROM/TO	PROCEDURE CODE	AMOUNT CHARGED	ALLOWED AMOUNT	DEDUCTIBLE /CO-PAYMENT	AMOUNT PAID
Practice, Harvey	03/03/2006-03/03/2006	99201	$46.00	$ 40.00	$15.00	$ 25.00

FIGURE 13-11
From the remittance advice for Harvey Practice.

Now enter the amount paid to your office for Mr. Harvey Practice's second procedure code 45378. When you have finished and hit the Enter key, this section of your screen should look like (Figure 13-12).

FIGURE 13-12
Insurance payments applied to Harvey Practice's account.

In the upper right-hand corner of your screen, you should see that the unapplied amount is now $0.00. This means that you have accounted for every dollar that was sent to you from the insurance company in this payment. However, Mr. Practice does not have a zero balance because of the difference between the amount charged and the allowed amounts. Some offices will have you bill the patient for this difference. This is called **Balance Billing**. Other offices will instruct you to enter an adjustment (into the adjustment column) so the account will zero out. Participating providers will generally have you adjust to zero once the insurance company has paid.

Across the bottom of the dialog box, to the right of the middle, is a button that reads Save Payments/Adjustments (Figure 13-13). Click on this button to save your work. A small dialog box should come up in the center of your screen that reads Claim number(s): 5 have been marked "done" for the primary insurance (Figure 13-14). This box is telling you that the computer has marked this claim that you created and sent to the insurance company for Harvey Practice as "done." This is the same thing as marking it paid. Click on OK.

Key Term

Balance Billing: The custom of invoicing patients for the difference between the amount charged and the allowed amount.

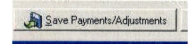

FIGURE 13-13
Save Payments/Adjustments button.

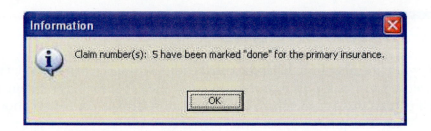

FIGURE 13-14
This box means the computer has marked this claim "PAID".

If you had more money from the insurance company to apply to other patients you would simply go up to the field in the upper left, choose another patient's file and go through this same process.

Now click the CLOSE button in the lower right-hand corner of the dialog box. This will take you back to the Deposit List.

Good job! You have now

- Entered the entire insurance company payment to your office, so that you will be able to match it with the bank statement
- Credited the patient's account to show that the insurance company has paid part or the entire balance of the charges

To double-check your work, close the Deposit List and go to Transaction Entry (under the ACTIVITIES Menu). Bring up Mr. Harvey Practice's chart. You should see the two procedure codes that you entered in the top portion under Charges. Nothing has changed there. However, if you look at the lower portion of the screen, under Payments, Adjustments and Comments, where you had previously entered the patient's co-payment of $15.00, you should see a change. Now you should see the additional entries, dated 3/20/06 from McGraw Hill Insurance Co., #00055468—one for $25.00, one for $145.00 and those for the adjustments. In the upper portion of this dialog box, you should see the accounting totals for this patient. It should look like the following:

Charges:	$201.00
Adjustments:	$ 31.00
Subtotal:	$170.00
Payment:	$170.00
Balance:	0.00
Account Total:	0.00

This tells you that Mr. Harvey Practice's account has been paid in full and that you have entered everything correctly. Excellent!

CAPITATION PAYMENTS

You will remember from Chapter 1 that there are times when a physician's office is paid not for each procedure performed (fee-for-service) but for each patient that is a member of a particular insurance plan (capitation).

With a capitation plan, the physician's office receives a certain amount of money for each patient belonging to a certain insurance plan each month. This means that the money received from that insurance carrier would not/could not be applied to a particular procedure or service provided to an individual patient. In any case, if the physician's office is receiving money, it must be recorded.

> **IMPORTANT NOTE**
>
> The specific amount of every dollar received, along with who paid and why, must be a part of the office's official financial records.

Different physicians' offices handle these payments in varying manners. You may remember that NDCMedisoft Advanced has an option for capitation payments in the New Deposit list screen. However, most insurance plans that engage in a capitation agreement with a physician's office contain a cap, or maximum level of service before additional monies will be paid. In other words, the agreement holds that the physician will provide a certain number and/or certain level of services that will be included in the monthly payment agreement. For example, the agreement might include all office visits and consultations, standard checkups, evaluations, and vaccinations. Should the physician provide services of a higher level (such as minor surgery), or services above a certain number of visits or treatments (for example, the agreement includes four office visits a year and the patient requires nine visits in one year), then a claim will be issued for the extra money.

> **IMPORTANT NOTE**
>
> Each insurance carrier that has a capitation agreement with your office will provide instructions regarding the billing of services to be paid above the basic monthly amount.

The services provided by a physician must be documented in all cases for every patient, whether or not the payment for these services will be made under a fee-for-service, a capitation plan or any other type of contract. Therefore, the process of creating the superbill/encounter form for the patient visit and having the codes entered into the patient accounting system must be done regardless of whether or not a CMS-1500 claim form is to be created. In addition, you might create a CMS-1500 that is sent to the insurance carrier or filed for the record.

CHAPTER SUMMARY

Depositing revenues in your health care facility's bank account is the equivalent of crossing the finish line of a race. It is a wonderful accomplishment. Remember, in order for it to count, you must register the payment properly and accurately into the company's accounting system. Just as this entire textbook has led you to this chapter, the process of this job position is all about getting to this point—depositing the money. Great job!

Chapter Review

In Chapter 11, you created the CMS-1500 health insurance claim forms for some of the patients for whom you coded services at the end of Chapter 9:

1. Marvin Doe

2. Patience Loyal

3. Mary Lou Sweet

4. Tex T. Books

5. Sarah Student

On the following page, you will see a remittance advice from McGraw Insurance Company for the claims that you submitted for these five patients (Figure 13-15). Using your patient accounting software program, enter the information about the insurance payment, make adjustments as necessary, and apply credit to the patients' accounts appropriately. Print receipts or a suitable report to show the status of these patients' accounts.

McGraw Insurance Company
P.O. Box 5544
Wilson, OH 45533
800-555-6654

To:
Family Doctors Associates
123 Main Street
Anytown, FL 32711
407-555-1200

Practice ID# 6654321   RA# 00055468

PATIENT NAME	DATES OF SERVICE FROM/TO	PROCEDURE CODE	AMOUNT CHARGED	ALLOWED AMOUNT	DEDUCTIBLE /CO-PAYMENT	AMOUNT PAID
DOE, MARVIN	02/27/06-02/27/06	99215	135.00	115.00	15.00	100.00
DOE, MARVIN	02/27/06-02/27/06	82947	30.00	25.00	0	25.00
DOE, MARVIN	02/27/06-02/27/06	92081	35.00	33.00	0	33.00
DOE, MARVIN	02/27/06-02/27/06	99173	35.00	29.00	0	29.00
LOYAL, PATIENCE	03/01/06-03/01/06	99214	83.00	76.00	15.00	61.00
LOYAL, PATIENCE	03/01/06-03/01/06	80050	81.00	61.00	0	61.00
LOYAL, PATIENCE	03/01/06-03/01/06	93000	65.00	55.00	0	55.00
SWEET, MARY LOU	02/24/06-02/24/06	99202	59.00	56.00	15.00	41.00
SWEET, MARY LOU	02/24/06-02/24/06	73100	65.00	63.00	0	63.00
SWEET, MARY LOU	02/24/06-02/24/06	29125	68.00	63.00	0	63.00
STUDENT, SARAH	02/27/06-02/27/06	99281	110.00	103.00	15.00	98.00
STUDENT, SARAH	02/27/06-02/27/06	73590	87.00	83.00	0	83.00
STUDENT, SARAH	02/27/06-02/27/06	29355	175.00	169.00	0	169.00
TOTAL:	**CHECK 728557**					**$881.00**

Questions regarding this remittance should be directed to:
McGraw Insurance Company • P.O. Box 5544 • Wilson, OH 45533
800-555-6654

FIGURE 13-15
McGraw Insurance remittance advice.

14 Complete Coding and Claims Practice

OBJECTIVES

To experience all aspects of insurance coding and electronic billing for a medical office by

- Reviewing patient files
- Finding the key words to use for coding the encounter
- Finding the best, most accurate diagnosis codes
- Finding the best, most accurate procedure codes
- Linking procedure codes to diagnosis codes to confirm medical necessity
- Entering patient data accurately into a patient accounting computer program
- Completing a clean CMS-1500 health insurance claim form for each patient encounter
- Entering payments from the third-party payer accurately
- Correctly crediting each patient's account with the amount paid by the third-party payer on behalf of that patient
- Reviewing a denied claim to find errors, correct them, and resubmit the claim
- Reviewing a denial notice, investigating the cause for the denial, and writing a persuasive letter for appeal

PART I: CODING PRACTICE

Congratulations! You've come full circle in the world of insurance coding and electronic billing. Now you will apply what you have learned and will deal with real-life challenges, such as claim rejection. In this chapter, you will find a patient registration form and physician's notes for five patients:

1. Bette Brothenheim
2. Margaret Mathison
3. Elise Dawson
4. Zachery Zolman
5. Keith Jackson

Review their information, along with the physician's notes. Then, for each patient,

1. Find the best, most accurate diagnosis codes.
2. Find the best, most accurate procedure (CPT) codes.
3. Link the procedure codes to the diagnosis codes.
4. Enter the information for each of these patients into NDCMedisoft Advanced or whichever patient accounting software application you are using.
5. Create and print the CMS-1500 claim form for each of these patients.

IMPORTANT NOTE
Watch your dates carefully!

Don't forget to *CHECK, DOUBLE-CHECK, and TRIPLE-CHECK* what you have entered into every field on every screen in comparison with what you see on the registration forms and physician's notes. Capitals, lowercase letters, numbers, punctuation, and spaces are all important. It must match *exactly*.

Bette Brothenheim

PATIENT REGISTRATION FORM

RESPONSIBLE PARTY			DATE *February 27, 2006*	
LAST NAME *Brothenheim*	FIRST NAME *Bette*	MI	SOCIAL SECURITY # *387-49-5987*	DATE OF BIRTH *July 13, 1978*
ADDRESS *8712 Career Circle*	CITY *Cityville*	STATE *FL*	ZIP CODE *32901*	SEX *F*	MARITAL STATUS *Single*
HOME PHONE *407-555-8843*	WORK PHONE *407-555-4451*		REFERRED BY: *Mark C. Welby, M.D.*	

EMPLOYER INFORMATION	WORK STATUS: (FULL-TIME) PART-TIME STUDENT	
COMPANY NAME *Prime Incorporated*	ADDRESS *5580 Rehearsal Lane*	CITY, STATE, ZIP *Our Town, FL 32704*

DEPENDENT INFORMATION					
DEPENDENT'S NAME		DEPENDENT'S NAME		DEPENDENT'S NAME	
RELATIONSHIP	DATE OF BIRTH	RELATIONSHIP	DATE OF BIRTH	RELATIONSHIP	DATE OF BIRTH
SOC. SEC. #	SEX	SOC. SEC. #	SEX	SOC. SEC. #	SEX
EMPLOYER	WORK PHONE	EMPLOYER	WORK PHONE	EMPLOYER	WORK PHONE

INSURANCE INFORMATION–PRIMARY POLICY		
COMPANY NAME *McGraw Insurance Co.*	ADDRESS *P.O. Box 5544*	CITY, STATE, ZIP *Wilson, OH 45533*
PHONE NUMBER *800-555-6654*	ID OR POLICY NUMBER *387495987A*	GROUP NUMBER OR NAME *PTI029*
INSURED'S NAME (IF DIFFERENT)	SOCIAL SECURITY #	RELATIONSHIP TO RESPONSIBLE PARTY
INSURED'S ADDRESS (IF DIFFERENT)	INSURED'S CITY, STATE, ZIP	INSURED'S PHONE NUMBER

INSURANCE INFORMATION–SECONDARY POLICY		
COMPANY NAME	ADDRESS	CITY, STATE, ZIP
PHONE NUMBER	ID OR POLICY NUMBER	GROUP NUMBER OR NAME
INSURED'S NAME (IF DIFFERENT)	SOCIAL SECURITY #	RELATIONSHIP TO RESPONSIBLE PARTY
INSURED'S ADDRESS (IF DIFFERENT)	INSURED'S CITY, STATE, ZIP	INSURED'S PHONE NUMBER

OTHER INFORMATION	
ALLERGIES	REASON FOR TODAY'S VISIT *Severe leg pain, possible fracture*
PATIENT'S SIGNATURE *Bette Brothenheim*	DATE *2/27/06*

FOR OFFICE USE ONLY		
CO-PAY $ *15.00*	CO-INSURANCE $ _____	DEDUCTIBLE $ _____
CHECK ☒ # *5719* CASH ☐ CHARGE ☐ PAID IN FULL ☐		
ASSIGNED PROVIDER ____ *J. Healer, MD*		

Family Doctors Associates
123 Main Street • Anytown, FL 32711
(407) 555-1200

Date: *April 13, 2006*   Attending Physician: *J. Healer, MD*

Patient Name: *Bette Brothenheim*

S: Patient is a 27 yo female seen by her regular physician after her car was struck from behind when she was driving down the highway on her way home. Patient is complaining of severe neck pain and difficulty turning her head since the accident two days ago. Patient states that the pain has become more intense over the last few days.

O: PE reveals tightness upon palpitation of neck and shoulder ligaments, most pronounced C3 to C5. X-rays are taken of the cervical vertebrae (2 views). Radiological review denies any fracture.

A: Anterior longitudinal cervical sprain

P: 1. Cervical collar to be worn during all waking hours.

2. Rx Vicodin (hydrocodone) 500 mg po prn.

3. 1,000 mg aspirin q.i.d.

4. Pt to return in 2 weeks for follow-up.

James Healer, MD

JHW/mg   D: 4/13/06 09:50:16   T: 4/18/06 12:55:01

The best, most appropriate diagnosis code(s): _____.
The best, most appropriate E/M code is _____.
The best, most appropriate procedure code(s): _____.
Link the procedure codes to the diagnosis codes. _____

Scotty Mathison

PATIENT REGISTRATION FORM

RESPONSIBLE PARTY			DATE *February 28, 2006*	
LAST NAME *Mathison*	FIRST NAME *Scotty*	MI	SOCIAL SECURITY # *513-33-5313*	DATE OF BIRTH *April 7, 1946*
ADDRESS *417 Getajob Way*	CITY *Cityville*	STATE *FL*	ZIP CODE *32901*	SEX *M* / MARITAL STATUS *Married*
HOME PHONE *407-555-9521*	WORK PHONE *407-555-5115*		REFERRED BY: *Mark C. Welby, M.D.*	

EMPLOYER INFORMATION	WORK STATUS:	(FULL-TIME) PART-TIME STUDENT
COMPANY NAME *University College*	ADDRESS *1359 Education Path*	CITY, STATE, ZIP *Our Town, FL 32704*

DEPENDENT INFORMATION

DEPENDENT'S NAME *Margaret Mathison*		DEPENDENT'S NAME		DEPENDENT'S NAME	
RELATIONSHIP *Wife*	DATE OF BIRTH *5/23/51*	RELATIONSHIP	DATE OF BIRTH	RELATIONSHIP	DATE OF BIRTH
SOC. SEC. # *535-67-1121*	SEX *Female*	SOC. SEC. #	SEX	SOC. SEC. #	SEX
EMPLOYER *none*	WORK PHONE	EMPLOYER	WORK PHONE	EMPLOYER	WORK PHONE

INSURANCE INFORMATION–PRIMARY POLICY

COMPANY NAME *McGraw Insurance Co.*	ADDRESS *P.O. Box 5544*	CITY, STATE, ZIP *Wilson, OH 45533*
PHONE NUMBER *800-555-6654*	ID OR POLICY NUMBER *RT513335313*	GROUP NUMBER OR NAME *9947G*
INSURED'S NAME (IF DIFFERENT)	SOCIAL SECURITY #	RELATIONSHIP TO RESPONSIBLE PARTY
INSURED'S ADDRESS (IF DIFFERENT)	INSURED'S CITY, STATE, ZIP	INSURED'S PHONE NUMBER

INSURANCE INFORMATION–SECONDARY POLICY

COMPANY NAME	ADDRESS	CITY, STATE, ZIP
PHONE NUMBER	ID OR POLICY NUMBER	GROUP NUMBER OR NAME
INSURED'S NAME (IF DIFFERENT)	SOCIAL SECURITY #	RELATIONSHIP TO RESPONSIBLE PARTY
INSURED'S ADDRESS (IF DIFFERENT)	INSURED'S CITY, STATE, ZIP	INSURED'S PHONE NUMBER

OTHER INFORMATION

ALLERGIES	REASON FOR TODAY'S VISIT *Stomach cramps*
PATIENT'S SIGNATURE *Scotty Mathison*	DATE *2/28/06*

FOR OFFICE USE ONLY		
CO-PAY $ *15.00*	CO-INSURANCE $ _____	DEDUCTIBLE $ _____
CHECK ☒ # *542*	CASH ☐ CHARGE ☐ PAID IN FULL ☐	
ASSIGNED PROVIDER *J. Healer, MD*		

Family Doctors Associates
123 Main Street • Anytown, FL 32711
(407) 555-1200

Date: *May 29, 2006*   Attending Physician: *J. Healer, MD*

Patient Name: *Margaret Mathison*

S: Pt is a 55-year-old female seen in the emergency room. Daughter, who accompanied pt to hospital, states pt was found unconscious in her bedroom, a bottle of Nytol found empty on the nightstand. Pt exhibited signs of severe depression over the course of the last 3–4 days after being served with divorce papers.

O: Pt is listless and unresponsive. Respiration labored, BP 80/65, P slow and erratic. Skin pale and moist. Stomach pumped. Pt responding to treatment but still exhibiting transient alteration of consciousness.

A: Poisoning by Nytol due to attempted suicide

P: Admit to hospital for observation

James Healer, MD

JHW/mg   D: 05/29/06 09:50:16   T: 06/02/06 12:55:01

The best, most appropriate diagnosis code(s): _____.
The best, most appropriate E/M code is _____.
The best, most appropriate procedure code(s): _____.
Link the procedure codes to the diagnosis codes. _____

Elise Dawson

PATIENT REGISTRATION FORM

RESPONSIBLE PARTY			DATE *May 4, 2006*		
LAST NAME *Dawson*	FIRST NAME *Elise*	MI	SOCIAL SECURITY # *617-73-1649*		DATE OF BIRTH *Feb. 23, 1985*
ADDRESS *145 Lakeside Circle*	CITY *Orlando*	STATE *FL*	ZIP CODE *32701*	SEX *F*	MARITAL STATUS *Single*
HOME PHONE *407-555-9763*	WORK PHONE *407-555-3233*		REFERRED BY: *Mark C. Welby, M.D.*		

EMPLOYER INFORMATION	WORK STATUS:	(FULL-TIME) PART-TIME STUDENT
COMPANY NAME *Cutie-Pie Pet Services*	ADDRESS *3 Tail Wagging Way*	CITY, STATE, ZIP *Casselberry, FL 32707*

DEPENDENT INFORMATION					
DEPENDENT'S NAME		DEPENDENT'S NAME		DEPENDENT'S NAME	
RELATIONSHIP	DATE OF BIRTH	RELATIONSHIP	DATE OF BIRTH	RELATIONSHIP	DATE OF BIRTH
SOC. SEC. #	SEX	SOC. SEC. #	SEX	SOC. SEC. #	SEX
EMPLOYER	WORK PHONE	EMPLOYER	WORK PHONE	EMPLOYER	WORK PHONE

INSURANCE INFORMATION–PRIMARY POLICY		
COMPANY NAME *McGraw Insurance Co.*	ADDRESS *P.O. Box 5544*	CITY, STATE, ZIP *Wilson, OH 45533*
PHONE NUMBER *800-555-6654*	ID OR POLICY NUMBER *XE617531649*	GROUP NUMBER OR NAME *CPP9755*
INSURED'S NAME (IF DIFFERENT)	SOCIAL SECURITY #	RELATIONSHIP TO RESPONSIBLE PARTY
INSURED'S ADDRESS (IF DIFFERENT)	INSURED'S CITY, STATE, ZIP	INSURED'S PHONE NUMBER

INSURANCE INFORMATION–SECONDARY POLICY		
COMPANY NAME	ADDRESS	CITY, STATE, ZIP
PHONE NUMBER	ID OR POLICY NUMBER	GROUP NUMBER OR NAME
INSURED'S NAME (IF DIFFERENT)	SOCIAL SECURITY #	RELATIONSHIP TO RESPONSIBLE PARTY
INSURED'S ADDRESS (IF DIFFERENT)	INSURED'S CITY, STATE, ZIP	INSURED'S PHONE NUMBER

OTHER INFORMATION	
ALLERGIES	REASON FOR TODAY'S VISIT *Earache*
PATIENT'S SIGNATURE *Elise Dawson*	DATE *5/4/06*

FOR OFFICE USE ONLY		
CO-PAY $ *15.00*	CO-INSURANCE $ _____	DEDUCTIBLE $ _____
CHECK ☒ # *5427* CASH ☐ CHARGE ☐ PAID IN FULL ☐		
ASSIGNED PROVIDER *J. Healer, MD*		

Family Doctors Associates
123 Main Street • Anytown, FL 32711
(407) 555-1200

Date: *May 14, 2006*   Attending Physician: *J. Healer, MD*

Patient Name: *Elise Dawson*

S: Pt is a 21-year-old female seen in her physician's office for burns on her right forearm and

hand. She was at a nightclub two days prior and reached across the table, over the centerpiece,

which had a lit candle in its center.

O: BP 120/85. P normal. R normal. Ht 5′6″. Wt 135 lbs. HEENT: unremarkable. Heart and lung

sounds unremarkable. Blistering observed on both the right forearm above the wrist and the heel of the

right hand. Burned area was cleansed, ointment was applied, and area was covered with a sterile bandage.

A: Second-degree burns, forearm and hand

P: 1. Return for bandage change in 3 days.

 2. Rx aspirin prn

James Healer, MD

JHW/mg   D: 05/14/06 09:50:16   T: 05/17/06 12:55:01

The best, most appropriate diagnosis code(s): _____.
The best, most appropriate E/M code is _____.
The best, most appropriate procedure code(s): _____.
Link the procedure codes to the diagnosis codes. _____

Gregory H. Zolman

PATIENT REGISTRATION FORM

RESPONSIBLE PARTY			DATE *April 25, 2006*	
LAST NAME *Zolman*	FIRST NAME *Gregory*	MI *H*	SOCIAL SECURITY # *231-44-8897*	DATE OF BIRTH *Aug. 19, 1970*

ADDRESS *3201 Maison Street*	CITY *Cityville*	STATE *FL*	ZIP CODE *32901*	SEX *M*	MARITAL STATUS *Divorced*

HOME PHONE *407-555-7715*	WORK PHONE *407-555-5858*	REFERRED BY:

EMPLOYER INFORMATION	WORK STATUS:	(FULL-TIME)	PART-TIME	STUDENT

COMPANY NAME *Coding Incorporated*	ADDRESS *21 Reimbursement Lane*	CITY, STATE, ZIP *Casselberry, FL 32707*

DEPENDENT INFORMATION

DEPENDENT'S NAME *Zachery Zolman*		DEPENDENT'S NAME		DEPENDENT'S NAME	
RELATIONSHIP *Son*	DATE OF BIRTH *10/27/2000*	RELATIONSHIP	DATE OF BIRTH	RELATIONSHIP	DATE OF BIRTH
SOC. SEC. # *154-99-7643*	SEX *Male*	SOC. SEC. #	SEX	SOC. SEC. #	SEX
EMPLOYER	WORK PHONE	EMPLOYER	WORK PHONE	EMPLOYER	WORK PHONE

INSURANCE INFORMATION–PRIMARY POLICY

COMPANY NAME *McGraw Insurance Co.*	ADDRESS *P.O. Box 5544*	CITY, STATE, ZIP *Wilson, OH 45533*
PHONE NUMBER *800-555-6654*	ID OR POLICY NUMBER *231448897*	GROUP NUMBER OR NAME *CI4411*
INSURED'S NAME (IF DIFFERENT)	SOCIAL SECURITY #	RELATIONSHIP TO RESPONSIBLE PARTY
INSURED'S ADDRESS (IF DIFFERENT)	INSURED'S CITY, STATE, ZIP	INSURED'S PHONE NUMBER

INSURANCE INFORMATION–SECONDARY POLICY

COMPANY NAME	ADDRESS	CITY, STATE, ZIP
PHONE NUMBER	ID OR POLICY NUMBER	GROUP NUMBER OR NAME
INSURED'S NAME (IF DIFFERENT)	SOCIAL SECURITY #	RELATIONSHIP TO RESPONSIBLE PARTY
INSURED'S ADDRESS (IF DIFFERENT)	INSURED'S CITY, STATE, ZIP	INSURED'S PHONE NUMBER

OTHER INFORMATION

ALLERGIES *Eggs*	REASON FOR TODAY'S VISIT *Employment health exam*
PATIENT'S SIGNATURE *Gregory Zolman*	DATE *4/25/06*

FOR OFFICE USE ONLY

CO-PAY $ _15.00_	CO-INSURANCE $ _____	DEDUCTIBLE $ _____

CHECK ☒ # _9821_____   CASH ☐   CHARGE ☐   PAID IN FULL ☐

ASSIGNED PROVIDER _____ *J. Healer, MD*

Family Doctors Associates
123 Main Street • Anytown, FL 32711
(407) 555-1200

Date: *May 20, 2006*   Attending Physician: *J. Healer, MD*

Patient Name: *Zachery Zolman*

S: Pt is a 5-year-old male brought to the emergency department by his father. Father stated that he found the child sitting on the garage floor, drooling, coughing, and having difficulty breathing. An empty bottle of drain cleaner was found nearby. Hx unremarkable. Father states nothing like this has happened before. NKA.

O: On HEENT exam, inside of boy's mouth and throat were burned by the lye-based drain cleaner. Endoscope inserted to determine severity of injury to esophagus. Vital signs: T 99°, R 20, Ht 3'2", Wt 51 lbs. Pulse rapid. Skin moist.

A: Chemical burn of larynx and trachea

P: 1. Rx pain meds, corticosteroids, and antibiotics to prevent strictures and infections

2. Referral to burn specialist

James Healer, MD

JHW/mg   D: 05/21/06 09:50:16   T: 05/22/06 12:55:01

The best, most appropriate diagnosis code(s): _____.
The best, most appropriate E/M code is _____.
The best, most appropriate procedure code(s): _____.
Link the procedure codes to the diagnosis codes. _____

Halle A. Jackson

PATIENT REGISTRATION FORM

RESPONSIBLE PARTY			DATE *April 30, 2006*	
LAST NAME *Jackson*	FIRST NAME *Halle*	MI *A*	SOCIAL SECURITY # *693-75-4973*	DATE OF BIRTH *Feb. 27, 1954*

ADDRESS *6155 Guardian Way*	CITY *Cityville*	STATE *FL*	ZIP CODE *32901*	SEX *F*	MARITAL STATUS *Married*

HOME PHONE *407-555-6431*	WORK PHONE *407-555-5858*	REFERRED BY:

EMPLOYER INFORMATION	WORK STATUS:	(FULL-TIME) PART-TIME STUDENT
COMPANY NAME *Coding Incorporated*	ADDRESS *21 Reimbursement Lane*	CITY, STATE, ZIP *Casselberry, FL 32707*

DEPENDENT INFORMATION

DEPENDENT'S NAME *Keith Jackson*		DEPENDENT'S NAME *Alex Jackson*		DEPENDENT'S NAME	
RELATIONSHIP *Grandson*	DATE OF BIRTH *8/13/1991*	RELATIONSHIP *Husband*	DATE OF BIRTH *8/13/53*	RELATIONSHIP	DATE OF BIRTH
SOC. SEC. # *546-98-5569*	SEX *Male*	SOC. SEC. # *546-98-5574*	SEX *Male*	SOC. SEC. #	SEX
EMPLOYER *Fig High*	WORK PHONE *407-555-4237*	EMPLOYER *Retired*	WORK PHONE	EMPLOYER	WORK PHONE

INSURANCE INFORMATION–PRIMARY POLICY

COMPANY NAME *McGraw Insurance Co.*	ADDRESS *P.O. Box 5544*	CITY, STATE, ZIP *Wilson, OH 45533*
PHONE NUMBER *800-555-6654*	ID OR POLICY NUMBER *693754973A*	GROUP NUMBER OR NAME *CI4415*
INSURED'S NAME (IF DIFFERENT)	SOCIAL SECURITY #	RELATIONSHIP TO RESPONSIBLE PARTY
INSURED'S ADDRESS (IF DIFFERENT)	INSURED'S CITY, STATE, ZIP	INSURED'S PHONE NUMBER

INSURANCE INFORMATION–SECONDARY POLICY

COMPANY NAME	ADDRESS	CITY, STATE, ZIP
PHONE NUMBER	ID OR POLICY NUMBER	GROUP NUMBER OR NAME
INSURED'S NAME (IF DIFFERENT)	SOCIAL SECURITY #	RELATIONSHIP TO RESPONSIBLE PARTY
INSURED'S ADDRESS (IF DIFFERENT)	INSURED'S CITY, STATE, ZIP	INSURED'S PHONE NUMBER

OTHER INFORMATION

ALLERGIES *None*	REASON FOR TODAY'S VISIT *Swollen ankle*
PATIENT'S SIGNATURE *Halle Jackson*	DATE *4/30/06*

FOR OFFICE USE ONLY

CO-PAY $ _*15.00*_   CO-INSURANCE $ _____   DEDUCTIBLE $ _____

CHECK ☒ # _*5467*_   CASH ☐   CHARGE ☐   PAID IN FULL ☐

ASSIGNED PROVIDER _____ *J. Healer, MD*

Family Doctors Associates
123 Main Street • Anytown, FL 32711
(407) 555-1200

Date: *June 13, 2006*   Attending Physician: *J. Healer, MD*

Patient Name: *Keith Jackson*

S: Pt is a 14-year-old male who was involved in a fistfight at the baseball field near his school.

He complained of an ache in the area of his left eye, as well as severe pain around his left ear, and

exhibited an inability to open his jaw.

O: Ht 5'11". Wt. 229 lbs. R 19. Surface hematoma evident in the area surrounding the left eye

socket reaching to the upper cheekbone. X-ray of the left side of the temporomandibular joint

confirmed a closed fracture of the left mandible. PE shows no other remarkable issues of

musculoskeletal system, or HEENT.

A: Black eye; fracture of the left mandible, angle (closed)

P: 1. Wire right jaw

2. NPO except liquids for three weeks

3. Cold, wet compresses on eye prn

4. Return for follow-up in three weeks

James Healer, MD

JHW/mg   D: 06/13/06 09:50:16   T: 06/15/06 12:55:01

The best, most appropriate diagnosis code(s): _____.

The best, most appropriate E/M code is _____.

The best, most appropriate procedure code(s): _____.

Link the procedure codes to the diagnosis codes. _____

PART II: CLAIMS PRACTICE

Now that you have created and "submitted" the claims for these patients, you are ready for the responses from the insurance carrier. On the following pages, you will find remittance advices and denial notices (Figures 14-1, 14-2, 14-3, and 14-4) for

- Bette Brothenheim
- Margaret Mathison
- Elise Dawson
- Zachery Zolman
- Keith Jackson

1. If your "office" received a payment for a claim or claims submitted, then enter the deposit into your patient accounting software program. Remember to credit the accounts of your patients for whom the insurance carrier sent you remittance. Print a receipt or statement showing all charges and payments for each patient after you have completed all the entries.
2. If your "office" received a denial notice, research the denial and the claim. Once you discover the problem, either
   a. Correct the original claim and "resubmit" it, *or*
   b. Write a letter of appeal to the insurance carrier, explaining, in as much detail as possible, why the denial should be reversed and the claim paid as originally filed. Print out your letter.

**McGraw Insurance Company
P.O. Box 5544
Wilson, OH 45533
800-555-6654**

To:
Family Doctors Associates
123 Main Street
Anytown, FL 32711
407-555-1200

Practice ID# 6654321

RA# 0008722411

PATIENT NAME	DATES OF SERVICE FROM/TO	PROCEDURE CODE	AMOUNT CHARGED	ALLOWED AMOUNT	DEDUCTIBLE /CO-PAYMENT	AMOUNT PAID
Zolman, Zachery	05/20/06-05/20/06	99284	$305.00	$ 256.35	$15.00	$ 241.35
Zolman, Zachery	05/20/06-05/20/06	43200	$155.00	$ 125.07	$ 0	$ 125.07
Mathison, Margaret	05/29/06-05/29/06	99285	$379.55	$ 289.95	$15.00	$ 274.95
Mathison, Margaret	05/29/06-05/29/06	91105	$ 65.65	$ 49.35	$ 0	$ 49.35
Total: Check # 872-99113						$ 690.72

Questions regarding this remittance should be directed to:

McGraw Insurance Company

P.O. Box 5544

Wilson, OH 45533

Customer Service: 888-555-6654

FIGURE 14-1
Remittance advice.

McGraw Insurance Company
P.O. Box 5544
Wilson, OH 45533
800-555-6654

To:
Family Doctors Associates
123 Main Street
Anytown, FL 32711
407-555-1200

Practice ID# 6654321   RA# 0008729167

CLAIM # 426064009415

PATIENT NAME	DATES OF SERVICE FROM/TO	PROCEDURE CODE	AMOUNT CHARGED	ALLOWED AMOUNT	DEDUCTIBLE /CO-PAYMENT	AMOUNT PAID
Brothenheim, Betty	04/13/06-04/13/06	99214	$105.00	$ 99.35	$15.00	$ 0[1]
Brothenheim, Betty	04/13/06-04/13/06	72040	$55.00	$ 44.79	$ 0	$ 0[1]
Total: Check # ---						$ 0[1]

NOTES:

1 Claim denied due to lack of coverage.

Questions regarding this remittance should be directed to:

McGraw Insurance Company

P.O. Box 5544

Wilson, OH 45533

Customer Service: 888-555-6654

FIGURE 14-2
Denial notice.

McGraw Insurance Company
P.O. Box 5544
Wilson, OH 45533
800-555-6654

To:
Family Doctors Associates
123 Main Street
Anytown, FL 32711
407-555-1200

Practice ID# 6654321   RA# 0008729167

CLAIM # 426064009415

PATIENT NAME	DATES OF SERVICE FROM/TO	PROCEDURE CODE	AMOUNT CHARGED	ALLOWED AMOUNT	DEDUCTIBLE /CO-PAYMENT	AMOUNT PAID
Dawson, Elise	05/14/06-05/14/06	99214	$105.00	$ 99.35	$15.00	$ 0[1]
Dawson, Elise	05/14/06-05/14/06	16001x2	$97.99	$ 71.79	$ 0	$ 0[1]
Total: Check # ---						$ 0[1]

NOTES:

1 Claim denied—code(s) invalid

Questions regarding this remittance should be directed to:

McGraw Insurance Company

P.O. Box 5544

Wilson, OH 45533

Customer Service: 888-555-6654

FIGURE 14-3
Denial notice.

McGraw Insurance Company
P.O. Box 5544
Wilson, OH 45533
800-555-6654

To:
Family Doctors Associates
123 Main Street
Anytown, FL 32711
407-555-1200

Practice ID# 6654321   RA# 0008721593

CLAIM # 4260640097533

PATIENT NAME	DATES OF SERVICE FROM/TO	PROCEDURE CODE	AMOUNT CHARGED	ALLOWED AMOUNT	DEDUCTIBLE /CO-PAYMENT	AMOUNT PAID
Jackson, Keith	06/13/06-06/13/06	99213	$105.00	$ 99.35	$15.00	$ 0[1]
Jackson, Keith	06/13/06-06/13/06	70328	$47.91	$ 43.33	$ 0	$ 0[1]
Jackson, Keith	06/13/06-06/13/06	21453	$ 693.47	$ 627.85	$ 0	$ 0[1]
Total: Check # ---						$ 0[1]

NOTES:

1 Claim denied due to lack of medical necessity

Questions regarding this remittance should be directed to:

McGraw Insurance Company

P.O. Box 5544

Wilson, OH 45533

Customer Service: 800-555-6654

FIGURE 14-4
Denial notice.

BOOK OVERVIEW

Throughout this book, you learned and experienced the sequence of responsibilities of an insurance coding and billing specialist. You learned about the types of insurance and about your responsibilities with regard to patient privacy. You also learned how to apply your knowledge of diagnosis and procedure coding. You then entered the information for each patient into the computer application designed to handle patient accounting and billing, created claim forms, supported your work with proper documentation when you received a denied claim, and received the payments for the services provided by your physician's office.

Congratulations! You are going to have a great career.

Appendix A

Abbreviations

Professionals in the health care industry use many abbreviations and acronyms. After you have spent time in the field, some of these will become second nature to you. In the meantime, read through this appendix and keep it handy for reference, particularly while you read physician's notes in preparing to code a patient encounter.

You can see that there are several different abbreviations that mean the same thing, some that come from Latin, and some that come from commonly used English. In addition, some physicians develop their own shorthand. Unless you are certain you know what is meant in the notes, always ask the person who wrote them to confirm. A misunderstanding can create a bad situation for a patient.

Abbreviation	Meaning
$\bar{a}$	before
$\bar{c}$	with
$\bar{p}$	after
$\bar{s}$	without

A

abdom or abd.	abdomen
a.c.	before meals
AD	advance directive
a.d.	right ear
ad lib.	as much as needed
AF	atrial fibrillation
AM	morning
AMA	against medical advice
ant	anterior
AP	anterior posterior
ap	before dinner
A&P	auscultation and percussion
AP&L	anterior posterior and lateral
aq	water
ARC	AIDS-related complex

A.S. or a.s.	left ear
ASCVD	arteriosclerotic cardiovascular disease
ASD	atrial septal defect
ASHD	arteriosclerotic heart disease
A.U. or a.u.	both ears
auto	automobile

B

Ba	barium
BAC	blood alcohol concentration
BI or BX	biopsy
b.i.d.	two times per day
b.i.n.	two times per night
BK	below the knee
BM	bowel movement
BP or B/P	blood pressure
BPH	benign prostatic hypertrophy
bpm	beats per minute
BR	bathroom
BRP	bathroom privileges
BSA	body surface area
BW	birth weight
Bx	biopsy

C

C	cervical, centigrade, or Celsius
C&S	culture and sensitivity
Ca or CA	cancer or carcinoma
caps	capsules
cath	catheter
CBC	complete blood count
CC	chief complaint or complications
CCU	coronary care unit
CHF	congestive heart failure
CI	cardiac index
CK	creatine kinase
ck	check
c.m.s.	to be taken tomorrow morning
c.n.	tomorrow night

CNS	central nervous system
c.n.s.	to be taken tomorrow night
CO, C/O, or c/o	complains of
comp	comprehensive or compound
compl	complete
Con or Cons	consultation
Cont. or cont.	continue
COPD	chronic obstructive pulmonary disease
CPX or CPE	complete physical examination
CR	conditioned reflex
CS or C section	cesarean section
CSF	cerebrospinal fluid
CT	computerized tomography
CV	cardiovascular
CVA	cardiovascular accident
CVP	central venous pressure
CXR	chest X-ray
Cysto	cystoscopy

D

d	day
D&C	dilatation and curettage
DC	discharge
dc	discontinue
dil	dilute
DNA	does not apply
DNR	do not resuscitate
DNS	does not show
DOB	date of birth
dos	dose
DPT	diphtheria/pertussis/tetanus vaccine
DRG	diagnosis-related group
Dx or Dg	diagnosis

E

E	emergency
ECG or EKG	electrocardiogram
ECT	electroconvulsive therapy
ED	emergency department

EEG	electroencephalogram
EENT	eye, ear, nose, and throat
elix	elixir
EMG	electromyogram
emul	emulsion
ENT	ear, nose, throat
EOM	extraocular muscles
ER	emergency room
EU	etiology unknown
EX or exam	examination
exc.	excision
ext	external

F

FBS	fasting blood sugar
FD	fatal dose
FH	family history
FHS	fetal heart sounds
Fld	fluid
fluor	fluoroscopy
ft	foot or feet
FU	follow-up
FUO	fever of unknown origin
Fx	fracture

G

G	gravida (number of pregnancies)
g or gm	gram
GA	gastric analysis
garg	gargle
GB	gallbladder
GC	gonorrhea
GGE	generalized glandular enlargement
GI	gastrointestinal
gr	grain
gt	drop
GTT	glucose tolerance test
GU	genitourinary
GYN or Gyn	gynecology

H

H or HC	hospital consultation
h	hour
HA or H/A	headache
HBP	high blood pressure
HCT or hct	hematocrit
HCVD	hypertensive cardiovascular disease
HEENT	head, eyes, ears, nose, throat
Hgb or Hb	hemoglobin
HPI	history of present illness
h.s.	hour of sleep (before bedtime)
HTN	hypertension
HX, hist, or h/o	history

I

I, inj, or INJ	injection
I&D	incision and drainage
I&O	intake and output
IBW	ideal body weight
IC	initial consultation
ICU	intensive care unit
ID	intradermal
IM	intramuscular
inc	include
inf or INF	infected
inflam or INFL	inflammation
int or INT	internal
IOP	intraocular pressure
IPPB	intermittent positive pressure breathing
IUD	intrauterine device
IUFD	intrauterine fetal death
IV	intravenous
IVP	intravenous pyelogram

K

K	potassium or kidney
k	kilo
kg	kilogram
KUB	kidney/ureter/bladder

L

l	liter
lbs	pounds
lig	ligament
liq	liquid
LLE	left lower extremity
LLL	left lower lobe
LLQ	left lower quadrant
LMP	last menstrual period
LOC	loss of consciousness or level of consciousness
LP	lumbar puncture
LT or lt	left
LTD	lowest tolerated dose
LUE	left upper extremity
LUL	left upper lobe
LUQ	left upper quadrant
LV	left ventricle
LVH	left ventricular hypertrophy

M

MA	mental age
MAP	mean arterial pressure
mcg	microgram
MDI	metered dose inhaler
MDM	medical decision making
MED	minimum effective dose
MH	marital history
ml	milliliter
MM	mucous membrane
mm	millimeter
MMR	measles, mumps, rubella
MRA	magnetic resonance angiography
MRI	magnetic resonance imaging
mV	millivolt
MVA	motor vehicle accident
My	myopia

N

NA or N/A	not applicable
NAD	no appreciable disease or acute distress

Neg or ne	negative
NG or ng	nasogastric
NICU	neonatal intensive care unit
NKA	no known allergies
NMR	nuclear magnetic resonance
nn	nerves
noct	in the night
NP	new patient
NPO or n.p.o.	nothing by mouth
NSAID	nonsteroidal anti-inflammatory drug
NSR	normal sinus rhythm
N&V	nausea and vomiting
NYD	not yet diagnosed

O

O_2	oxygen
OC	office consultation
O.D.	right eye
o.d.	once a day
OH	occupational history
o.h.	every hour
oint	ointment
o.m.	every morning
o.n.	every night
OOB	out of bed
OPD	outpatient department
OR	operating room
os	mouth
O.S.	office surgery
O.S. or o.s.	left eye
OT	occupational therapy
OTC	over-the-counter
OU	each eye or both eyes
oz	ounce

P

P	pulse
PA	posterior anterior
P&A	percussion and auscultation

PAP or Pap	Papanicolaou test
Para I	woman having borne one child (Para II = two children, etc.)
PC	present complaint
p.c.	after meals
PCA	patient-controlled analgesia
PCO_2	carbon dioxide pressure
PCWP	pulmonary capillary wedge pressure
PD	permanent disability
PE, Ph ex, or phys.	physical examination
PEFR	peak expiratory flow rate
per	by or through
PET	positron emission tomography
PH	past history
pH	hydrogen ion concentration
PI	present illness
PICC	peripherally inserted central catheter
PID	pelvic inflammatory disease
PM	afternoon or evening
PMH	past medical history
PND	postnasal drip
PO or postop	postoperative
p.o.	by mouth
pos.	positive
Post.	posterior
PPD	purified protein derivative (TB test)
p.r.	per rectum
PRN or p.r.n.	as necessary
PSP	phenolsulfonphthalein
Pt or pt	patient
PT	physical therapy
PTR	patient to return
p.v.	through the vagina

Q

Q	every
q.a.m.	every morning
q.d.	one time daily, every day
q.h.	every hour

q.h.s.	every night
q.i.d.	four times a day, not at night
q.l.	as much as wanted
q.n.	every night
q.o.d.	every other day
q.p.	as much as desired
q.p.m.	every night
q.s.	as much as needed
q.2.h.	every two hours
q.3.h.	every three hours
q.4.h.	every four hours
quotid	daily

R

rad	radiation absorbed dose
RBC	red blood count
RDA	recommended daily/dietary allowance
RE	right eye
re ch	recheck
re-exam or reex	reexamination
REM	rapid eye movement
REP or rep	let it be repeated
RHD	rheumatic heart disease
RLE	right lower extremity
RLL	right lower lobe
RLQ	right lower quadrant
RML	right middle lobe of lung
RO or R/O	rule out
ROM	range of motion
RPM	revolutions per minute
RQ	respiratory quotient
RR	recovery room or respiratory rate
RT	respiratory therapy
rt.	right
R/T	related to
RUE	right upper extremity
RUL	right upper lobe
RUQ	right upper quadrant
Rx or RX	prescription

S

sat.	saturated
SC or subq or sq	subcutaneous (under the skin)
Sig.	write on label; give directions on prescription
SL	sublingual
SOB	shortness of breath
sol	solution
s.o.s.	if necessary
S/P	no change after
SR	suture removal
ss	a half
st.	let it (them) stand
STAT or stat	immediately
STD	sexually transmitted disease
STU	skin test unit
Sx	symptoms
syr.	syrup

T

T	temperature
T&A	tonsillectomy and adenoidectomy
tab	tablet
TB, Tb, or tbc	tuberculosis
TD	temporary disability
Te	tetanus
TENS	transcutaneous electrical nerve stimulation
TIA	transient ischemic attack
t.i.d. or t.d.s.	three times daily
t.i.n.	three times a night
tinc or Tr	tincture
TLC	total lung capacity or thin-layer chromatography
TMs	tympanic membranes
top	topically
TPR	temperature/pulse/respiration
tsp	teaspoon
TURB	transurethral resection of bladder
TURP	transurethral resection of prostate
TX or Tx	treatment

U

U	unit
UA or U/A	urinalysis
UCR	usual, customary, and reasonable
UE	upper extremity
UGI	upper gastrointestinal
UPJ	ureteropelvic junction or point
UR or ur	urine
URI	upper respiratory infection
UTI	urinary tract infection
UV	ultraviolet

V

V	vein
VA	visual acuity
vac	vaccine
vag	vagina
VC	vital capacity
VD	venereal disease
VDRL	test for syphilis
Vf	field of vision
VLBW	very low birth weight
vol.	Volume

W

WBC	white blood count
WH	well hydrated
WNL	within normal limits
WR	Wassermann reaction
Wt or wt	weight

X

X	times (multiply by)
XR or X	X-ray(s)

Y

yo	years old

Appendix B

ICD-9-CM Official Guidelines for Coding and Reporting

**EFFECTIVE APRIL 1, 2005
NARRATIVE CHANGES APPEAR IN BOLD TEXT
THE GUIDELINES HAVE BEEN UPDATED TO
INCLUDE THE V CODE TABLE**

The Centers for Medicare and Medicaid Services (CMS) and the National Center for Health Statistics (NCHS), two departments within the U.S. Federal Government's Department of Health and Human Services (DHHS) provide the following guidelines for coding and reporting using the International Classification of Diseases, 9th Revision, Clinical Modification (ICD-9-CM). These guidelines should be used as a companion document to the official version of the ICD-9-CM book as published on CD-ROM by the U.S. Government Printing Office (GPO).

These guidelines have been approved by the four organizations that make up the Cooperating Parties for the ICD-9-CM book: the American Hospital Association (AHA), the American Health Information Management Association (AHIMA), CMS, and NCHS. These guidelines are included on the official government version of the ICD-9-CM book, and also appear in *"Coding Clinic for ICD-9-CM"* published by the AHA.

These guidelines are a set of rules that have been developed to accompany and complement the official conventions and instructions provided within the ICD-9-CM book itself. These guidelines are based on the coding and sequencing instructions in Volumes I, II and III of ICD-9-CM, but provide additional instruction. **Adherence to these guidelines when assigning ICD-9-CM diagnosis and procedure codes is required under the Health Insurance Portability and Accountability Act (HIPAA). The diagnosis codes (Volumes 1-2) have been adopted under HIPAA for all healthcare settings. Volume 3 procedure codes have been adopted for inpatient procedures reported by hospitals.** A joint effort between the healthcare provider and the coder is essential to achieve complete and accurate documentation, code assignment, and reporting of diagnoses and procedures. These guidelines have been developed to assist both the healthcare provider and the coder in identifying those diagnoses and procedures that are to be reported. The importance of consistent, complete documentation in the medical record cannot be overemphasized. Without such documentation accurate coding cannot be achieved. **The entire record should be reviewed to determine the specific reason for the encounter and the conditions treated.**

The term encounter is used for all settings, including hospital admissions. **In the context of these guidelines, the term provider is used throughout the guidelines to mean physician or any qualified health care practitioner who is legally accountable for establishing the patient's diagnosis.** Only this set of guidelines, approved by the Cooperating Parties, is official.

The guidelines are organized into sections. Section I includes the structure and conventions of the classification and general guidelines that apply to the entire classification, and chapter-specific guidelines that correspond to the chapters as they are arranged in the classification. Section II includes guidelines for selection of principal diagnosis for non-outpatient settings. Section III includes guidelines for reporting additional diagnoses in non-outpatient settings. Section IV is for outpatient coding and reporting.

ICD-9-CM Official Guidelines for Coding and Reporting

SECTION I.   CONVENTIONS, GENERAL CODING GUIDELINES, AND CHAPTER SPECIFIC GUIDELINES

The conventions, general guidelines, and chapter-specific guidelines are applicable to all health care settings unless otherwise indicated.

A. Conventions for the ICD-9-CM Book

The conventions for the ICD-9-CM book are the general rules for use of the classification independent of the guidelines. These conventions are incorporated within the index and tabular of the ICD-9-CM book as instructional notes. The conventions are as follows:

1. Format:

The ICD-9-CM book uses an indented format for ease in reference

2. Abbreviations

a. Index abbreviations

NEC   "Not elsewhere classifiable"

This abbreviation in the index represents "other specified" when a specific code is not available for a condition the index directs the coder to the "other specified" code in the tabular.

b. Tabular abbreviations

NEC   "Not elsewhere classifiable"

This abbreviation in the tabular represents "other specified". When a specific code is not available for a condition the tabular includes an NEC entry under a code to identify the code as the "other specified" code (See Section I.A.5.a. "Other" codes).

NOS   "Not otherwise specified"

This abbreviation is the equivalent of unspecified (See Section I.A.5.b., "Unspecified" codes).

3. Punctuation

[] Brackets are used in the tabular list to enclose synonyms, alternative wording, or explanatory phrases. Brackets are used in the index to identify manifestation codes (See Section I.A.6. "Etiology/manifestations").

() Parentheses are used in both the index and tabular to enclose supplementary words that may be present or absent in the statement of a disease or procedure without affecting the code number to which it is assigned. The terms within the parentheses are referred to as nonessential modifiers.

: Colons are used in the Tabular List after an incomplete term which needs one or more of the modifiers following the colon to make it assignable to a given category.

4. Includes and excludes notes and inclusion terms

Includes: This note appears immediately under a three-digit code title to further define, or give examples of, the content of the category.

Excludes:
An excludes note under a code indicates that the terms excluded from the code are to be coded elsewhere. In some cases the codes for the excluded terms should not be used in conjunction with the code from which it is excluded. An example of this is a congenital condition excluded from an acquired form of the same condition. The congenital and acquired codes should not be used together. In other cases, the excluded terms may be used together with an excluded code. An example of this is when fractures of different bones are coded to different codes. Both codes may be used together if both types of fractures are present.

Inclusion terms:
List of terms are included under certain four and five digit codes. These terms are the conditions for which that code number is to be used. The terms may be synonyms of the code title, or, in the case of "other specified" codes, the terms are a list of the various conditions assigned to that code. The inclusion terms are not necessarily exhaustive. Additional terms found only in the index may also be assigned to a code.

5. **Other and unspecified codes**

   a. **"Other" codes**

   Codes titled "other" or "other specified" (usually a code with a 4th digit 8 or fifth-digit 9 for diagnosis codes) are for use when the information in the medical record provides detail for which a specific code does not exist. Index entries with NEC in the line designate "other" codes in the tabular. These index entries represent specific disease entities for which no specific code exists so the term is included within an "other" code.

   b. **"Unspecified" codes**

   Codes (usually a code with a 4th digit 9 or 5th digit 0 for diagnosis codes) titled "unspecified" are for use when the information in the medical record is insufficient to assign a more specific code.

6. **Etiology/manifestation convention ("code first," "use additional code" and "in diseases classified elsewhere" notes)**

   Certain conditions have both an underlying etiology and multiple body system manifestations due to the underlying etiology. For such conditions, the ICD-9-CM book has a coding convention that requires the underlying condition be sequenced first followed by the manifestation. Wherever such a combination exists, there is a "use additional code" note at the etiology code, and a "code first" note at the manifestation code. These instructional notes indicate the proper sequencing order of the codes, etiology followed by manifestation.

   In most cases, the manifestation codes will have in the code title, "in diseases classified elsewhere." Codes with this title are a component of the etiology/manifestation convention. The code title indicates that it is a manifestation code. "In diseases classified elsewhere" codes are never permitted to be used as first listed or principal diagnosis codes. They must be used in conjunction with an underlying condition code and they must be listed following the underlying condition.

   There are manifestation codes that do not have "in diseases classified elsewhere" in the title. For such codes a "use additional code" note will still be present and the rules for sequencing apply.

   In addition to the notes in the tabular, these conditions also have a specific index entry structure. In the index both conditions are listed together with the etiology code first followed by the manifestation codes in brackets. The code in brackets is always to be sequenced second.

The most commonly used etiology/manifestation combinations are the codes for Diabetes mellitus, category 250. For each code under category 250 there is a use additional code note for the manifestation that is specific for that particular diabetic manifestation. Should a patient have more than one manifestation of diabetes, more than one code from category 250 may be used with as many manifestation codes as are needed to fully describe the patient's complete diabetic condition. The **category** 250 diabetes codes should be sequenced first, followed by the manifestation codes.

"Code first" and "Use additional code" notes are also used as sequencing rules in the classification for certain codes that are not part of an etiology/manifestation combination. See - Section I.B.9. "Multiple coding for a single condition."

7. "And"

The word "and" should be interpreted to mean either "and" or "or" when it appears in a title.

8. "With"

The word "with" in the alphabetic index is sequenced immediately following the main term, not in alphabetical order.

9. "See" and "See Also"

The "see" instruction following a main term in the index indicates that another term should be referenced. It is necessary to go to the main term referenced with the "see" note to locate the correct code.

A "see also" instruction following a main term in the index instructs that there is another main term that may also be referenced that may provide additional index entries that may be useful. It is not necessary to follow the "see also" note when the original main term provides the necessary code.

B. General Coding Guidelines

1. **Use of both Alphabetic Index and Tabular List**

   Use both the Alphabetic Index and the Tabular List when locating and assigning a code. Reliance on only the Alphabetic Index or the Tabular List leads to errors in code assignments and less specificity in code selection.

2. **Locate each term in the Alphabetic Index**

   Locate each term in the Alphabetic Index and verify the code selected in the Tabular List. Read and be guided by instructional notations that appear in both the Alphabetic Index and the Tabular List.

3. **Level of detail in coding**

   Diagnosis and procedure codes are to be used at their highest number of digits available.

   ICD-9-CM diagnosis codes are composed of codes with either 3, 4, or 5 digits. Codes with three digits are included in ICD-9-CM as the heading of a category of codes that may be further subdivided by the use of fourth and/or fifth digits, which provide greater detail.

   A three-digit code is to be used only if it is not further subdivided. Where fourth-digit subcategories and/or fifth-digit subclassifications are provided, they must be assigned. A code is invalid if it has not been coded to the full number of digits required for that code. For example, Acute myocardial infarction, code 410, has fourth digits that describe the location of the infarction (e.g., 410.2, Of inferolateral wall), and fifth digits that identify the episode of care. It would be incorrect to report a code in category 410 without a fourth and fifth digit.

   ICD-9-CM, Volume 3 procedure codes are composed of codes with either 3 or 4 digits. Codes with two digits are included in ICD-9-CM as the heading of a category of codes that may be further subdivided by the use of third and/or fourth digits, which provide greater detail.

4. **Code or codes from 001.0 through V84.8**

   The appropriate code or codes from 001.0 through V84.8 must be used to identify diagnoses, symptoms, conditions, problems, complaints or other reason(s) for the encounter/visit.

5. **Selection of codes 001.0 through 999.9**

   The selection of codes 001.0 through 999.9 will frequently be used to describe the reason for the admission/encounter. These codes are from the section of ICD-9-CM for the classification of diseases and injuries (e.g., infectious and parasitic diseases; neoplasms; symptoms, signs, and ill-defined conditions, etc.).

6. **Signs and symptoms**

   Codes that describe symptoms and signs, as opposed to diagnoses, are acceptable for reporting purposes when a related definitive diagnosis has not been established (confirmed) by the provider. Chapter 16 of ICD-9-CM, Symptoms, Signs, and Ill-defined conditions (codes 780.0–799.9) contains many, but not all codes for symptoms.

7. **Conditions that are an integral part of a disease process**

   Signs and symptoms that are integral to the disease process should not be assigned as additional codes.

8. **Conditions that are not an integral part of a disease process**

   Additional signs and symptoms that may not be associated routinely with a disease process should be coded when present.

9. **Multiple coding for a single condition**

   In addition to the etiology/manifestation convention that requires two codes to fully describe a single condition that affects multiple body systems, there are other single conditions that also require more than one code. "Use additional code" notes are found in the tabular list at codes that are not part of an etiology/manifestation pair where a secondary code is useful to fully describe a condition. The sequencing rule is the same as the etiology/manifestation pair, "use additional code" indicates that a secondary code should be added.

   For example, for infections that are not included in Chapter 1, a secondary code from category 041, Bacterial infection in conditions classified elsewhere and of unspecified site, may be required to identify the bacterial organism causing the infection. A "use additional code" note will normally be found at the infectious disease code, indicating a need for the organism code to be added as a secondary code.

   "Code first" notes are also under certain codes that are not specifically manifestation codes but may be due to an underlying cause. When a "code first" note is present and an underlying condition is present the underlying condition should be sequenced first.

   "Code, if applicable, any causal condition first," notes indicate that this code may be assigned as a principal diagnosis when the causal condition is unknown or not applicable. If a causal condition is known, then the code for that condition should be sequenced as the principal or first-listed diagnosis.

   Multiple codes may be needed for late effects, complication codes and obstetric codes to more fully describe a condition. See the specific guidelines for these conditions for further instruction.

10. **Acute and chronic conditions**

    If the same condition is described as both acute (subacute) and chronic, and separate subentries exist in the Alphabetic Index at the same indentation level, code both and sequence the acute (subacute) code first.

11. **Combination code**

A combination code is a single code used to classify:
Two diagnoses, or
A diagnosis with an associated secondary process (manifestation)
A diagnosis with an associated complication

Combination codes are identified by referring to subterm entries in the Alphabetic Index and by reading the inclusion and exclusion notes in the Tabular List.

Assign only the combination code when that code fully identifies the diagnostic conditions involved or when the Alphabetic Index so directs. Multiple coding should not be used when the classification provides a combination code that clearly identifies all of the elements documented in the diagnosis. When the combination code lacks necessary specificity in describing the manifestation or complication, an additional code should be used as a secondary code.

12. **Late effects**

A late effect is the residual effect (condition produced) after the acute phase of an illness or injury has terminated. There is no time limit on when a late effect code can be used. The residual may be apparent early, such as in cerebrovascular accident cases, or it may occur months or years later, such as that due to a previous injury. Coding of late effects generally requires two codes sequenced in the following order: The condition or nature of the late effect is sequenced first. The late effect code is sequenced second.

An exception to the above guidelines are those instances where the code for late effect is followed by a manifestation code identified in the Tabular List and title, or the late effect code has been expanded (at the fourth and fifth-digit levels) to include the manifestation(s). The code for the acute phase of an illness or injury that led to the late effect is never used with a code for the late effect.

13. **Impending or threatened condition**

Code any condition described at the time of discharge as "impending" or "threatened" as follows:

If it did occur, code as confirmed diagnosis.

If it did not occur, reference the Alphabetic Index to determine if the condition has a subentry term for "impending" or "threatened" and also reference main term entries for "Impending" and for "Threatened."

If the subterms are listed, assign the given code.

If the subterms are not listed, code the existing underlying condition(s) and not the condition described as impending or threatened.

C. **Chapter-Specific Coding Guidelines**

In addition to general coding guidelines, there are guidelines for specific diagnoses and/or conditions in the classification. Unless otherwise indicated, these guidelines apply to all health care settings. Please refer to Section II for guidelines on the selection of principal diagnosis.

1. **Chapter 1: Infectious and Parasitic Diseases (001–139)**

a. **Human Immunodeficiency Virus (HIV) Infections**

1) **Code only confirmed cases**

Code only confirmed cases of HIV infection/illness. This is an exception to the hospital inpatient guideline Section II, H.

In this context, "confirmation" does not require documentation of positive serology or culture for HIV; the provider's diagnostic statement that the patient is HIV positive, or has an HIV-related illness is sufficient.

2) **Selection and sequencing of HIV codes**

   (a) **Patient admitted for HIV-related condition**

   If a patient is admitted for an HIV-related condition, the principal diagnosis should be 042, followed by additional diagnosis codes for all reported HIV-related conditions.

   (b) **Patient with HIV disease admitted for unrelated condition**

   If a patient with HIV disease is admitted for an unrelated condition (such as a traumatic injury), the code for the unrelated condition (e.g., the nature of injury code) should be the principal diagnosis. Other diagnoses would be 042 followed by additional diagnosis codes for all reported HIV-related conditions.

   (c) **Whether the patient is newly diagnosed**

   Whether the patient is newly diagnosed or has had previous admissions/encounters for HIV conditions is irrelevant to the sequencing decision.

   (d) **Asymptomatic human immunodeficiency virus**

   V08 Asymptomatic human immunodeficiency virus [HIV] infection, is to be applied when the patient without any documentation of symptoms is listed as being "HIV positive," "known HIV," "HIV test positive," or similar terminology. Do not use this code if the term "AIDS" is used or if the patient is treated for any HIV-related illness or is described as having any condition(s) resulting from his/her HIV positive status; use 042 in these cases.

   (e) **Patients with inconclusive HIV serology**

   Patients with inconclusive HIV serology, but no definitive diagnosis or manifestations of the illness, may be assigned code 795.71, Inconclusive serologic test for Human Immunodeficiency Virus [HIV].

   (f) **Previously diagnosed HIV-related illness**

   Patients with any known prior diagnosis of an HIV-related illness should be coded to 042. Once a patient has developed an HIV-related illness, the patient should always be assigned code 042 on every subsequent admission/encounter. Patients previously diagnosed with any HIV illness (042) should never be assigned to 795.71 or V08.

   (g) **HIV Infection in pregnancy, childbirth and the puerperium**

   During pregnancy, childbirth or the puerperium, a patient admitted (or presenting for a health care encounter) because of an HIV-related illness should receive a principal diagnosis code of 647.6X. Other specified infectious and parasitic diseases in the mother classifiable elsewhere, but complicating the pregnancy, childbirth or the puerperium, followed by 042 and the code(s) for the HIV-related illness(es). Codes from Chapter 15 always take sequencing priority.

   Patients with asymptomatic HIV infection status admitted (or presenting for a health care encounter) during pregnancy, childbirth, or the puerperium should receive codes of 647.6X and V08.

(h) **Encounters for testing for HIV**

If a patient is being seen to determine his/her HIV status, use code V73.89, Screening for other specified viral disease. Use code V69.8, Other problems related to lifestyle, as a secondary code if an asymptomatic patient is in a known high risk group for HIV. Should a patient with signs or symptoms or illness, or a confirmed HIV related diagnosis be tested for HIV, code the signs and symptoms or the diagnosis. An additional counseling code V65.44 may be used if counseling is provided during the encounter for the test.

When a patient returns to be informed of his/her HIV test results use code V65.44, HIV counseling, if the results of the test are negative.

If the results are positive but the patient is asymptomatic use code V08, Asymptomatic HIV infection. If the results are positive and the patient is symptomatic use code 042, HIV infection, with codes for the HIV related symptoms or diagnosis. The HIV counseling code may also be used if counseling is provided for patients with positive test results.

b. **Septicemia, Systemic Inflammatory Response Syndrome (SIRS), Sepsis, Severe Sepsis, and Septic Shock**

1) **Sepsis as principal diagnosis or secondary diagnosis**

(a) **Sepsis as principal diagnosis**

If sepsis is present on admission, and meets the definition of principal diagnosis, the underlying systemic infection code (e.g., 038.xx, 112.5, etc.) should be assigned as the principal diagnosis, followed by code 995.91, Systemic inflammatory response syndrome due to infectious process without organ dysfunction, as required by the sequencing rules in the Tabular List. Codes from subcategory 995.9 can never be assigned as a principal diagnosis.

(b) **Sepsis as secondary diagnoses**

When sepsis develops during the encounter (it was not present on admission), the sepsis codes may be assigned as secondary diagnoses, following the sequencing rules provided in the Tabular List.

(c) **Documentation unclear as to whether sepsis present on admission**

If the documentation is not clear whether the sepsis was present on admission, the provider should be queried. After provider query, if sepsis is determined at that point to have met the definition of principal diagnosis, the underlying systemic infection (038.xx, 112.5, etc.) may be used as principal diagnosis along with code 995.91, Systemic inflammatory response syndrome due to infectious process without organ dysfunction.

2) **Septicemia/Sepsis**

In most cases, it will be a code from category 038, Septicemia, that will be used in conjunction with a code from subcategory 995.9 such as the following:

(a) **Streptococcal sepsis**

If the documentation in the record states streptococcal sepsis, codes 038.0 and code 995.91 should be used, in that sequence.

(b) **Streptococcal septicemia**

If the documentation states streptococcal septicemia, only code 038.0 should be assigned, however, the provider should be queried whether the patient has sepsis, an infection with SIRS.

(c) **Sepsis or SIRS must be documented**

Either the term sepsis or SIRS must be documented, to assign a code from subcategory 995.9.

3) **Terms sepsis, severe sepsis, or SIRS**

If the terms sepsis, severe sepsis, or SIRS are used with an underlying infection other than septicemia, such as pneumonia, cellulitis or a nonspecified urinary tract infection, a code from category 038 should be assigned first, then code 995.91, followed by the code for the initial infection. The use of the terms sepsis or SIRS indicates that the patient's infection has advanced to the point of a systemic infection so the systemic infection should be sequenced before the localized infection. The instructional note under subcategory 995.9 instructs to assign the underlying systemic infection first.

Note: The term urosepsis is a non-specific term. If that is the only term documented then only code 599.0 should be assigned based on the default for the term in the ICD-9-CM index, in addition to the code for the causal organism if known.

4) **Severe sepsis**

For patients with severe sepsis, the code for the systemic infection (e.g., 038.xx, 112.5, etc.) or trauma should be sequenced first, followed by either code 995.92, Systemic inflammatory response syndrome due to infectious process with organ dysfunction, or code 995.94, Systemic inflammatory response syndrome due to noninfectious process with organ dysfunction. Codes for the specific organ dysfunctions should also be assigned.

5) **Septic shock**

(a) **Sequencing of septic shock**

Septic shock is a form of organ dysfunction associated with severe sepsis. A code for the initiating underlying systemic infection followed by a code for SIRS (code 995.92) must be assigned before the code for septic shock. As noted in the sequencing instructions in the Tabular List, the code for septic shock cannot be assigned as a principal diagnosis.

(b) **Septic shock without documentation of severe sepsis**

Septic shock cannot occur in the absence of severe sepsis. A code from subcategory 995.9 must be sequenced before the code for septic shock. The use additional code notes and the code first note provide sequencing instructions.

6) **Sepsis and septic shock associated with abortion**

Sepsis and septic shock associated with abortion, ectopic pregnancy, and molar pregnancy are classified to category codes in Chapter 11 (630–639).

7) **Negative or inconclusive blood cultures**

Negative or inconclusive blood cultures do not preclude a diagnosis of septicemia or sepsis in patients with clinical evidence of the condition, however, the provider should be queried.

8) **Newborn sepsis**

See Section I.C.15.j for information on the coding of newborn sepsis.

9) **Sepsis due to a Postprocedural Infection**

Sepsis resulting from a postprocedural infection is a complication of care. For such cases code 998.59, Other postoperative infections, should be coded first followed by the appropriate codes for the sepsis. The other guidelines for coding sepsis should then be followed for the assignment of additional codes.

10) **External cause of injury codes with SIRS**

An external cause code is not needed with codes 995.91, Systemic inflammatory response syndrome due to infectious process without organ dysfunction, or code 995.92, Systemic inflammatory response syndrome due to infectious process with organ dysfunction.

Refer to Section I.C.19.a.7 for instruction on the use of external cause of injury codes with codes for SIRS resulting from trauma.

2. **Chapter 2: Neoplasms (140–239)**

<u>General guidelines</u>

Chapter 2 of the ICD-9-CM book contains the codes for most benign and all malignant neoplasms. Certain benign neoplasms, such as prostatic adenomas, may be found in the specific body system chapters. To properly code a neoplasm it is necessary to determine from the record if the neoplasm is benign, in-situ, malignant, or of uncertain histologic behavior. If malignant, any secondary (metastatic) sites should also be determined.

The Neoplasm Table in the Alphabetic Index should be referenced first. However, if the histological term is documented, that term should be referenced first, rather than going immediately to the Neoplasm Table, in order to determine which column in the Neoplasm Table is appropriate. For example, if the documentation indicates "adenoma," refer to the term in the Alphabetic Index to review the entries under this term and the instructional note to "see also neoplasm, by site, benign." The table provides the proper code based on the type of neoplasm and the site. It is important to select the proper column in the table that corresponds to the type of neoplasm. The tabular should then be referenced to verify that the correct code has been selected from the table and that a more specific site code does not exist.

See Section I.C.18.d.4. for information regarding V codes for genetic susceptibility to cancer.

a. **Treatment directed at the malignancy**

If the treatment is directed at the malignancy, designate the malignancy as the principal diagnosis.

b. **Treatment of secondary site**

When a patient is admitted because of a primary neoplasm with metastasis and treatment is directed toward the secondary site only, the secondary neoplasm is designated as the principal diagnosis even though the primary malignancy is still present.

c. **Coding and sequencing of complications**

Coding and sequencing of complications associated with the malignancies or with the therapy thereof are subject to the following guidelines:

1) **Anemia associated with malignancy**

When admission/encounter is for management of an anemia associated with the malignancy, and the treatment is only for anemia, the anemia is designated at the principal diagnosis and is followed by the appropriate code(s) for the malignancy.

2) **Anemia associated with chemotherapy**

When the admission/encounter is for management of an anemia associated with chemotherapy or radiotherapy and the only treatment is for the anemia, the anemia is sequenced first followed by the appropriate code(s) for the malignancy.

3) **Management of dehydration due to the malignancy**

When the admission/encounter is for management of dehydration due to the malignancy or the therapy, or a combination of both, and only the dehydration is being treated (intravenous rehydration), the dehydration is sequenced first, followed by the code(s) for the malignancy.

4) **Treatment of a complication resulting from a surgical procedure**

When the admission/encounter is for treatment of a complication resulting from a surgical procedure, designate the complication as the principal or first-listed diagnosis if treatment is directed at resolving the complication.

d. **Primary malignancy previously excised**

When a primary malignancy has been previously excised or eradicated from its site and there is no further treatment directed to that site and there is no evidence of any existing primary malignancy, a code from category V10, Personal history of malignant neoplasm, should be used to indicate the former site of the malignancy. Any mention of extension, invasion, or metastasis to another site is coded as a secondary malignant neoplasm to that site. The secondary site may be the principal or first-listed with the V10 code used as a secondary code.

e. **Admissions/encounters involving chemotherapy and radiation therapy**

1) **Episode of care involves surgical removal of neoplasm**

When an episode of care involves the surgical removal of a neoplasm, primary or secondary site, followed by adjunct chemotherapy or radiation treatment, the neoplasm code should be assigned as principal or first-listed diagnosis, using codes in the 140–198 series or where appropriate in the 200–203 series.

2) **Patient admission/encounter solely for administration of chemotherapy**

If a patient admission/encounter is solely for the administration of chemotherapy or radiation therapy, code V58.0, Encounter for radiation therapy, or V58.1, Encounter for chemotherapy, should be the first-listed or principal diagnosis. If a patient receives both chemotherapy and radiation therapy both codes should be listed, in either order of sequence.

3) **Patient admitted for radiotherapy/chemotherapy and develops complications**

When a patient is admitted for the purpose of radiotherapy or chemotherapy and develops complications such as uncontrolled nausea and vomiting or dehydration, the principal or first-listed diagnosis is V58.0, Encounter for radiotherapy, or V58.1, Encounter for chemotherapy, followed by any codes for the complications.

See Section I.C.18.d.8. for additional information regarding aftercare V codes.

f. **Admission/encounter to determine extent of malignancy**

When the reason for admission/encounter is to determine the extent of the malignancy, or for a procedure such as paracentesis or thoracentesis, the primary malignancy or appropriate metastatic site is designated as the principal or first-listed diagnosis, even though chemotherapy or radiotherapy is administered.

g. **Symptoms, signs, and ill-defined conditions listed in Chapter 16**

Symptoms, signs, and ill-defined conditions listed in Chapter 16 characteristic of, or associated with, an existing primary or secondary site malignancy cannot be used to replace the malignancy as principal or first-listed diagnosis, regardless of the number of admissions or encounters for treatment and care of the neoplasm.

h. **Encounter for prophylactic organ removal**

For encounters specifically for prophylactic removal of breasts, ovaries, or another organ due to a genetic susceptibility to cancer or a family history of cancer, the principal or first listed code should be a code from subcategory V50.4, Prophylactic organ removal, followed by the appropriate genetic susceptibility code and the appropriate family history code.

If the patient has a malignancy of one site and is having prophylactic removal of another site to prevent either a new primary malignancy or metastatic disease, a code for the malignancy should also be assigned in addition to a code from subcategory V50.4. A V50.4 code should not be assigned if the patient is having organ removal for treatment of a malignancy, such as the removal of the testes for the treatment of prostate cancer.

3. **Chapter 3: Endocrine, Nutritional, and Metabolic Diseases and Immunity Disorders (240–279)**

a. Diabetes mellitus

Codes under category 250, Diabetes mellitus, identify complications/manifestations associated with diabetes mellitus. A fifth-digit is required for all category 250 codes to identify the type of diabetes mellitus and whether the diabetes is controlled or uncontrolled.

1) Fifth-digits for category 250:

The following are the fifth-digits for the codes under category 250:

0   type II or unspecified type, not stated as uncontrolled
1   type I, [juvenile type], not stated as uncontrolled
2   type II or unspecified type, uncontrolled
3   type I, [juvenile type], uncontrolled

The age of a patient is not the sole determining factor, though most type I diabetics develop the condition before reaching puberty. For this reason type I diabetes mellitus is also referred to as juvenile diabetes.

2) Type of diabetes mellitus not documented

If the type of diabetes mellitus is not documented in the medical record the default is type II.

3) Diabetes mellitus and the use of insulin

All type I diabetics must use insulin to replace what their bodies do not produce. However, the use of insulin does not mean that a patient is a type I diabetic. Some patients with type II diabetes mellitus are unable to control their blood sugar through diet and oral medication alone and do require insulin. If the documentation in a medical record does not indicate the type of diabetes but does indicate that the patient uses insulin, the appropriate fifth-digit for type II must be used. For type II patients who routinely use insulin, code V58.67, Long-term (current) use of insulin, should also be assigned to indicate that the patient uses insulin. Code V58.67 should not be assigned if insulin is given temporarily to bring a type II patient's blood sugar under control during an encounter.

4) Assigning and sequencing diabetes codes and associated conditions

When assigning codes for diabetes and its associated conditions, the code(s) from category 250 must be sequenced before the codes for the associated conditions. The diabetes codes and the secondary codes that correspond to them are paired codes that follow the etiology/manifestation convention of the classification (See Section I.A.6., Etiology/manifestation convention). Assign as many codes from category 250 as needed to identify all of the associated conditions that the patient has. The corresponding secondary codes are listed under each of the diabetes codes.

5) Diabetes mellitus in pregnancy and gestational diabetes

(a) For diabetes mellitus complicating pregnancy, see Section I.C.11.f., Diabetes mellitus in pregnancy.

(b) For gestational diabetes, see Section I.C.11,g., Gestational diabetes.

6) Insulin pump malfunction

(a) Underdose of insulin due insulin pump failure. An underdose of insulin due to an insulin pump failure should be assigned 996.57, Mechanical complication due to insulin pump, as the principal or first listed code, followed by the appropriate diabetes mellitus code based on documentation.

(b) Overdose of insulin due to insulin pump failure. The principal or first listed code for an encounter due to an insulin pump malfunction resulting in an overdose of insulin, should also be 996.57, Mechanical complication due to insulin pump, followed by code 962.3, Poisoning by insulins and antidiabetic agents, and the appropriate diabetes mellitus code based on documentation.

4. **Chapter 4: Diseases of Blood and Blood Forming Organs (280–289)**

Reserved for future guideline expansion

5. **Chapter 5: Mental Disorders (290–319)**

Reserved for future guideline expansion

6. **Chapter 6: Diseases of Nervous System and Sense Organs (320–389)**

Reserved for future guideline expansion

7. **Chapter 7: Diseases of Circulatory System (390–459)**

a. **Hypertension**

Hypertension Table

The Hypertension Table, found under the main term, "Hypertension," in the Alphabetic Index, contains a complete listing of all conditions due to or associated with hypertension and classifies them according to malignant, benign, and unspecified.

1) **Hypertension, Essential, or NOS**

Assign hypertension (arterial) (essential) (primary) (systemic) (NOS) to category code 401 with the appropriate fourth digit to indicate malignant (.0), benign (.1), or unspecified (.9). Do not use either .0 malignant or .1 benign unless medical record documentation supports such a designation.

2) **Hypertension with Heart Disease**

Heart conditions (425.8, 429.0–429.3, 429.8, 429.9) are assigned to a code from category 402 when a causal relationship is stated (due to hypertension) or implied (hypertensive). Use an additional code from category 428 to identify the type of heart failure in those patients with heart failure. More than one code from category 428 may be assigned if the patient has systolic or diastolic failure and congestive heart failure.

The same heart conditions (425.8, 429.0–429.3, 429.8, 429.9) with hypertension, but without a stated casual relationship, are coded separately. Sequence according to the circumstances of the admission/encounter.

3) Hypertensive Renal Disease with Chronic Renal Failure

Assign codes from category 403, Hypertensive renal disease, when conditions classified to categories 585–587 are present. Unlike hypertension with heart disease, ICD-9-CM presumes a cause-and-effect relationship and classifies renal failure with hypertension as hypertensive renal disease.

4) Hypertensive Heart and Renal Disease

Assign codes from combination category 404, Hypertensive heart and renal disease, when both hypertensive renal disease and hypertensive heart disease are stated in the diagnosis. Assume a relationship between the hypertension and the renal disease, whether or not the condition is so designated. Assign an additional code from category 428, to identify the type of heart failure. More than one code from category 428 may be assigned if the patient has systolic or diastolic failure and congestive heart failure.

5) Hypertensive Cerebrovascular Disease

First assign codes from 430–438, Cerebrovascular disease, then the appropriate hypertension code from categories 401–405.

6) Hypertensive Retinopathy

Two codes are necessary to identify the condition. First assign the code from subcategory 362.11, Hypertensive retinopathy, then the appropriate code from categories 401–405 to indicate the type of hypertension.

7) Hypertension, Secondary

Two codes are required: one to identify the underlying etiology and one from category 405 to identify the hypertension. Sequencing of codes is determined by the reason for admission/encounter.

8) Hypertension, Transient

Assign code 796.2, Elevated blood pressure reading without diagnosis of hypertension, unless patient has an established diagnosis of hypertension. Assign code 642.3x for transient hypertension of pregnancy.

9) Hypertension, Controlled

Assign appropriate code from categories 401–405. This diagnostic statement usually refers to an existing state of hypertension under control by therapy.

10) Hypertension, Uncontrolled

Uncontrolled hypertension may refer to untreated hypertension or hypertension not responding to current therapeutic regimen. In either case, assign the appropriate code from categories 401–405 to designate the stage and type of hypertension. Code to the type of hypertension.

11) Elevated Blood Pressure

For a statement of elevated blood pressure without further specificity, assign code 796.2, Elevated blood pressure reading without diagnosis of hypertension, rather than a code from category 401.

b. Cerebral infarction/stroke/cerebrovascular accident (CVA)

The terms stroke and CVA are often used interchangeably to refer to a cerebral infarction. The terms stroke, CVA, and cerebral infarction NOS are all indexed to the default code 434.91, Cerebral artery occlusion, unspecified, with infarction. Code 436, Acute, but ill-defined, cerebrovascular disease, should not be used when the documentation states stroke or CVA.

c. Postoperative cerebrovascular accident

A cerebrovascular hemorrhage or infarction that occurs as a result of medical intervention is coded to 997.02, Iatrogenic cerebrovascular infarction or hemorrhage. Medical record documentation should clearly specify the cause-and-effect relationship between the medical intervention and the cerebrovascular accident in order to assign this code. A secondary code from the code range 430–432 or from a code from subcategories 433 or 434 with a fifth digit of "1" should also be used to identify the type of hemorrhage or infarct.

This guideline conforms to the use additional code note instruction at category 997. Code 436, Acute, but ill-defined, cerebrovascular disease, should not be used as a secondary code with code 997.02.

d. Late effects of cerebrovascular disease

1) Category 438, Late Effects of Cerebrovascular disease

Category 438 is used to indicate conditions classifiable to categories 430–437 as the causes of late effects (neurologic deficits), themselves classified elsewhere. These "late effects" include neurologic deficits that persist after initial onset of conditions classifiable to 430–437. The neurologic deficits caused by cerebrovascular disease may be present from the onset or may arise at any time after the onset of the condition classifiable to 430–437.

2) Codes from category 438 with codes from 430–437

Codes from category 438 may be assigned on a health care record with codes from 430–437, if the patient has a current cerebrovascular accident (CVA) and deficits from an old CVA.

3) Code V12.59

Assign code V12.59 (and not a code from category 438) as an additional code for history of cerebrovascular disease when no neurologic deficits are present.

8. Chapter 8: Diseases of Respiratory System (460–519)

a. Chronic Obstructive Pulmonary Disease [COPD] and Asthma

1) Conditions that comprise COPD and Asthma

The conditions that comprise COPD are obstructive chronic bronchitis, subcategory 491.2, and emphysema, category 492. All asthma codes are under category 493, Asthma. Code 496, Chronic airway obstruction, not elsewhere classified, is a nonspecific code that should only be used when the documentation in a medical record does not specify the type of COPD being treated.

2) Acute exacerbation of chronic obstructive bronchitis and asthma

The codes for chronic obstructive bronchitis and asthma distinguish between uncomplicated cases and those in acute exacerbation. An acute exacerbation is a worsening or a decompensation of a chronic condition. An acute exacerbation is not equivalent to an infection superimposed on a chronic condition, though an exacerbation may be triggered by an infection.

3) Overlapping nature of the conditions that comprise COPD and asthma

Due to the overlapping nature of the conditions that make up COPD and asthma, there are many variations in the way these conditions are documented. Code selection must be based on the terms as documented. When selecting the correct code for the documented type of COPD and asthma, it is essential to first review the index, and then verify the code in the tabular list. There are many instructional notes under the different COPD subcategories and codes. It is important that all such notes be reviewed to assure correct code assignment.

4) Acute exacerbation of asthma and status asthmaticus

An acute exacerbation of asthma is an increased severity of the asthma symptoms, such as wheezing and shortness of breath. Status asthmaticus refers to a patient's failure to respond to therapy administered during an asthmatic episode and is a life threatening complication that requires emergency care. If status asthmaticus is documented by the provider with any type of COPD or with acute bronchitis, the status asthmaticus should be sequenced first. It supersedes any type of COPD including that with acute exacerbation or acute bronchitis. It is inappropriate to assign an asthma code with 5th digit 2, with acute exacerbation, together with an asthma code with 5th digit 1, with status asthmatics. Only the 5th digit 1 should be assigned.

b. Chronic Obstructive Pulmonary Disease [COPD] and Bronchitis

1) Acute bronchitis with COPD

Acute bronchitis, code 466.0, is due to an infectious organism. When acute bronchitis is documented with COPD, code 491.22, Obstructive chronic bronchitis with acute bronchitis, should be assigned. It is not necessary to also assign code 466.0. If a medical record documents acute bronchitis with COPD with acute exacerbation, only code 491.22 should be assigned. The acute bronchitis included in code 491.22 supersedes the acute exacerbation. If a medical record documents COPD with acute exacerbation without mention of acute bronchitis, only code 491.21 should be assigned.

9. Chapter 9: Diseases of Digestive System (520–579)

Reserved for future guideline expansion

10. Chapter 10: Diseases of Genitourinary System (580–629)

Reserved for future guideline expansion

11. Chapter 11: Complications of Pregnancy, Childbirth, and the Puerperium (630–677)

a. General Rules for Obstetric Cases

1) Codes from Chapter 11 and sequencing priority

Obstetric cases require codes from Chapter 11, codes in the range 630–677, Complications of Pregnancy, Childbirth, and the Puerperium. Chapter 11 codes have sequencing priority over codes from other chapters. Additional codes from other chapters may be used in conjunction with Chapter 11 codes to further specify conditions. Should the provider document that the pregnancy is incidental to the encounter, then code V22.2 should be used in place of any Chapter 11 codes. It is the provider's responsibility to state that the condition being treated is not affecting the pregnancy.

2) Chapter 11 codes used only on the maternal record

Chapter 11 codes are to be used only on the maternal record, never on the record of the newborn.

3) **Chapter 11 fifth-digits**

Categories 640–648, 651–676 have required fifth-digits, which indicate whether the encounter is antepartum, postpartum and whether a delivery has also occurred.

4) **Fifth-digits, appropriate for each code**

The fifth-digits, which are appropriate for each code number, are listed in brackets under each code. The fifth-digits on each code should all be consistent with each other. That is, should a delivery occur all of the fifth-digits should indicate the delivery.

b. **Selection of OB Principal or First-listed Diagnosis**

1) **Routine outpatient prenatal visits**

For routine outpatient prenatal visits when no complications are present codes V22.0, Supervision of normal first pregnancy, and V22.1, Supervision of other normal pregnancy, should be used as the first-listed diagnoses. These codes should not be used in conjunction with Chapter 11 codes.

2) **Prenatal outpatient visits for high-risk patients**

For prenatal outpatient visits for patients with high-risk pregnancies, a code from category V23, Supervision of high-risk pregnancy, should be used as the principal or first-listed diagnosis. Secondary Chapter 11 codes may be used in conjunction with these codes if appropriate.

3) **Episodes when no delivery occurs**

In episodes when no delivery occurs, the principal diagnosis should correspond to the principal complication of the pregnancy, which necessitated the encounter. Should more than one complication exist, all of which are treated or monitored, any of the complications codes may be sequenced first.

4) **When a delivery occurs**

When a delivery occurs, the principal diagnosis should correspond to the main circumstances or complication of the delivery. In cases of cesarean delivery, the selection of the principal diagnosis should correspond to the reason the cesarean delivery was performed unless the reason for admission/encounter was unrelated to the condition resulting in the cesarean delivery.

5) **Outcome of delivery**

An outcome of delivery code, V27.0–V27.9, should be included on every maternal record when a delivery has occurred. These codes are not to be used on subsequent records or on the newborn record.

c. **Fetal Conditions Affecting the Management of the Mother**

1) **Codes from category 655**

Known or suspected fetal abnormality affecting management of the mother, and category 656, Other fetal and placental problems affecting the management of the mother, are assigned only when the fetal condition is actually responsible for modifying the management of the mother, i.e., by requiring diagnostic studies, additional observation, special care, or termination of pregnancy. The fact that the fetal condition exists does not justify assigning a code from this series to the mother's record.

2) In utero surgery

In cases when surgery is performed on the fetus, a diagnosis code from category 655, Known or suspected fetal abnormalities affecting management of the mother, should be assigned identifying the fetal condition. Procedure code 75.36, Correction of fetal defect, should be assigned on the hospital inpatient record.

No code from Chapter 15, the perinatal codes, should be used on the mother's record to identify fetal conditions. Surgery performed in utero on a fetus is still to be coded as an obstetric encounter.

d. HIV infection in pregnancy, childbirth, and the puerperium

During pregnancy, childbirth, or the puerperium, a patient admitted because of an HIV-related illness should receive a principal diagnosis of 647.6X, Other specified infectious and parasitic diseases in the mother classifiable elsewhere, but complicating the pregnancy, childbirth, or the puerperium, followed by 042 and the code(s) for the HIV-related illness(es).

Patients with asymptomatic HIV infection status admitted during pregnancy, childbirth, or the puerperium should receive codes of 647.6X and V08.

e. Current conditions complicating pregnancy

Assign a code from subcategory 648.x for patients that have current conditions when the condition affects the management of the pregnancy, childbirth, or the puerperium. Use additional secondary codes from other chapters to identify the conditions, as appropriate.

f. Diabetes mellitus in pregnancy

Diabetes mellitus is a significant complicating factor in pregnancy. Pregnant women who are diabetic should be assigned code 648.0x, Diabetes mellitus complicating pregnancy, and a secondary code from category 250, Diabetes mellitus, to identify the type of diabetes.

Code V58.67, Long-term (current) use of insulin, should also be assigned if the diabetes mellitus is being treated with insulin.

g. Gestational diabetes

Gestational diabetes can occur during the second and third trimester of pregnancy in women who were not diabetic prior to pregnancy. Gestational diabetes can cause complications in the pregnancy similar to those of pre-existing diabetes mellitus. It also puts the woman at greater risk of developing diabetes after the pregnancy. Gestational diabetes is coded to 648.8x, Abnormal glucose tolerance. Codes 648.0x and 648.8x should never be used together on the same record.

Code V58.67, Long-term (current) use of insulin, should also be assigned if the gestational diabetes is being treated with insulin.

h. Normal delivery, Code 650

1) Normal delivery

Code 650 is for use in cases when a woman is admitted for a full-term normal delivery and delivers a single, healthy infant without any complications antepartum, during the delivery, or postpartum during the delivery episode. Code 650 is always a principal diagnosis. It is not to be used if any other code from Chapter 11 is needed to describe a current complication of the antenatal, delivery, or perinatal period. Additional codes from other chapters may be used with code 650 if they are not related to or are in any way complicating the pregnancy.

2) Normal delivery with resolved antepartum complication

Code 650 may be used if the patient had a complication at some point during her pregnancy, but the complication is not present at the time of the admission for delivery.

3) V27.0, Single liveborn, outcome of delivery

V27.0, Single liveborn, is the only outcome of delivery code appropriate for use with 650.

i. The Postpartum and Peripartum Periods

1) Postpartum and peripartum periods

The postpartum period begins immediately after delivery and continues for six weeks following delivery. The peripartum period is defined as the last month of pregnancy to five months postpartum.

2) Postpartum complication

A postpartum complication is any complication occurring within the six-week period.

3) Pregnancy-related complications after 6 week period

Chapter 11 codes may also be used to describe pregnancy-related complications after the six-week period should the provider document that a condition is pregnancy related.

4) Postpartum complications occurring during the same admission as delivery

Postpartum complications that occur during the same admission as the delivery are identified with a fifth digit of "2." Subsequent admissions/encounters for postpartum complications should be identified with a fifth digit of "4."

5) Admission for routine postpartum care following delivery outside hospital

When the mother delivers outside the hospital prior to admission and is admitted for routine postpartum care and no complications are noted, code V24.0, Postpartum care and examination immediately after delivery, should be assigned as the principal diagnosis.

6) Admission following delivery outside hospital with postpartum conditions

A delivery diagnosis code should not be used for a woman who has delivered prior to admission to the hospital. Any postpartum conditions and/or postpartum procedures should be coded.

j. Code 677, Late effect of complication of pregnancy

1) Code 677

Code 677, Late effect of complication of pregnancy, childbirth, and the puerperium is for use in those cases when an initial complication of a pregnancy develops a sequelae requiring care or treatment at a future date.

2) After the initial postpartum period

This code may be used at any time after the initial postpartum period.

3) Sequencing of Code 677

This code, like all late effect codes, is to be sequenced following the code describing the sequelae of the complication.

k. Abortions

1) Fifth-digits required for abortion categories

Fifth-digits are required for abortion categories 634–637. Fifth-digit 1, incomplete, indicates that all of the products of conception have not been expelled from the uterus. Fifth-digit 2, complete, indicates that all products of conception have been expelled from the uterus prior to the episode of care.

2) Code from categories 640–648 and 651–659

A code from categories 640–648 and 651–659 may be used as additional codes with an abortion code to indicate the complication leading to the abortion.

Fifth digit 3 is assigned with codes from these categories when used with an abortion code because the other fifth digits will not apply. Codes from the 660–669 series are not to be used for complications of abortion.

3) Code 639 for complications

Code 639 is to be used for all complications following abortion. Code 639 cannot be assigned with codes from categories 634–638.

4) Abortion with liveborn fetus

When an attempted termination of pregnancy results in a liveborn fetus assign code 644.21, Early onset of delivery, with an appropriate code from category V27, Outcome of Delivery. The procedure code for the attempted termination of pregnancy should also be assigned.

5) Retained products of conception following an abortion

Subsequent admissions for retained products of conception following a spontaneous or legally induced abortion are assigned the appropriate code from category 634, Spontaneous abortion, or 635 Legally induced abortion, with a fifth digit of "I" (incomplete). This advice is appropriate even when the patient was discharged previously with a discharge diagnosis of complete abortion.

12. **Chapter 12: Diseases of Skin and Subcutaneous Tissue (680–709)**

Reserved for future guideline expansion

13. **Chapter 13: Diseases of Musculoskeletal and Connective Tissue (710–739)**

Reserved for future guideline expansion

14. **Chapter 14: Congenital Anomalies (740–759)**

a. **Codes in categories 740–759, Congenital Anomalies**

Assign an appropriate code(s) from categories 740–759, Congenital Anomalies, when an anomaly is documented. A congenital anomaly may be the principal/first listed diagnosis on a record or a secondary diagnosis. Use additional secondary codes from other chapters to specify conditions associated with the anomaly, if applicable. Codes from Chapter 14 may be used throughout the life of the patient. If a congenital anomaly has been corrected, a personal history code should be used to identify the history of the anomaly.

For the birth admission, the appropriate code from category V30, Liveborn infants, according to type of birth should be sequenced as the principal diagnosis, followed by any congenital anomaly codes, 740–759.

15. **Chapter 15: Newborn (Perinatal) Guidelines (760–779)**

For coding and reporting purposes the perinatal period is defined as birth through the 28th day following birth. The following guidelines are provided for reporting purposes. Hospitals may record other diagnoses as needed for internal data use.

a. **General Perinatal Rules**

1) **Chapter 15 Codes**

They are <u>never</u> for use on the maternal record. Codes from Chapter 11, the obstetric chapter, are never permitted on the newborn record. Chapter 15 code may be used throughout the life of the patient if the condition is still present.

2) Sequencing of perinatal codes

Generally, codes from Chapter 15 should be sequenced as the principal/first-listed diagnosis on the newborn record, with the exception of the appropriate V30 code for the birth episode, followed by codes from any other chapter that provide additional detail. The "use additional code" note at the beginning of the chapter supports this guideline. If the index does not provide a specific code for a perinatal condition, assign code 779.89, Other specified conditions originating in the perinatal period, followed by the code from another chapter that specifies the condition. Codes for signs and symptoms may be assigned when a definitive diagnosis has not been established.

3) Birth process or community acquired conditions

If a newborn has a condition that may be either due to the birth process or community acquired and the documentation does not indicate which it is, the default is due to the birth process and the code from Chapter 15 should be used. If the condition is community-acquired, a code from Chapter 15 should not be assigned.

4) Code all clinically significant conditions

All clinically significant conditions noted on routine newborn examination should be coded. A condition is clinically significant if it requires:

- clinical evaluation; or
- therapeutic treatment; or
- diagnostic procedures; or
- extended length of hospital stay; or
- increased nursing care and/or monitoring; or
- has implications for future health care needs

Note: The perinatal guidelines listed above are the same as the general coding guidelines for "additional diagnoses", except for the final point regarding implications for future health care needs. **Codes should be assigned for conditions that have been specified by the provider as having implications for future health care needs. Codes from the perinatal chapter should not be assigned unless the provider has established a definitive diagnosis.**

b. **Use of codes V30–V39**

When coding the birth of an infant, assign a code from categories V30–V39, according to the type of birth. A code from this series is assigned as a principal diagnosis, and assigned only once to a newborn at the time of birth.

c. **Newborn transfers**

If the newborn is transferred to another institution, the V30 series is not used at the receiving hospital.

d. **Use of category V29**

1) **Assigning a code from category V29**

Assign a code from category V29, Observation and evaluation of newborns and infants for suspected conditions not found, to identify those instances when a healthy newborn is evaluated for a suspected condition that is determined after study not to be present. Do not use a code from category V29 when the patient has identified signs or symptoms of a suspected problem; in such cases, code the sign or symptom.

A code from category V29 may also be assigned as a principal code for readmissions or encounters when the V30 code no longer applies. Codes from category V29 are for use only for healthy newborns and infants for which no condition after study is found to be present.

2) **V29 code on a birth record**

A V29 code is to be used as a secondary code after the V30, Outcome of delivery, code.

e. **Use of other V codes on perinatal records**

V codes other than V30 and V29 may be assigned on a perinatal or newborn record code. The codes may be used as a principal or first-listed diagnosis for specific types of encounters or for readmissions or encounters when the V30 code no longer applies.

See Section I.C.18 for information regarding the assignment of V codes.

f. **Maternal causes of perinatal morbidity**

Codes from categories 760–763, Maternal causes of perinatal morbidity and mortality, are assigned only when the maternal condition has actually affected the fetus or newborn. The fact that the mother has an associated medical condition or experiences some complication of pregnancy, labor, or delivery does not justify the routine assignment of codes from these categories to the newborn record.

g. **Congenital anomalies in newborns**

For the birth admission, the appropriate code from category V30, Liveborn infants according to type of birth, should be used, followed by any congenital anomaly codes, categories 740–759. **Use additional secondary codes from other chapters to specify conditions associated with the anomaly, if applicable.**

Also, see Section I.C.14 for information on the coding of congenital anomalies.

h. **Coding additional perinatal diagnoses**

1) **Assigning codes for conditions that require treatment**

Assign codes for conditions that require treatment or further investigation, prolong the length of stay, or require resource utilization.

2) **Codes for conditions specified as having implications for future health care needs**

Assign codes for conditions that have been specified by the provider as having implications for future health care needs.

Note: This guideline should not be used for adult patients.

3) **Codes for newborn conditions originating in the perinatal period**

Assign a code for newborn conditions originating in the perinatal period (categories 760–779); as well as complications arising during the current episode of care classified in other chapters, only if the diagnoses have been documented by the responsible provider at the time of transfer or discharge as having affected the fetus or newborn.

i. **Prematurity and fetal growth retardation**

Providers utilize different criteria in determining prematurity. A code for prematurity should not be assigned unless it is documented. The 5th digit assignment for codes from category 764 and subcategories 765.0 and 765.1 should be based on the recorded birth weight and estimated gestational age.

A code from subcategory 765.2, Weeks of gestation, should be assigned as an additional code with category 764 and codes from 765.0 and 765.1 to specify weeks of gestation as documented by the provider in the record.

j. **Newborn sepsis**

Code 771.81, Septicemia [sepsis] of newborn, should be assigned with a secondary code from category 041, Bacterial infections in conditions classified elsewhere and of unspecified site, to identify the organism. It is not necessary to use a code from subcategory 995.9, Systemic inflammatory response syndrome (SIRS), on a newborn record. A code from category 038, Septicemia, should not be used on a newborn record. Code 771.81 describes the sepsis.

16. **Chapter 16: Signs, Symptoms, and Ill-Defined Conditions (780–799)**

Reserved for future guideline expansion

17. **Chapter 17: Injury and Poisoning (800–999)**

a. **Coding of injuries**

When coding injuries, assign separate codes for each injury unless a combination code is provided, in which case the combination code is assigned. Multiple injury codes are provided in ICD-9-CM, but should not be assigned unless information for a more specific code is not available. These codes are not to be used for normal, healing surgical wounds or to identify complications of surgical wounds.

The code for the most serious injury, as determined by the provider and the focus of treatment, is sequenced first.

1) **Superficial injuries**

Superficial injuries such as abrasions or contusions are not coded when associated with more severe injuries of the same site.

2) **Primary injury with damage to nerves/blood vessels**

When a primary injury results in minor damage to peripheral nerves or blood vessels, the primary injury is sequenced first with additional code(s) from categories 950–957, Injury to nerves and spinal cord, and/or 900–904, Injury to blood vessels. When the primary injury is to the blood vessels or nerves, that injury should be sequenced first.

b. **Coding of fractures**

The principles of multiple coding of injuries should be followed in coding fractures. Fractures of specified sites are coded individually by site in accordance with both the provisions within categories 800–829 and the level of detail furnished by medical record content. Combination categories for multiple fractures are provided for use when there is insufficient detail in the medical record (such as trauma cases transferred to another hospital), when the reporting form limits the number of codes that can be used in reporting pertinent clinical data, or when there is insufficient specificity at the fourth-digit or fifth-digit level. More specific guidelines are as follows:

1) **Multiple fractures of same limb**

Multiple fractures of same limb classifiable to the same three-digit or four-digit category are coded to that category.

2) **Multiple unilateral or bilateral fractures of same bone**

Multiple unilateral or bilateral fractures of same bone(s) but classified to different fourth-digit subdivisions (bone part) within the same three-digit category are coded individually by site.

3) **Multiple fracture categories 819 and 828**

Multiple fracture categories 819 and 828 classify bilateral fractures of both upper limbs (819) and both lower limbs (828), but without any detail at the fourth-digit level other than open and closed type of fractures.

4) Multiple fractures sequencing

Multiple fractures are sequenced in accordance with the severity of the fracture. The provider should be asked to list the fracture diagnoses in the order of severity.

c. **Coding of burns**

Current burns (940–948) are classified by depth, extent, and by agent (E code). Burns are classified by depth as first degree (erythema), second degree (blistering), and third degree (full-thickness involvement).

1) Sequencing of burn codes

Sequence first the code that reflects the highest degree of burn when more than one burn is present.

2) Burns of the same local site

Classify burns of the same local site (three-digit category level, 940–947) but of different degrees to the subcategory identifying the highest degree recorded in the diagnosis.

3) Non-healing burns

Non-healing burns are coded as acute burns.

Necrosis of burned skin should be coded as a non-healed burn.

4) Code 958.3, Posttraumatic wound infection

Assign code 958.3, Posttraumatic wound infection, not elsewhere classified, as an additional code for any documented infected burn site.

5) Assign separate codes for each burn site

When coding burns, assign separate codes for each burn site. Category 946 Burns of Multiple specified sites, should only be used if the location of the burns are not documented. Category 949, Burn, unspecified, is extremely vague and should rarely be used.

6) Assign codes from category 948, Burns

Burns classified according to extent of body surface involved, when the site of the burn is not specified or when there is a need for additional data. It is advisable to use category 948 as additional coding when needed to provide data for evaluating burn mortality, such as that needed by burn units. It is also advisable to use category 948 as an additional code for reporting purposes when there is mention of a third-degree burn involving 20 percent or more of the body surface.

In assigning a code from category 948:

Fourth-digit codes are used to identify the percentage of total body surface involved in a burn (all degree).

Fifth-digits are assigned to identify the percentage of body surface involved in third-degree burn.

Fifth-digit zero (0) is assigned when less than 10 percent or when no body surface is involved in a third-degree burn.

Category 948 is based on the classic "rule of nines" in estimating body surface involved: head and neck are assigned nine percent, each arm nine percent, each leg 18 percent, the anterior trunk 18 percent, posterior trunk 18 percent, and genitalia one percent. Providers may change these percentage assignments where necessary to accommodate infants and children who have proportionately larger heads than adults and patients who have large buttocks, thighs, or abdomen that involve burns.

7) Encounters for treatment of late effects of burns

Encounters for the treatment of the late effects of burns (i.e., scars or joint contractures) should be coded to the residual condition (sequelae) followed by the appropriate late effect code (906.5–906.9). A late effect E code may also be used, if desired.

8) Sequelae with a late effect code and current burn

When appropriate, both a sequelae with a late effect code, and a current burn code may be assigned on the same record (**when both a current burn and sequelae of an old burn exist**).

d. Coding of debridement of wound, infection, or burn

Excisional debridement involves an excisional debridement (surgical removal or cutting away), as opposed to a mechanical (brushing, scrubbing, washing) debridement.

For coding purposes, excisional debridement **is assigned to code** 86.22.

Nonexcisional debridement is assigned to **code** 86.28.

e. Adverse effects, poisoning and toxic effects

The properties of certain drugs, medicinal and biological substances or combinations of such substances, may cause toxic reactions. The occurrence of drug toxicity is classified in ICD-9-CM as follows:

1) Adverse effect

When the drug was correctly prescribed and properly administered, code the reaction plus the appropriate code from the E930–E949 series. Codes from the E930–E949 series must be used to identify the causative substance for an adverse effect of drug, medicinal and biological substances, correctly prescribed and properly administered. The effect, such as tachycardia, delirium, gastrointestinal hemorrhaging, vomiting, hypokalemia, hepatitis, renal failure, or respiratory failure, is coded and followed by the appropriate code from the E930–E949 series.

Adverse effects of therapeutic substances correctly prescribed and properly administered (toxicity, synergistic reaction, side effect, and idiosyncratic reaction) may be due to (1) differences among patients, such as age, sex, disease, and genetic factors, and (2) drug-related factors, such as type of drug, route of administration, duration of therapy, dosage, and bioavailability.

2) Poisoning

(a) Error was made in drug prescription

Errors made in drug prescription or in the administration of the drug by provider, nurse, patient, or other person, use the appropriate poisoning code from the 960–979 series.

(b) Overdose of a drug intentionally taken

If an overdose of a drug was intentionally taken or administered and resulted in drug toxicity, it would be coded as a poisoning (960–979 series).

(c) Nonprescribed drug taken with correctly prescribed and properly administered drug

If a nonprescribed drug or medicinal agent was taken in combination with a correctly prescribed and properly administered drug, any drug toxicity or other reaction resulting from the interaction of the two drugs would be classified as a poisoning.

(d) Sequencing of poisoning

When coding a poisoning or reaction to the improper use of a medication (e.g., wrong dose, wrong substance, wrong route of administration) the poisoning code is sequenced first, followed by a code for the manifestation. If there is also a diagnosis of drug abuse or dependence to the substance, the abuse or dependence is coded as an additional code.

See Section I.C.3.a.6.b. if poisoning is the result of insulin pump malfunctions and Section 1.C.19 for general use of E codes.

3) Toxic effects

(a) Toxic effect codes

When a harmful substance is ingested or comes in contact with a person, this is classified as a toxic effect. The toxic effect codes are in categories 980–989.

(b) Sequencing toxic effect codes

A toxic effect code should be sequenced first, followed by the code(s) that identify the result of the toxic effect.

(c) External cause codes for toxic effects

An external cause code from categories E860–E869 for accidental exposure, codes E950.6 or E950.7 for intentional self-harm, category E962 for assault, or categories E980–E982, for undetermined, should also be assigned to indicate intent.

18. Classification of Factors Influencing Health Status and Contact with Health Service (Supplemental V01–V84)

Note: The chapter specific guidelines provide additional information about the use of V codes for specified encounters.

a. Introduction

ICD-9-CM provides codes to deal with encounters for circumstances other than a disease or injury. The Supplementary Classification of Factors Influencing Health Status and Contact with Health Services (V01.0–V84.8) is provided to deal with occasions when circumstances other than a disease or injury (codes 001–999) are recorded as a diagnosis or problem.

There are four primary circumstances for the use of V codes:

1) A person who is not currently sick encounters the health services for some specific reason, such as to act as an organ donor, to receive prophylactic care, such as inoculations or health screenings, or to receive counseling on health related issues.

2) A person with a resolving disease or injury, or a chronic, longterm condition requiring continuous care, encounters the health care system for specific aftercare of that disease or injury (e.g., dialysis for renal disease; chemotherapy for malignancy; cast change). A diagnosis/symptom code should be used whenever a current, acute, diagnosis is being treated or a sign or symptom is being studied.

3) Circumstances or problems influence a person's health status but are not in themselves a current illness or injury.

4) Newborns, to indicate birth status

b. V codes use in any healthcare setting

V codes are for use in any healthcare setting. V codes may be used as either a first listed (principal diagnosis code in the inpatient setting) or secondary code, depending on the circumstances of the encounter. Certain V codes may only be used as first listed, others only as secondary codes. See Section I.C.18.e, **V Code Table.**

c. **V codes indicate a reason for an encounter**

They are not procedure codes. A corresponding procedure code must accompany a V code to describe the procedure performed.

d. **Categories of V codes**

1) **Contact/exposure**

   Category V01 indicates contact with or exposure to communicable diseases. These codes are for patients who do not show any sign or symptom of a disease but have been exposed to it by close personal contact with an infected individual or are in an area where a disease is epidemic. These codes may be used as a first listed code to explain an encounter for testing, or, more commonly, as a secondary code to identify a potential risk.

2) **Inoculations and vaccinations**

   Categories V03–V06 are for encounters for inoculations and vaccinations. They indicate that a patient is being seen to receive a prophylactic inoculation against a disease. The injection itself must be represented by the appropriate procedure code. A code from V03–V06 may be used as a secondary code if the inoculation is given as a routine part of preventive health care, such as a well-baby visit.

3) **Status**

   Status codes indicate that a patient is either a carrier of a disease or has the sequelae or residual of a past disease or condition. This includes such things as the presence of prosthetic or mechanical devices resulting from past treatment. A status code is informative, because the status may affect the course of treatment and its outcome. A status code is distinct from a history code. The history code indicates that the patient no longer has the condition.

   A status code should not be used with a diagnosis code from one of the body system chapters, if the diagnosis code includes the information provided by the status code. For example, code V42.1, Heart transplant status, should not be used with code 996.83, Complications of transplanted heart. The status code does not provide additional information. The complication code indicates that the patient is a heart transplant patient.

   The status V codes/categories are:

V02	Carrier or suspected carrier of infectious diseases
	Carrier status indicates that a person harbors the specific organisms of a disease without manifest symptoms and is capable of transmitting the infection.
V08	Asymptomatic HIV infection status
	This code indicates that a patient has tested positive for HIV but has manifested no signs or symptoms of the disease.
V09	Infection with drug-resistant microorganisms
	This category indicates that a patient has an infection that is resistant to drug treatment.
	Sequence the infection code first.
V21	Constitutional states in development
V22.2	Pregnant state, incidental
	This code is a secondary code only for use when the pregnancy is in no way complicating the reason for visit. Otherwise, a code from the obstetric chapter is required.
V26.5x	Sterilization status
V42	Organ or tissue replaced by transplant
V43	Organ or tissue replaced by other means

V44   Artificial opening status
V45   Other postsurgical states
V46   Other dependence on machines
V49.6   Upper limb amputation status
V49.7   Lower limb amputation status
V49.81   Postmenopausal status
V49.82   Dental sealant status
V49.83   Awaiting organ transplant status
V58.6   Long-term (current) drug use
           This subcategory indicates a patient's continuous use of a prescribed drug (including such things as aspirin therapy) for the long-term treatment of a condition or for prophylactic use. It is not for use for patients who have addictions to drugs.
V83   Genetic carrier status
           Genetic carrier status indicates that a person carries a gene, associated with a particular disease, which may be passed to offspring who may develop that disease. The person does not have the disease and is not at risk of developing the disease.
V84   **Genetic susceptibility status**
           Genetic susceptibility indicates that a person has a gene that increases the risk of that person developing the disease.

Note: Categories V42–V46, and subcategories V49.6, V49.7 are for use only if there are no complications or malfunctions of the organ or tissue replaced, the amputation site, or the equipment on which the patient is dependent. These are always secondary codes.

4) **History (of)**

There are two types of history V codes, personal and family. Personal history codes explain a patient's past medical condition that no longer exists and is not receiving any treatment, but that has the potential for recurrence, and therefore may require continued monitoring. The exceptions to this general rule are category V14, Personal history of allergy to medicinal agents, and subcategory V15.0, Allergy, other than to medicinal agents. A person who has had an allergic episode to a substance or food in the past should always be considered allergic to the substance.

Family history codes are for use when a patient has a family member(s) who has had a particular disease that causes the patient to be at higher risk of also contracting the disease.

Personal history codes may be used in conjunction with followup codes and family history codes may be used in conjunction with screening codes to explain the need for a test or procedure. History codes are also acceptable on any medical record regardless of the reason for visit. A history of an illness, even if no longer present, is important information that may alter the type of treatment ordered.

The history V code categories are:
V10   Personal history of malignant neoplasm
V12   Personal history of certain other diseases
V13   Personal history of other diseases
      Except: V13.4, Personal history of arthritis, and V13.6, Personal history of congenital malformations. These conditions are life-long so are not true history codes.

V14   Personal history of allergy to medicinal agents

V15   Other personal history presenting hazards to health Except: V15.7, Personal history of contraception.

V16   Family history of malignant neoplasm

V17   Family history of certain chronic disabling diseases

V18   Family history of certain other specific diseases

V19   Family history of other conditions

5) **Screening**

Screening is the testing for disease or disease precursors in seemingly well individuals so that early detection and treatment can be provided for those who test positive for the disease. Screenings that are recommended for many subgroups in a population include: routine mammograms for women over 40, a fecal occult blood test for everyone over 50, an amniocentesis to rule out a fetal anomaly for pregnant women over 35, because the incidence of breast cancer and colon cancer in these subgroups is higher than in the general population, as is the incidence of Down's syndrome in older mothers.

The testing of a person to rule out or confirm a suspected diagnosis because the patient has some sign or symptom is a diagnostic examination, not a screening. In these cases, the sign or symptom is used to explain the reason for the test.

A screening code may be a first listed code if the reason for the visit is specifically the screening exam. It may also be used as an additional code if the screening is done during an office visit for other health problems. A screening code is not necessary if the screening is inherent to a routine examination, such as a pap smear done during a routine pelvic examination. Should a condition be discovered during the screening then the code for the condition may be assigned as an additional diagnosis.

The V code indicates that a screening exam is planned. A procedure code is required to confirm that the screening was performed.

The screening V code categories:

V28   Antenatal screening

V73–V82   Special screening examinations

6) **Observation**

There are two observation V code categories. They are for use in very limited circumstances when a person is being observed for a suspected condition that is ruled out. The observation codes are not for use if an injury or illness or any signs or symptoms related to the suspected condition are present. In such cases the diagnosis/symptom code is used with the corresponding E code to identify any external cause.

The observation codes are to be used as principal diagnosis only. The only exception to this is when the principal diagnosis is required to be a code from the V30, Live born infant, category. Then the V29 observation code is sequenced after the V30 code. Additional codes may be used in addition to the observation code but only if they are unrelated to the suspected condition being observed.

The observation V code categories:

V29   Observation and evaluation of newborns for suspected condition not found
       For the birth encounter, a code from category V30 should be sequenced before the V29 code.

V71   Observation and evaluation for suspected condition not found

7) **Aftercare**

Aftercare visit codes cover situations when the initial treatment of a disease or injury has been performed and the patient requires continued care during the healing or recovery phase, or for the long-term consequences of the disease. The aftercare V code should not be used if treatment is directed at a current, acute disease or injury, the diagnosis code is to be used in these cases. Exceptions to this rule are codes V58.0, Radiotherapy, and V58.1, Chemotherapy. These codes are to be first listed, followed by the diagnosis code when a patient's encounter is solely to receive radiation therapy or chemotherapy for the treatment of a neoplasm. Should a patient receive both chemotherapy and radiation therapy during the same encounter code V58.0 and V58.1 may be used together on a record with either one being sequenced first.

The aftercare codes are generally first listed to explain the specific reason for the encounter. An aftercare code may be used as an additional code when some type of aftercare is provided in addition to the reason for admission and no diagnosis code is applicable. An example of this would be the closure of a colostomy during an encounter for treatment of another condition.

Certain aftercare V code categories need a secondary diagnosis code to describe the resolving condition or sequelae, for others, the condition is inherent in the code title.

Additional V code aftercare category terms include, fitting and adjustment, and attention to artificial openings.

Status V codes may be used with aftercare V codes to indicate the nature of the aftercare. For example code V45.81, Aortocoronary bypass status, may be used with code V58.73, Aftercare following surgery of the circulatory system, NEC, to indicate the surgery for which the aftercare is being performed. Also, a transplant status code may be used following code V58.44, Aftercare following organ transplant, to identify the organ transplanted. A status code should not be used when the aftercare code indicates the type of status, such as using V55.0, Attention to tracheostomy with V44.0, Tracheostomy status.

The aftercare V category/codes:

V52	Fitting and adjustment of prosthetic device and implant
V53	Fitting and adjustment of other device
V54	Other orthopedic aftercare
V55	Attention to artificial openings
V56	Encounter for dialysis and dialysis catheter care
V57	Care involving the use of rehabilitation procedures
V58.0	Radiotherapy
V58.1	Chemotherapy
V58.3	Attention to surgical dressings and sutures
V58.41	Encounter for planned post-operative wound closure
V58.42	Aftercare, surgery, neoplasm
V58.43	Aftercare, surgery, trauma
V58.44	**Aftercare involving organ transplant**
V58.49	Other specified aftercare following surgery
V58.7x	Aftercare following surgery
V58.81	Fitting and adjustment of vascular catheter
V58.82	Fitting and adjustment of non-vascular catheter
V58.83	Monitoring therapeutic drug
V58.89	Other specified aftercare

8) **Follow-up**

The follow-up codes are used to explain continuing surveillance following completed treatment of a disease, condition, or injury. They imply that the condition has been fully treated and no longer exists. They should not be confused with aftercare codes that explain current treatment for a healing condition or its sequelae. Follow-up codes may be used in conjunction with history codes to provide the full picture of the healed condition and its treatment. The follow-up code is sequenced first, followed by the history code.

A follow-up code may be used to explain repeated visits. Should a condition be found to have recurred on the follow-up visit, then the diagnosis code should be used in place of the follow-up code.

The follow-up V code categories:
V24   Postpartum care and evaluation
V67   Follow-up examination

9) **Donor**

Category V59 are the donor codes. They are used for living individuals who are donating blood or other body tissue. These codes are only for individuals donating for others, not for self donations. They are not for use to identify cadaveric donations.

10) **Counseling**

Counseling V codes are used when a patient or family member receives assistance in the aftermath of an illness or injury, or when support is required in coping with family or social problems. They are not necessary for use in conjunction with a diagnosis code when the counseling component of care is considered integral to standard treatment.

The counseling V categories/codes:
V25.0   General counseling and advice for contraceptive management
V26.3   Genetic counseling
V26.4   General counseling and advice for procreative management
V61   Other family circumstances
V65.1   Person consulted on behalf of another person
V65.3   Dietary surveillance and counseling
V65.4   Other counseling, not elsewhere classified

11) **Obstetrics and related conditions**

See Section I.C.11., the Obstetrics guidelines for further instruction on the use of these codes.

V codes for pregnancy are for use in those circumstances when none of the problems or complications included in the codes from the Obstetrics chapter exist (a routine prenatal visit or postpartum care). Codes V22.0, Supervision of normal first pregnancy, and V22.1, Supervision of other normal pregnancy, are always first listed and are not to be used with any other code from the OB chapter.

The outcome of delivery, category V27, should be included on all maternal delivery records. It is always a secondary code.

V codes for family planning (contraceptive) or procreative management and counseling should be included on an obstetric record either during the pregnancy or the postpartum stage, if applicable.

Obstetrics and related conditions V code categories:

V22   Normal pregnancy
V23   Supervision of high-risk pregnancy
       Except: V23.2, Pregnancy with history of abortion.
       Code 646.3, Habitual aborter, from the OB chapter is required to indicate a history
       of abortion during a pregnancy.
V24   Postpartum care and evaluation
V25   Encounter for contraceptive management
       Except V25.0x (See Section I.C.18.d.11, Counseling)
V26   Procreative management
       Except V26.5x, Sterilization status, V26.3 and V26.4 (See Section I.C.18.d.11.,
       Counseling)
V27   Outcome of delivery
V28   Antenatal screening (See Section I.C.18.d.6., Screening)

12) **Newborn, infant, and child**

See Section I.C.15, the Newborn guidelines for further instruction on the use of these codes.

Newborn V code categories:

V20   Health supervision of infant or child
V29   Observation and evaluation of newborns for suspected condition not found
            (See Section I.C.18.d.7, Observation)
V30–V39   Liveborn infant according to type of birth

13) **Routine and administrative examinations**

The V codes allow for the description of encounters for routine examinations, such as, a general check-up, or, examinations for administrative purposes, such as, a pre-employment physical. The codes are for use as first listed codes only, and are not to be used if the examination is for diagnosis of a suspected condition or for treatment purposes. In such cases the diagnosis code is used. During a routine exam, should a diagnosis or condition be discovered, it should be coded as an additional code. Pre-existing and chronic conditions and history codes may also be included as additional codes as long as the examination is for administrative purposes and not focused on any particular condition.

Preoperative examination V codes are for use only in those situations when a patient is being cleared for surgery and no treatment is given.

The V codes categories/code for routine and administrative examinations:

V20.2   Routine infant or child health check
        Any injections given should have a corresponding procedure code.
V70   General medical examination
V72   Special investigations and examinations
        Except V72.5 and V72.6

14) **Miscellaneous V codes**

The miscellaneous V codes capture a number of other health care encounters that do not fall into one of the other categories. Certain of these codes identify the reason for the encounter, others are for use as additional codes that provide useful information on circumstances that may affect a patient's care and treatment.

Miscellaneous V code categories/codes:

V07	Need for isolation and other prophylactic measures
V50	Elective surgery for purposes other than remedying health states
V58.5	Orthodontics
V60	Housing, household, and economic circumstances
V62	Other psychosocial circumstances
V63	Unavailability of other medical facilities for care
V64	Persons encountering health services for specific procedures, not carried out
V66	Convalescence and Palliative Care
V68	Encounters for administrative purposes
V69	Problems related to lifestyle

15) **Non-specific V codes**

Certain V codes are so non-specific, or potentially redundant with other codes in the classification, that there can be little justification for their use in the inpatient setting. Their use in the outpatient setting should be limited to those instances when there is no further documentation to permit more precise coding. Otherwise, any sign or symptom or any other reason for visit that is captured in another code should be used.

Non-specific V code categories/codes:

V11	Personal history of mental disorder
	A code from the mental disorders chapter, with an in remission fifth-digit, should be used.
V13.4	Personal history of arthritis
V13.6	Personal history of congenital malformations
V15.7	Personal history of contraception
V23.2	Pregnancy with history of abortion
V40	Mental and behavioral problems
V41	Problems with special senses and other special functions
V47	Other problems with internal organs
V48	Problems with head, neck, and trunk
V49	Problems with limbs and other problems

Exceptions:

V49.6	Upper limb amputation status
V49.7	Lower limb amputation status
V49.81	Postmenopausal status
V49.82	Dental sealant status
V49.83	**Awaiting organ transplant status**

V51	Aftercare involving the use of plastic surgery
V58.2	Blood transfusion, without reported diagnosis
V58.9	Unspecified aftercare
V72.5	Radiological examination, NEC
V72.6	Laboratory examination
	Codes V72.5 and V72.6 are not to be used if any sign or symptoms, or reason for a test is documented. See Section IV.K. and Section IV.L. of the Outpatient guidelines.

V CODE TABLE

Items in bold indicate a change from the October 2003 table

Items underlined have been moved within the table since October 2003

FIRST LISTED: V codes/categories/subcategories which are only acceptable as principal/first listed.

Codes:

V22.0	Supervision of normal first pregnancy
V22.1	Supervision of other normal pregnancy
V46.12	**Encounter for respirator dependence during power failure**
V56.0	<u>Extracorporeal dialysis</u>
V58.0	Radiotherapy
V58.1	Chemotherapy

V58.0 and V58.1 may be used together on a record with either one being sequenced first, when a patient receives both chemotherapy and radiation therapy during the same encounter code.

Categories/Subcategories:

V20	Health supervision of infant or child
V24	Postpartum care and examination
V29	Observation and evaluation of newborns for suspected condition not found

Exception: A code from the V30–V39 may be sequenced before the V29 if it is the newborn record.

V30–V39	Liveborn infants according to type of birth
V59	Donors
V66	Convalescence and palliative care

Exception: V66.7 Palliative care

V68	Encounters for administrative purposes
V70	General medical examination

Exception: V70.7 Examination of participant in clinical trial

V71	Observation and evaluation for suspected conditions not found
V72	Special investigations and examinations

Exceptions:

V22.5	Radiological examination, NEC
V72.6	Laboratory examination

FIRST OR ADDITIONAL: V code categories/subcategories which may be either principal/first listed or additional codes

Codes:

V43.22	Fully implantable artificial heart status
V49.81	Asymptomatic postmenopausal status (age-related) (natural)
V70.7	Examination of participant in clinical trial

Categories/Subcategories:

V01	Contact with or exposure to communicable diseases
V02	Carrier or suspected carrier of infectious diseases
V03–06	Need for prophylactic vaccination and inoculations
V07	Need for isolation and other prophylactic measures
V08	Asymptomatic HIV infection status
V10	Personal history of malignant neoplasm
V12	Personal history of certain other diseases
V13	Personal history of other diseases

Exception:
    V13.4 Personal history of arthritis
    V13.69 Personal history of other congenital malformations

V16–V19	Family history of disease
V23	Supervision of high-risk pregnancy
V25	Encounter for contraceptive management
V26	Procreative management

Exception: V26.5 Sterilization status

V28	Antenatal screening
V45.7	Acquired absence of organ
V50	Elective surgery for purposes other than remedying health states
V52	Fitting and adjustment of prosthetic device and implant
V53	Fitting and adjustment of other device
V54	Other orthopedic aftercare
V55	Attention to artificial openings
V56	Encounter for dialysis and dialysis catheter care

Exception: V56.0 Extracorporeal dialysis

V57	Care involving use of rehabilitation procedures
V58.3	Attention to surgical dressings and sutures
V58.4	Other aftercare following surgery
V58.6	Long-term (current) drug use
V58.7	Aftercare following surgery to specified body systems, not elsewhere classified
V58.8	Other specified procedures and aftercare
V61	Other family circumstances
V63	Unavailability of other medical facilities for care
V65	Other persons seeking consultation without complaint or sickness
V67	Follow-up examination
V69	Problems related to lifestyle
V73–V82	Special screening examinations
V83	Genetic carrier status

ADDITIONAL ONLY: V code categories/subcategories which may only be used as additional codes, not principal/first listed

Codes:

V13.61	Personal history of hypospadias
V22.2	Pregnancy state, incidental
V49.82	Dental sealant status
V49.83	**Awaiting organ transplant status**
V66.7	Palliative care

Categories/Subcategories:

V09	Infection with drug-resistant microorganisms
V14	Personal history of allergy to medicinal agents
V15	Other personal history presenting hazards to health

    Exception: V15.7   Personal history of contraception

V21	Constitutional states in development
V26.5	Sterilization status
V27	Outcome of delivery
V42	Organ or tissue replaced by transplant
V43	Organ or tissue replaced by other means

    Exception: V43.22   Fully implantable artificial heart status

V44	Artificial opening status
V45	Other postsurgical states

    Exception: Subcategory V45.7   Acquired absence of organ

V46	Other dependence on machines

    Exception: V46.12   Encounter for respirator dependence during power failure

V49.6x	Upper limb amputation status
V49.7x	Lower limb amputation status
V60	Housing, household, and economic circumstances
V62	Other psychosocial circumstances
V64	Persons encountering health services for specified procedure, not carried out
V84	**Genetic susceptibility to disease**

NONSPECIFIC CODES AND CATEGORIES:

V11	Personal history of mental disorder
V13.4	Personal history of arthritis
V13.69	Personal history of congenital malformations
V15.7	Personal history of contraception
V40	Mental and behavioral problems
V41	Problems with special senses and other special functions
V47	Other problems with internal organs
V48	Problems with head, neck, and trunk
V49	Problems with limbs and other problems

    Exceptions:

V49.6	Upper limb amputation status
V49.7	Lower limb amputation status
V49.81	Postmenopausal status (age-related) (natural)
V49.82	Dental sealant status
V49.83	**Awaiting organ transplant status**

V51	Aftercare involving the use of plastic surgery
V58.2	Blood transfusion, without reported diagnosis
V58.5	Orthodontics
V58.9	Unspecified aftercare
V72.5	Radiological examination, NEC
V72.6	Laboratory examination

19. **Supplemental Classification of External Causes of Injury and Poisoning (E codes, E800–E999)**

Introduction: These guidelines are provided for those who are currently collecting E codes in order that there will be standardization in the process. If your institution plans to begin collecting E codes, these guidelines are to be applied. The use of E codes is supplemental to the application of ICD-9-CM diagnosis codes. E codes are never to be recorded as principal diagnoses (first-listed in non-inpatient setting) and are not required for reporting to CMS.

External causes of injury and poisoning codes (E codes) are intended to provide data for injury research and evaluation of injury prevention strategies. E codes capture how the injury or poisoning happened (cause), the intent (unintentional or accidental; or intentional, such as suicide or assault), and the place where the event occurred.

Some major categories of E codes include:

> transport accidents
> poisoning and adverse effects of drugs, medicinal substances and biologicals
> accidental falls
> accidents caused by fire and flames
> accidents due to natural and environmental factors
> late effects of accidents, assaults, or self injury
> assaults or purposely inflicted injury
> suicide or self-inflicted injury

These guidelines apply for the coding and collection of E codes from records in hospitals, outpatient clinics, emergency departments, other ambulatory care settings and provider offices, and nonacute care settings, except when other specific guidelines apply.

a. **General E Code Coding Guidelines**

1) **Used with any code in the range of 001–V84.8**

An E code may be used with any code in the range of 001–V84.8, which indicates an injury, poisoning, or adverse effect due to an external cause.

2) **Assign the appropriate E code for all initial treatments**

Assign the appropriate E code for the initial encounter of an injury, poisoning, or adverse effect of drugs, **not for subsequent treatment.**

3) **Use the full range of E codes**

Use the full range of E codes to completely describe the cause, the intent, and the place of occurrence, if applicable, for all injuries, poisonings, and adverse effects of drugs.

4) **Assign as many E codes as necessary**

Assign as many E codes as necessary to fully explain each cause. If only one E code can be recorded, assign the E code most related to the principal diagnosis.

5) **The selection of the appropriate E code**

The selection of the appropriate E code is guided by the Index to External Causes, which is located after the alphabetical index to diseases and by Inclusion and Exclusion notes in the Tabular List.

6) **E code can never be a principal diagnosis**

An E code can never be a principal (first listed) diagnosis.

7) **External cause code(s) with systemic inflammatory response syndrome (SIRS)**

An external cause code(s) may be used with codes 995.93, Systemic inflammatory response syndrome due to noninfectious process without organ dysfunction, and 995.94, Systemic inflammatory response syndrome due to noninfectious process with organ dysfunction, if trauma was the initiating insult that precipitated the SIRS. The external cause(s) code should correspond to the most serious injury resulting from the trauma. The external cause code(s) should only be assigned if the trauma necessitated the admission in which the patient also developed SIRS. If a patient is admitted with SIRS but the trauma has been treated previously, the external cause codes should not be used.

b. **Place of Occurrence Guideline**

Use an additional code from category E849 to indicate the Place of Occurrence for injuries and poisonings. The Place of Occurrence describes the place where the event occurred and not the patient's activity at the time of the event.

Do not use E849.9 if the place of occurrence is not stated.

c. **Adverse Effects of Drugs, Medicinal and Biological Substances Guidelines**

1) **Do not code directly from the Table of Drugs**

Do not code directly from the Table of Drugs and Chemicals. Always refer back to the Tabular List.

2) **Use as many codes as necessary to describe**

Use as many codes as necessary to describe completely all drugs, medicinal or biological substances.

3) **If the same E code would describe the causative agent**

If the same E code would describe the causative agent for more than one adverse reaction, assign the code only once.

4) **If two or more drugs, medicinal or biological substances**

If two or more drugs, medicinal or biological substances are reported, code each individually unless the combination code is listed in the Table of Drugs and Chemicals. In that case, assign the E code for the combination.

5) **When a reaction results from the interaction of a drug(s)**

When a reaction results from the interaction of a drug(s) and alcohol, use poisoning codes and E codes for both.

6) **If the reporting format limits the number of E codes**

If the reporting format limits the number of E codes that can be used in reporting clinical data, code the one most related to the principal diagnosis. Include at least one from each category (cause, intent, place) if possible.

If there are different fourth digit codes in the same three digit category, use the code for "Other specified" of that category. If there is no "Other specified" code in that category, use the appropriate "Unspecified" code in that category.

If the codes are in different three digit categories, assign the appropriate E code for other multiple drugs and medicinal substances.

7) Codes from the E930–E949 series

Codes from the E930–E949 series must be used to identify the causative substance for an adverse effect of drug, medicinal and biological substances, correctly prescribed and properly administered. The effect, such as tachycardia, delirium, gastrointestinal hemorrhaging, vomiting, hypokalemia, hepatitis, renal failure, or respiratory failure, is coded and followed by the appropriate code from the E930–E949 series.

d. Multiple Cause E Code Coding Guidelines

If two or more events cause separate injuries, an E code should be assigned for each cause. The first listed E code will be selected in the following order:

E codes for child and adult abuse take priority over all other E codes. See Section I.C.19.e., Child and Adult abuse guidelines

E codes for terrorism events take priority over all other E codes except Child and Adult abuse

E codes for cataclysmic events take priority over all other E codes except Child and Adult abuse and terrorism.

E codes for transport accidents take priority over all other E codes except cataclysmic events and Child and Adult abuse and terrorism.

The first-listed E code should correspond to the cause of the most serious diagnosis due to an assault, accident, or self-harm, following the order of hierarchy listed above.

e. Child and Adult Abuse Guideline

1) Intentional injury

When the cause of an injury or neglect is intentional child or adult abuse, the first listed E code should be assigned from categories E960–E968, Homicide and injury purposely inflicted by other persons, (except category E967). An E code from category E967, Child and adult battering and other maltreatment, should be added as an additional code to identify the perpetrator, if known.

2) Accidental intent

In cases of neglect when the intent is determined to be accidental E code E904.0, Abandonment or neglect of infant and helpless person, should be the first listed E code.

f. Unknown or Suspected Intent Guideline

1) If the intent (accident, self-harm, assault) of the cause of an injury or poisoning is unknown

If the intent (accident, self-harm, assault) of the cause of an injury or poisoning is unknown or unspecified, code the intent as undetermined E980–E989.

2) If the intent (accident, self-harm, assault) of the cause of an injury or poisoning is questionable

If the intent (accident, self-harm, assault) of the cause of an injury or poisoning is questionable, probable or suspected, code the intent as undetermined E980–E989.

g. Undetermined Cause

When the intent of an injury or poisoning is known, but the cause is unknown, use codes: E928.9, Unspecified accident, E958.9, Suicide and self-inflicted injury by unspecified means, and E968.9, Assault by unspecified means.

These E codes should rarely be used, as the documentation in the medical record, in both the inpatient outpatient and other settings, should normally provide sufficient detail to determine the cause of the injury.

h. Late Effects of External Cause Guidelines

1) Late effect E codes

Late effect E codes exist for injuries and poisonings but not for adverse effects of drugs, misadventures, and surgical complications.

2) Late effect E codes (E929, E959, E969, E977, E989, or E999.1)

A late effect E code (E929, E959, E969, E977, E989, or E999.1) should be used with any report of a late effect or sequela resulting from a previous injury or poisoning (905–909).

3) Late effect E code with a related current injury

A late effect E code should never be used with a related current nature of injury code.

4) Use of late effect E codes for subsequent visits

Use a late effect E code for subsequent visits when a late effect of the initial injury or poisoning is being treated. There is no late effect E code for adverse effects of drugs. Do not use a late effect E code for subsequent visits for follow-up care (e.g., to assess healing, to receive rehabilitative therapy) of the injury or poisoning when no late effect of the injury has been documented.

i. Misadventures and Complications of Care Guidelines

1) Code range E870–E876

Assign a code in the range of E870–E876 if misadventures are stated by the provider.

2) Code range E878–E879

Assign a code in the range of E878–E879 if the provider attributes an abnormal reaction or later complication to a surgical or medical procedure, but does not mention misadventure at the time of the procedure as the cause of the reaction.

j. Terrorism Guidelines

1) Cause of injury identified by the Federal Government (FBI) as terrorism

When the cause of an injury is identified by the Federal Government (FBI) as terrorism, the first-listed E-code should be a code from category E979, Terrorism. The definition of terrorism employed by the FBI is found at the inclusion note at E979. The terrorism E-code is the only E-code that should be assigned. Additional E codes from the assault categories should not be assigned.

2) Cause of an injury is suspected to be the result of terrorism

When the cause of an injury is suspected to be the result of terrorism a code from category E979 should not be assigned. Assign a code in the range of E codes based circumstances on the documentation of intent and mechanism.

3) Code E979.9, Terrorism, secondary effects

Assign code E979.9, Terrorism, secondary effects, for conditions occurring subsequent to the terrorist event. This code should not be assigned for conditions that are due to the initial terrorist act.

4) Statistical tabulation of terrorism codes

For statistical purposes these codes will be tabulated within the category for assault, expanding the current category from E960–E969 to include E979 and E999.1.

SECTION II.   SELECTION OF PRINCIPAL DIAGNOSIS

The circumstances of inpatient admission always govern the selection of principal diagnosis. The principal diagnosis is defined in the Uniform Hospital Discharge Data Set (UHDDS) as "that condition established after study to be chiefly responsible for occasioning the admission of the patient to the hospital for care."

The UHDDS definitions are used by hospitals to report inpatient data elements in a standardized manner. These data elements and their definitions can be found in the July 31, 1985, Federal Register (Vol. 50, No, 147), pp. 31038–40.

Since that time the application of the UHDDS definitions has been expanded to include all non-outpatient settings (acute care, short term, long term care and psychiatric hospitals; home health agencies; rehab facilities; nursing homes, etc.).

In determining principal diagnosis, the coding conventions in the ICD-9-CM book, Volumes I and II take precedence over these official coding guidelines. (See Section I.A., Conventions for the ICD-9-CM book.)

The importance of consistent, complete documentation in the medical record cannot be overemphasized. Without such documentation the application of all coding guidelines is a difficult, if not impossible, task.

A. **Codes for symptoms, signs, and ill-defined conditions**

Codes for symptoms, signs, and ill-defined conditions from Chapter 16 are not to be used as principal diagnosis when a related definitive diagnosis has been established.

B. **Two or more interrelated conditions, each potentially meeting the definition for principal diagnosis.**

When there are two or more interrelated conditions (such as diseases in the same ICD-9-CM chapter or manifestations characteristically associated with a certain disease) potentially meeting the definition of principal diagnosis, either condition may be sequenced first, unless the circumstances of the admission, the therapy provided, the Tabular List, or the Alphabetic Index indicate otherwise.

C. **Two or more diagnoses that equally meet the definition for principal diagnosis**

In the unusual instance when two or more diagnoses equally meet the criteria for principal diagnosis as determined by the circumstances of admission, diagnostic workup and/or therapy provided, and the Alphabetic Index, Tabular List, or another coding guideline does not provide sequencing direction, any one of the diagnoses may be sequenced first.

D. **Two or more comparative or contrasting conditions**

In those rare instances when two or more contrasting or comparative diagnoses are documented as "either/or" (or similar terminology), they are coded as if the diagnoses were confirmed and the diagnoses are sequenced according to the circumstances of the admission. If no further determination can be made as to which diagnosis should be principal, either diagnosis may be sequenced first.

E. **A symptom(s) followed by contrasting/comparative diagnoses**

When a symptom(s) is followed by contrasting/comparative diagnoses, the symptom code is sequenced first. All the contrasting/comparative diagnoses should be coded as additional diagnoses.

F. **Original treatment plan not carried out**

Sequence as the principal diagnosis the condition, which after study occasioned the admission to the hospital, even though treatment may not have been carried out due to unforeseen circumstances.

G. **Complications of surgery and other medical care**

When the admission is for treatment of a complication resulting from surgery or other medical care, the complication code is sequenced as the principal diagnosis. If the complication is classified to the 996–999 series and the code lacks the necessary specificity in describing the complication, an additional code for the specific complication should be assigned.

H. **Uncertain Diagnosis**

If the diagnosis documented at the time of discharge is qualified as "probable", "suspected", "likely", "questionable", "possible", or "still to be ruled out", code the condition as if it existed or was established. The basis for these guidelines are the diagnostic workup, arrangements for further workup or observation, and initial therapeutic approach that correspond most closely with the established diagnosis.

Note: This guideline is applicable only to short-term, acute, long-term care and psychiatric hospitals.

SECTION III.   REPORTING ADDITIONAL DIAGNOSES

General Rules for other (Additional) Diagnoses

For reporting purposes the definition for "other diagnoses" is interpreted as additional conditions that affect patient care in terms of requiring:

clinical evaluation; or

therapeutic treatment; or

diagnostic procedures; or

extended length of hospital stay; or

increased nursing care and/or monitoring.

The UHDDS item # 11-b defines Other Diagnoses as "all conditions that coexist at the time of admission, that develop subsequently, or that affect the treatment received and/or the length of stay. Diagnoses that relate to an earlier episode which have no bearing on the current hospital stay are to be excluded." UHDDS definitions apply to inpatients in acute care, short-term, long term care and psychiatric hospital setting. The UHDDS definitions are used by acute care short-term hospitals to report inpatient data elements in a standardized manner. These data elements and their definitions can be found in the July 31, 1985, Federal Register (Vol. 50, No, 147), pp. 31038–40.

Since that time the application of the UHDDS definitions has been expanded to include all non-outpatient settings (acute care, short term, long term care and psychiatric hospitals; home health agencies; rehab facilities; nursing homes, etc.).

The following guidelines are to be applied in designating "other diagnoses" when neither the Alphabetic Index nor the Tabular List in ICD-9-CM provide direction. The listing of the diagnoses in the patient record is the responsibility of the attending provider.

A. Previous conditions

If the provider has included a diagnosis in the final diagnostic statement, such as the discharge summary or the face sheet, it should ordinarily be coded. Some providers include in the diagnostic statement resolved conditions or diagnoses and status-post procedures from a previous admission that have no bearing on the current stay. Such conditions are not to be reported and are coded only if required by hospital policy.

However, history codes (V10–V19) may be used as secondary codes if the historical condition or family history has an impact on current care or influences treatment.

B. Abnormal findings

Abnormal findings (laboratory, X-ray, pathologic, and other diagnostic results) are not coded and reported unless the provider indicates their clinical significance. If the findings are outside the normal range and the **attending** provider has ordered other tests to evaluate the condition or prescribed treatment, it is appropriate to ask the provider whether the abnormal finding should be added.

Please note: This differs from the coding practices in the outpatient setting for coding encounters for diagnostic tests that have been interpreted by a provider.

C. Uncertain diagnosis

If the diagnosis documented at the time of discharge is qualified as "probable," "suspected," "likely," "questionable," "possible," or "still to be ruled out," code the condition as if it existed or was established. The basis for these guidelines are the diagnostic workup, arrangements for further workup or observation, and initial therapeutic approach that correspond most closely with the established diagnosis.

Note: This guideline is applicable only to short-term, acute, long-term care and psychiatric hospitals.

SECTION IV.   DIAGNOSTIC CODING AND REPORTING GUIDELINES FOR OUTPATIENT SERVICES

These coding guidelines for outpatient diagnoses have been approved for use by hospitals/providers in coding and reporting hospital-based outpatient services and provider-based office visits.

Information about the use of certain abbreviations, punctuation, symbols, and other conventions used in the ICD-9-CM Tabular List (code numbers and titles), can be found in Section IA of these guidelines, under "Conventions Used in the Tabular List." Information about the correct sequence to use in finding a code is also described in Section I.

The terms encounter and visit are often used interchangeably in describing outpatient service contacts and, therefore, appear together in these guidelines without distinguishing one from the other.

Though the conventions and general guidelines apply to all settings, coding guidelines for outpatient and provider reporting of diagnoses will vary in a number of instances from those for inpatient diagnoses, recognizing that:

The Uniform Hospital Discharge Data Set (UHDDS) definition of principal diagnosis applies only to inpatients in acute, short-term, long-term care **and psychiatric** hospitals.

Coding guidelines for inconclusive diagnoses (probable, suspected, rule out, etc.) were developed for inpatient reporting and do not apply to outpatients.

A. **Selection of first-listed condition**

In the outpatient setting, the term first-listed diagnosis is used in lieu of principal diagnosis.

In determining the first-listed diagnosis the coding conventions of ICD-9-CM, as well as the general and disease specific guidelines take precedence over the outpatient guidelines.

Diagnoses often are not established at the time of the initial encounter/visit. It may take two or more visits before the diagnosis is confirmed.

The most critical rule involves beginning the search for the correct code assignment through the Alphabetic Index. Never begin searching initially in the Tabular List as this will lead to coding errors.

B. **Codes from 001.0 through V84.8**

The appropriate code or codes from 001.0 through V84.8 must be used to identify diagnoses, symptoms, conditions, problems, complaints, or other reason(s) for the encounter/visit.

C. **Accurate reporting of ICD-9-CM diagnosis codes**

For accurate reporting of ICD-9-CM diagnosis codes, the documentation should describe the patient's condition, using terminology which includes specific diagnoses as well as symptoms, problems, or reasons for the encounter. There are ICD-9-CM codes to describe all of these.

D. **Selection of codes 001.0 through 999.9**

The selection of codes 001.0 through 999.9 will frequently be used to describe the reason for the encounter. These codes are from the section of ICD-9-CM for the classification of diseases and injuries (e.g., infectious and parasitic diseases; neoplasms; symptoms, signs, and ill-defined conditions, etc.).

E. **Codes that describe symptoms and signs**

Codes that describe symptoms and signs, as opposed to diagnoses, are acceptable for reporting purposes when a diagnosis has not been established (confirmed) by the provider. Chapter 16 of ICD-9-CM, Symptoms, Signs, and III-defined conditions (codes 780.0–799.9) contains many, but not all codes for symptoms.

F. **Encounters for circumstances other than a disease or injury**

ICD-9-CM provides codes to deal with encounters for circumstances other than a disease or injury. The Supplementary Classification of factors Influencing Health Status and Contact with Health Services (V01.0–V84.8) is provided to deal with occasions when circumstances other than a disease or injury are recorded as diagnosis or problems.

G. **Level of Detail in Coding**

1. **ICD-9-CM codes with 3, 4, or 5 digits**

   ICD-9-CM is composed of codes with either 3, 4, or 5 digits. Codes with three digits are included in ICD-9-CM as the heading of a category of codes that may be further subdivided by the use of fourth and/or fifth digits, which provide greater specificity.

2. **Use of full number of digits required for a code**

   A three-digit code is to be used only if it is not further subdivided. Where fourth-digit subcategories and/or fifth-digit subclassifications are provided, they must be assigned. A code is invalid if it has not been coded to the full number of digits required for that code. See also discussion under Section I.b.3., General Coding Guidelines, Level of Detail in Coding.

H. **ICD-9-CM code for the diagnosis, condition, problem, or other reason for encounter/visit**

   List first the ICD-9-CM code for the diagnosis, condition, problem, or other reason for encounter/visit shown in the medical record to be chiefly responsible for the services provided. List additional codes that describe any coexisting conditions. **In some cases the first-listed diagnosis may be a symptom when a diagnosis has not been established (confirmed) by the physician.**

I. **"Probable," "suspected," "questionable," "rule out," or "working diagnosis"**

   Do not code diagnoses documented as "probable," "suspected," "questionable," "rule out," or "working diagnosis." Rather, code the condition(s) to the highest degree of certainty for that encounter/visit, such as symptoms, signs, abnormal test results, or other reason for the visit. **Please note:** This differs from the coding practices used by **short-term, acute care, long-term care and psychiatric** hospitals.

J. **Chronic diseases**

   Chronic diseases treated on an ongoing basis may be coded and reported as many times as the patient receives treatment and care for the condition(s)

K. **Code all documented conditions that coexist**

   Code all documented conditions that coexist at the time of the encounter/visit, and require or affect patient care treatment or management. Do not code conditions that were previously treated and no longer exist. However, history codes (V10–V19) may be used as secondary codes if the historical condition or family history has an impact on current care or influences treatment.

L. **Patients receiving diagnostic services only**

   For patients receiving diagnostic services only during an encounter/visit, sequence first the diagnosis, condition, problem, or other reason for encounter/visit shown in the medical record to be chiefly responsible for the outpatient services provided during the encounter/visit. Codes for other diagnoses (e.g., chronic conditions) may be sequenced as additional diagnoses.

   For outpatient encounters for diagnostic tests that have been interpreted by a physician, and the final report is available at the time of coding, code any confirmed or definitive diagnosis(es) documented in the interpretation. Do not code related signs and symptoms as additional diagnoses.

   Please note: This differs from the coding practice in the hospital inpatient setting regarding abnormal findings on test results.

M. **Patients receiving therapeutic services only**

   For patients receiving therapeutic services only during an encounter/visit, sequence first the diagnosis, condition, problem, or other reason for encounter/visit shown in the medical record to be chiefly responsible for the outpatient services provided during the encounter/visit. Codes for other diagnoses (e.g., chronic conditions) may be sequenced as additional diagnoses.

   The only exception to this rule is that when the primary reason for the admission/encounter is chemotherapy, radiation therapy, or rehabilitation, the appropriate V code for the service is listed first, and the diagnosis or problem for which the service is being performed listed second.

N. **Patients receiving preoperative evaluations only**

For patients receiving preoperative evaluations only, sequence **first** a code from category V72.8, Other specified examinations, to describe the pre-op consultations. Assign a code for the condition to describe the reason for the surgery as an additional diagnosis. Code also any findings related to the pre-op evaluation.

O. **Ambulatory surgery**

For ambulatory surgery, code the diagnosis for which the surgery was performed. If the postoperative diagnosis is known to be different from the preoperative diagnosis at the time the diagnosis is confirmed, select the postoperative diagnosis for coding, since it is the most definitive.

P. **Routine outpatient prenatal visits**

For routine outpatient prenatal visits when no complications are present, codes V22.0, Supervision of normal first pregnancy, **or** V22.1, Supervision of other normal pregnancy, should be used as **the** principal diagnosis. These codes should not be used in conjunction with Chapter 11 codes.

Appendix C

1997 Documentation Guidelines for Evaluation and Management Services

Table of Contents

I. INTRODUCTION

What Is Documentation and Why Is It Important?

Medical record documentation is required to record pertinent facts, findings, and observations about an individual's health history including past and present illnesses, examinations, tests, treatments, and outcomes. The medical record chronologically documents the care of the patient and is an important element contributing to high quality care. The medical record facilitates:

- the ability of the physician and other health care professionals to evaluate and plan the patient's immediate treatment, and to monitor his/her health care over time;
- communication and continuity of care among physicians and other health care professionals involved in the patient's care;
- accurate and timely claims review and payment;
- appropriate utilization review and quality of care evaluations; and
- collection of data that may be useful for research and education.

An appropriately documented medical record can reduce many of the "hassles" associated with claims processing and may serve as a legal document to verify the care provided, if necessary.

What Do Payers Want and Why?

Because payers have a contractual obligation to enrollees, they may require reasonable documentation that services are consistent with the insurance coverage provided. They may request information to validate:

- the site of service;
- the medical necessity and appropriateness of the diagnostic and/or therapeutic services provided; and/or
- that services provided have been accurately reported.

II. GENERAL PRINCIPLES OF MEDICAL RECORD DOCUMENTATION

The principles of documentation listed below are applicable to all types of medical and surgical services in all settings. For Evaluation and Management (E/M) services, the nature and amount of physician work and documentation varies by type of service, place of service, and the patient's status. The general principles listed below may be modified to account for these variable circumstances in providing E/M services.

1. The medical record should be complete and legible.
2. The documentation of each patient encounter should include:
   - reason for the encounter and relevant history, physical examination findings, and prior diagnostic test results;
   - assessment, clinical impression or diagnosis;
   - plan for care; and
   - date and legible identity of the observer.
3. If not documented, the rationale for ordering diagnostic and other ancillary services should be easily inferred.
4. Past and present diagnoses should be accessible to the treating and/or consulting physician.
5. Appropriate health risk factors should be identified.
6. The patient's progress, response to and changes in treatment, and revision of diagnosis should be documented.
7. The CPT and ICD-9-CM codes reported on the health insurance claim form or billing statement should be supported by the documentation in the medical record.

III. DOCUMENTATION OF E/M SERVICES

This publication provides definitions and documentation guidelines for the three key components of E/M services and for visits which consist predominately of counseling or coordination of care. The three *key* components—history, examination, and medical decision making—appear in the descriptors for office and other outpatient services, hospital observation services, hospital inpatient services, consultations, emergency department services, nursing facility services, domiciliary care services, and home services. While some of the text of CPT has been repeated in this publication, the reader should refer to CPT for the complete descriptors for E/M services and instructions for selecting a level of service. Documentation guidelines are identified by the symbol •*DG*.

The descriptors for the levels of E/M services recognize seven components which are used in defining the levels of E/M services. These components are:

- history;
- examination;
- medical decision making;
- counseling;
- coordination of care;
- nature of presenting problem; and
- time.

The first three of these components (i.e., history, examination, and medical decision making) are the key components in selecting the level of E/M services. In the case of visits which consist <u>predominantly</u> of counseling or coordination of care, time is the key or controlling factor to qualify for a particular level of E/M service.

Because the level of E/M service is dependent on two or three key components, performance and documentation of one component (e.g., examination) at the highest level does not necessarily mean that the encounter in its entirety qualifies for the highest level of E/M service.

These Documentation Guidelines for E/M Services reflect the needs of the typical adult population. For certain groups of patients, the recorded information may vary slightly from that described here. Specifically, the medical records of infants, children, adolescents, and pregnant women may have additional or modified information recorded in each history and examination area.

As an example, newborn records may include under history of the present illness (HPI) the details of the mother's pregnancy and the infant's status at birth; social history will focus on family structure; family history will focus on congenital anomalies and hereditary disorders in the family. In addition, the content of a pediatric examination will vary with the age and development of the child. Although not specifically defined in these documentation guidelines, these patient group variations on history and examination are appropriate.

A. Documentation of History

The levels of E/M services are based on four types of history (Problem-Focused, Expanded Problem-Focused, Detailed, and Comprehensive). Each type of history includes some or all of the following elements:

- Chief complaint (CC);
- History of present illness (HPI);
- Review of systems (ROS); and
- Past, family, and/or social history (PFSH).

The extent of history of present illness; review of systems; and past, family, and/or social history that is obtained and documented is dependent upon clinical judgement and the nature of the presenting problem(s).

The chart below shows the progression of the elements required for each type of history. To qualify for a given type of history all three elements in the table must be met. (A chief complaint is indicated at all levels.)

History of Present Illness (HPI)	Review of Systems (ROS)	Past, Family, and/or Social History (PFSH)	Type of History
Brief	N/A	N/A	Problem-Focused
Brief	Problem Pertinent	N/A	Expanded Problem-Focused
Extended	Extended	Pertinent	Detailed
Extended	Complete	Complete	Comprehensive

- *DG: The CC, ROS, and PFSH may be listed as separate elements of history, or they may be included in the description of the history of the present illness.*
- *DG: A ROS and/or a PFSH obtained during an earlier encounter does not need to be re-recorded if there is evidence that the physician reviewed and updated the previous information. This may occur when a physician updates his or her own record or in an institutional setting or group practice where many physicians use a common record. The review and update may be documented by:*
  - *describing any new ROS and/or PFSH information or noting there has been no change in the information; and*
  - *noting the date and location of the earlier ROS and/or PFSH.*
- *DG: The ROS and/or PFSH may be recorded by ancillary staff or on a form completed by the patient. To document that the physician reviewed the information, there must be a notation supplementing or confirming the information recorded by others.*
- *DG: If the physician is unable to obtain a history from the patient or other source, the record should describe the patient's condition or other circumstance which precludes obtaining a history.*

Definitions and specific documentation guidelines for each of the elements of history are listed below.

Chief Complaint (CC)

The CC is a concise statement describing the symptom, problem, condition, diagnosis, physician recommended return, or other factor that is the reason for the encounter, usually stated in the patient's words.

- *DG: The medical record should clearly reflect the chief complaint.*

History of Present Illness (HPI)

The HPI is a chronological description of the development of the patient's present illness from the first sign and/or symptom or from the previous encounter to the present. It includes the following elements:

- location,
- quality,
- severity,
- duration,
- timing,
- context,
- modifying factors, and
- associated signs and symptoms.

Brief and *extended* HPIs are distinguished by the amount of detail needed to accurately characterize the clinical problem(s).

A *brief* HPI consists of one to three elements of the HPI.

- *DG: The medical record should describe one to three elements of the present illness (HPI).*

An *extended* HPI consists of at least four elements of the HPI or the status of at least three chronic or inactive conditions.

- *DG: The medical record should describe at least four elements of the present illness (HPI), or the status of at least three chronic or inactive conditions.*

Review of Systems (ROS)

A ROS is an inventory of body systems obtained through a series of questions seeking to identify signs and/or symptoms which the patient may be experiencing or has experienced.

For purposes of ROS, the following systems are recognized:

- Constitutional symptoms (e.g., fever, weight loss)
- Eyes
- Ears, Nose, Mouth, Throat
- Cardiovascular
- Respiratory
- Gastrointestinal
- Genitourinary
- Musculoskeletal
- Integumentary (skin and/or breast)
- Neurological
- Psychiatric
- Endocrine
- Hematologic/Lymphatic
- Allergic/Immunologic

A *problem pertinent* ROS inquires about the system directly related to the problem(s) identified in the HPI.

- *DG: The patient's positive responses and pertinent negatives for the system related to the problem should be documented.*

An *extended* ROS inquires about the system directly related to the problem(s) identified in the HPI and a limited number of additional systems.

- *DG: The patient's positive responses and pertinent negatives for two to nine systems should be documented.*

A *complete* ROS inquires about the system(s) directly related to the problem(s) identified in the HPI *plus* all additional body systems.

- *DG: At least ten organ systems must be reviewed. Those systems with positive or pertinent negative responses must be individually documented. For the remaining systems, a notation indicating all other systems are negative is permissible. In the absence of such a notation, at least ten systems must be individually documented.*

Past, Family, and/or Social History (PFSH)

The PFSH consists of a review of three areas:

- past history (the patient's past experiences with illnesses, operations, injuries, and treatments);
- family history (a review of medical events in the patient's family, including diseases which may be hereditary or place the patient at risk); and
- social history (an age appropriate review of past and current activities).

For certain categories of E/M services that include only an interval history, it is not necessary to record information about the PFSH. Those categories are subsequent hospital care, follow-up inpatient consultations, and subsequent nursing facility care.

A *pertinent* PFSH is a review of the history area(s) directly related to the problem(s) identified in the HPI.

- *DG: At least one specific item from any of the three history areas must be documented for a pertinent PFSH.*

A *complete* PFSH is of a review of two or all three of the PFSH history areas, depending on the category of the E/M service. A review of all three history areas is required for services that by their nature include a comprehensive assessment or reassessment of the patient. A review of two of the three history areas is sufficient for other services.

- *DG: At least one specific item from two of the three history areas must be documented for a complete PFSH for the following categories of E/M services: office or other outpatient services, established patient; emergency department; domiciliary care, established patient; and home care, established patient.*
- *DG: At least one specific item from each of the three history areas must be documented for a complete PFSH for the following categories of E/M services: office or other outpatient services, new patient; hospital observation services; hospital inpatient services, initial care; consultations; comprehensive nursing facility assessments; domiciliary care, new patient; and home care, new patient.*

B. Documentation of Examination

The levels of E/M services are based on four types of examination:

- *Problem-Focused*—a limited examination of the affected body area or organ system.
- *Expanded Problem-Focused*—a limited examination of the affected body area or organ system and any other symptomatic or related body area(s) or organ system(s).
- *Detailed*—an extended examination of the affected body area(s) or organ system(s) and any other symptomatic or related body area(s) or organ system(s).
- *Comprehensive*—a general multisystem examination, or complete examination of a single organ system and other symptomatic or related body area(s) or organ system(s).

These types of examinations have been defined for general multisystem and the following single organ systems:

- Cardiovascular
- Ears, Nose, Mouth, and Throat
- Eyes
- Genitourinary (Female)
- Genitourinary (Male)
- Hematologic/Lymphatic/Immunologic
- Musculoskeletal
- Neurological
- Psychiatric
- Respiratory
- Skin

A general multisystem examination or a single organ system examination may be performed by any physician regardless of specialty. The type (general multisystem or single organ system) and content of examination are selected by the examining physician and are based upon clinical judgement, the patient's history, and the nature of the presenting problem(s).

The content and documentation requirements for each type and level of examination are summarized below and described in detail in tables beginning on page 405. In the tables, organ systems and body areas recognized by CPT for purposes of describing examinations are shown in the left column. The content, or individual elements, of the examination pertaining to that body area or organ system are identified by bullets (•) in the right column.

Parenthetical examples, "(e.g., . . .)," have been used for clarification and to provide guidance regarding documentation. Documentation for each element must satisfy any numeric requirements (such as "Measurement of *any three of the following seven . . .*") included in the description of the element. Elements with multiple components but with no specific numeric requirement (such as "Examination of *liver* and *spleen*") require documentation of at least one component. It is possible for a given examination to be expanded beyond what is defined here. When that occurs, findings related to the additional systems and/or areas should be documented.

- *DG: Specific abnormal and relevant negative findings of the examination of the affected or symptomatic body area(s) or organ system(s) should be documented. A notation of "abnormal" without elaboration is insufficient.*
- *DG: Abnormal or unexpected findings of the examination of any asymptomatic body area(s) or organ system(s) should be described.*
- *DG: A brief statement or notation indicating "negative" or "normal" is sufficient to document normal findings related to unaffected area(s) or asymptomatic organ system(s).*

General Multisystem Examinations

General multisystem examinations are described in detail beginning on page 405. To qualify for a given level of multisystem examination, the following content and documentation requirements should be met:

- *Problem-Focused Examination*—should include performance and documentation of one to five elements identified by a bullet (•) in one or more organ system(s) or body area(s).
- *Expanded Problem-Focused Examination*—should include performance and documentation of at least six elements identified by a bullet (•) in one or more organ system(s) or body area(s).
- *Detailed Examination*—should include at least six organ systems or body areas. For each system/area selected, performance and documentation of at least two elements identified by a bullet (•) is expected. Alternatively, a detailed examination may include performance and documentation of at least twelve elements identified by a bullet (•) in two or more organ systems or body areas.
- *Comprehensive Examination*—should include at least nine organ systems or body areas. For each system/area selected, all elements of the examination identified by a bullet (•) should be performed, unless specific directions limit the content of the examination. For each area/system, documentation of at least two elements identified by a bullet is expected.

Single Organ System Examinations

The single organ system examinations recognized by CPT are described in detail beginning on page 407. Variations among these examinations in the organ systems and body areas identified in the left columns and in the elements of the examinations described in the right columns reflect differing emphases among specialties. To qualify for a given level of single organ system examination, the following content and documentation requirements should be met:

- *Problem-Focused Examination*—should include performance and documentation of one to five elements identified by a bullet (•), whether in a box with a shaded or unshaded border.
- *Expanded Problem-Focused Examination*—should include performance and documentation of at least six elements identified by a bullet (•), whether in a box with a shaded or unshaded border.
- *Detailed Examination*—examinations other than the eye and psychiatric examinations should include performance and documentation of at least twelve elements identified by a bullet (•), whether in box with a shaded or unshaded border.

    Eye and psychiatric examinations should include the performance and documentation of at least nine elements identified by a bullet (•), whether in a box with a shaded or unshaded border.

- *Comprehensive Examination*—should include performance of all elements identified by a bullet (•), whether in a shaded or unshaded box. Documentation of every element in each box with a shaded border and at least one element in each box with an unshaded border is expected.

Content and Documentation Requirements

GENERAL MULTISYSTEM EXAMINATION	
System/Body Area	**Elements of Examination**
Constitutional	• Measurement of **any three of the following seven** vital signs: 1) sitting or standing blood pressure, 2) supine blood pressure, 3) pulse rate and regularity, 4) respiration, 5) temperature, 6) height, 7) weight (May be measured and recorded by ancillary staff) • General appearance of patient (e.g., development, nutrition, body habitus, deformities, attention to grooming)
Eyes	• Inspection of conjunctivae and lids • Examination of pupils and irises (e.g., reaction to light and accommodation, size and symmetry) • Ophthalmoscopic examination of optic discs (e.g., size, C/D ratio, appearance) and posterior segments (e.g., vessel changes, exudates, hemorrhages)
Ears, Nose, Mouth, and Throat	• External inspection of ears and nose (e.g., overall appearance, scars, lesions, masses) • Otoscopic examination of external auditory canals and tympanic membranes • Assessment of hearing (e.g., whispered voice, finger rub, tuning fork) • Inspection of nasal mucosa, septum and turbinates • Inspection of lips, teeth, and gums • Examination of oropharynx: oral mucosa, salivary glands, hard and soft palates, tongue, tonsils and posterior pharynx
Neck	• Examination of neck (e.g., masses, overall appearance, symmetry, tracheal position, crepitus) • Examination of thyroid (e.g., enlargement, tenderness, mass)
Respiratory	• Assessment of respiratory effort (e.g., intercostal retractions, use of accessory muscles, diaphragmatic movement) • Percussion of chest (e.g., dullness, flatness, hyperresonance) • Palpation of chest (e.g., tactile fremitus) • Auscultation of lungs (e.g., breath sounds, adventitious sounds, rubs)
Cardiovascular	• Palpation of heart (e.g., location, size, thrills) • Auscultation of heart with notation of abnormal sounds and murmurs Examination of: • carotid arteries (e.g., pulse amplitude, bruits) • abdominal aorta (e.g., size, bruits) • femoral arteries (e.g., pulse amplitude, bruits) • pedal pulses (e.g., pulse amplitude) • extremities for edema and/or varicosities
Chest (Breasts)	• Inspection of breasts (e.g., symmetry, nipple discharge) • Palpation of breasts and axillae (e.g., masses or lumps, tenderness)

(*continued*)

GENERAL MULTISYSTEM EXAMINATION (*CONTINUED*)

System/Body Area	Elements of Examination
Gastrointestinal (Abdomen)	• Examination of abdomen with notation of presence of masses or tenderness • Examination of liver and spleen • Examination for presence or absence of hernia • Examination (when indicated) of anus, perineum, and rectum, including sphincter tone, presence of hemorrhoids, rectal masses • Obtain stool sample for occult blood test when indicated
Genitourinary	**MALE:** • Examination of the scrotal contents (e.g., hydrocele, spermatocele, tenderness of cord, testicular mass) • Examination of the penis • Digital rectal examination of prostate gland (e.g., size, symmetry, nodularity, tenderness) **FEMALE:** Pelvic examination (with or without specimen collection for smears and cultures), including • Examination of external genitalia (e.g., general appearance, hair distribution, lesions) and vagina (e.g., general appearance, estrogen effect, discharge, lesions, pelvic support, cystocele, rectocele) • Examination of urethra (e.g., masses, tenderness, scarring) • Examination of bladder (e.g., fullness, masses, tenderness) • Cervix (e.g., general appearance, lesions, discharge) • Uterus (e.g., size, contour, position, mobility, tenderness, consistency, descent or support) • Adnexa/parametria (e.g., masses, tenderness, organomegaly, nodularity)
Lymphatic	Palpation of lymph nodes in **two or more** areas: • Neck • Axillae • Groin • Other
Musculoskeletal	• Examination of gait and station • Inspection and/or palpation of digits and nails (e.g., clubbing, cyanosis, inflammatory conditions, petechiae, ischemia, infections, nodes) Examination of joints, bones, and muscles of **one or more of the following six** areas: 1) head and neck; 2) spine, ribs, and pelvis; 3) right upper extremity; 4) left upper extremity; 5) right lower extremity; and 6) left lower extremity. The examination of a given area includes: • Inspection and/or palpation with notation of presence of any misalignment, asymmetry, crepitation, defects, tenderness, masses, effusions • Assessment of range of motion with notation of any pain, crepitation, or contracture • Assessment of stability with notation of any dislocation (luxation), subluxation, or laxity • Assessment of muscle strength and tone (e.g., flaccid, cog wheel, spastic) with notation of any atrophy or abnormal movements

Skin	• Inspection of skin and subcutaneous tissue (e.g., rashes, lesions, ulcers)
	• Palpation of skin and subcutaneous tissue (e.g., induration, subcutaneous nodules, tightening)
Neurologic	• Test cranial nerves with notation of any deficits
	• Examination of deep tendon reflexes with notation of pathological reflexes (e.g., Babinski)
	• Examination of sensation (e.g., by touch, pin, vibration, proprioception)
Psychiatric	• Description of patient's judgment and insight
	Brief assessment of mental status including:
	• orientation to time, place, and person
	• recent and remote memory
	• mood and affect (e.g., depression, anxiety, agitation)

Content and Documentation Requirements

Level of Exam	*Perform and Document:*
Problem-Focused	**One to five** elements identified by a bullet.
Expanded Problem-Focused	**At least six** elements identified by a bullet.
Detailed	**At least two** elements identified by a bullet **from each of six areas/ systems** OR **at least twelve** elements identified by a bullet **in two or more areas/systems.**
Comprehensive	Perform **all elements** identified by a bullet in **at least nine** organ systems or body areas and document **at least two** elements identified by a bullet **from each of nine areas/systems.**

CARDIOVASCULAR EXAMINATION

System/Body Area	Elements of Examination
Constitutional	• Measurement of **any three of the following seven** vital signs: 1) sitting or standing blood pressure, 2) supine blood pressure, 3) pulse rate and regularity, 4) respiration, 5) temperature, 6) height, 7) weight (May be measured and recorded by ancillary staff)
	• General appearance of patient (e.g., development, nutrition, body habitus, deformities, attention to grooming)
Head and Face	
Eyes	• Inspection of conjunctivae and lids (e.g., xanthelasma)
Ears, Nose, Mouth, and Throat	• Inspection of teeth, gums, and palate
	• Inspection of oral mucosa with notation of presence of pallor or cyanosis
Neck	• Examination of jugular veins (e.g., distension; a, v or cannon a waves)
	• Examination of thyroid (e.g., enlargement, tenderness, mass)

(continued)

CARDIOVASCULAR EXAMINATION (*CONTINUED*)

System/Body Area	Elements of Examination
Respiratory	• Assessment of respiratory effort (e.g., intercostal retractions, use of accessory muscles, diaphragmatic movement) • Auscultation of lungs (e.g., breath sounds, adventitious sounds, rubs)
Cardiovascular	• Palpation of heart (e.g., location, size and forcefulness of the point of maximal impact; thrills; lifts; palpable S3 or S4) • Auscultation of heart including sounds, abnormal sounds and murmurs • Measurement of blood pressure in two or more extremities when indicated (e.g., aortic dissection, coarctation) Examination of: • Carotid arteries (e.g., waveform, pulse amplitude, bruits, apical-carotid delay) • Abdominal aorta (e.g., size, bruits) • Femoral arteries (e.g., pulse amplitude, bruits) • Pedal pulses (e.g., pulse amplitude) • Extremities for peripheral edema and/or varicosities
Chest (Breasts)	
Gastrointestinal (Abdomen)	• Examination of abdomen with notation of presence of masses or tenderness • Examination of liver and spleen • Obtain stool sample for occult blood from patients who are being considered for thrombolytic or anticoagulant therapy
Genitourinary (Abdomen)	
Lymphatic	
Musculoskeletal	• Examination of the back with notation of kyphosis or scoliosis • Examination of gait with notation of ability to undergo exercise testing and/or participation in exercise programs • Assessment of muscle strength and tone (e.g., flaccid, cog wheel, spastic) with notation of any atrophy and abnormal movements
Extremities	• Inspection and palpation of digits and nails (e.g., clubbing, cyanosis, inflammation, petechiae, ischemia, infections, Osler's nodes)
Skin	• Inspection and/or palpation of skin and subcutaneous tissue (e.g., stasis dermatitis, ulcers, scars, xanthomas)
Neurological/ Psychiatric	Brief assessment of mental status including • Orientation to time, place, and person • Mood and affect (e.g., depression, anxiety, agitation)

Content and Documentation Requirements

Level of Exam	*Perform and Document:*
Problem-Focused	**One to five** elements identified by a bullet.
Expanded Problem-Focused	**At least six** elements identified by a bullet.
Detailed	**At least twelve** elements identified by a bullet.
Comprehensive	Perform **all** elements identified by a bullet; document every element in each box with a shaded border and at least one element in each box with an unshaded border.

EAR, NOSE, AND THROAT EXAMINATION

System/Body Area	Elements of Examination
Constitutional	• Measurement of **any three of the following seven** vital signs: 1) sitting or standing blood pressure, 2) supine blood pressure, 3) pulse rate and regularity, 4) respiration, 5) temperature, 6) height, 7) weight (May be measured and recorded by ancillary staff) • General appearance of patient (e.g., development, nutrition, body habitus, deformities, attention to grooming) • Assessment of ability to communicate (e.g., use of sign language or other communication aids) and quality of voice
Head and Face	• Inspection of head and face (e.g., overall appearance, scars, lesions, and masses) • Palpation and/or percussion of face with notation of presence or absence of sinus tenderness • Examination of salivary glands • Assessment of facial strength
Eyes	• Test ocular motility including primary gaze alignment
Ears, Nose, Mouth, and Throat	• Otoscopic examination of external auditory canals and tympanic membranes including pneumo-otoscopy with notation of mobility of membranes • Assessment of hearing with tuning forks and clinical speech reception thresholds (e.g., whispered voice, finger rub) • External inspection of ears and nose (e.g., overall appearance, scars, lesions, and masses) • Inspection of nasal mucosa, septum and turbinates • Inspection of lips, teeth, and gums • Examination of oropharynx: oral mucosa, hard and soft palates, tongue, tonsils and posterior pharynx (e.g., asymmetry, lesions, hydration of mucosal surfaces) • Inspection of pharyngeal walls and pyriform sinuses (e.g., pooling of saliva, asymmetry, lesions) • Examination by mirror of larynx including the condition of the epiglottis, false vocal cords, true vocal cords, and mobility of larynx (Use of mirror not required in children) • Examination by mirror of nasopharynx including appearance of the mucosa, adenoids, posterior choanae, and eustachian tubes (Use of mirror not required in children)

(*continued*)

EAR, NOSE, AND THROAT EXAMINATION (*CONTINUED*)

System/Body Area	Elements of Examination
Neck	• Examination of neck (e.g., masses, overall appearance, symmetry, tracheal position, crepitus) • Examination of thyroid (e.g., enlargement, tenderness, mass)
Respiratory	• Inspection of chest including symmetry, expansion and/or assessment of respiratory effort (e.g., intercostal retractions, use of accessory muscles, diaphragmatic movement) • Auscultation of lungs (e.g., breath sounds, adventitious sounds, rubs)
Cardiovascular	• Auscultation of heart with notation of abnormal sounds and murmurs • Examination of peripheral vascular system by observation (e.g., swelling, varicosities) and palpation (e.g., pulses, temperature, edema, tenderness)
Chest (Breasts)	
Gastrointestinal (Abdomen)	
Genitourinary	
Lymphatic	• Palpation of lymph nodes in neck, axillae, groin and/or other location
Musculoskeletal	
Extremities	
Skin	
Neurological/ Psychiatric	• Test cranial nerves with notation of any deficits Brief assessment of mental status including • Orientation to time, place, and person • Mood and affect (e.g., depression, anxiety, agitation)

Content and Documentation Requirements

Level of Exam	Perform and Document:
Problem-Focused	**One to five** elements identified by a bullet.
Expanded Problem-Focused	**At least six** elements identified by a bullet.
Detailed	**At least twelve** elements identified by a bullet.
Comprehensive	Perform **all** elements identified by a bullet; document every element in each box with a shaded border and at least one element in each box with an unshaded border.

EYE EXAMINATION

System/Body Area	Elements of Examination
Constitutional	
Head and Face	
Eyes	• Test visual acuity (Does not include determination of refractive error) • Gross visual field testing by confrontation • Test ocular motility including primary gaze alignment • Inspection of bulbar and palpebral conjunctivae • Examination of ocular adnexae including lids (e.g., ptosis or lagophthalmos), lacrimal glands, lacrimal drainage, orbits, and preauricular lymph nodes • Examination of pupils and irises including shape, direct and consensual reaction (afferent pupil), size (e.g., anisocoria), and morphology • Slit lamp examination of the corneas including epithelium, stroma, endothelium, and tear film • Slit lamp examination of the anterior chambers including depth, cells, and flare • Slit lamp examination of the lenses including clarity, anterior and posterior capsule, cortex, and nucleus • Measurement of intraocular pressures (except in children and patients with trauma or infectious disease) Ophthalmoscopic examination through dilated pupils (unless contraindicated) of • Optic discs including size, C/D ratio, appearance (e.g., atrophy, cupping, tumor elevation), and nerve fiber layer • Posterior segments including retina and vessels (e.g., exudates and hemorrhages)
Ears, Nose, Mouth, and Throat	
Neck	
Respiratory	
Cardiovascular	
Chest (Breasts)	
Gastrointestinal (Abdomen)	
Genitourinary	
Lymphatic	
Musculoskeletal	
Extremities	
Skin	
Neurological/ Psychiatric	Brief assessment of mental status including • Orientation to time, place, and person • Mood and affect (e.g., depression, anxiety, agitation)

Content and Documentation Requirements

Level of Exam	Perform and Document:
Problem-Focused	**One to five** elements identified by a bullet.
Expanded Problem-Focused	**At least six** elements identified by a bullet.
Detailed	**At least nine** elements identified by a bullet.
Comprehensive	Perform **all** elements identified by a bullet; document every element in each box with a shaded border and at least one element in each box with an unshaded border.

GENITOURINARY EXAMINATION

System/Body Area	Elements of Examination
Constitutional	• Measurement of **any three of the following seven** vital signs: 1) sitting or standing blood pressure, 2) supine blood pressure, 3) pulse rate and regularity, 4) respiration, 5) temperature, 6) height, 7) weight (May be measured and recorded by ancillary staff) • General appearance of patient (e.g., development, nutrition, body habitus, deformities, attention to grooming)
Head and Face	
Eyes	
Ears, Nose, Mouth, and Throat	
Neck	• Examination of neck (e.g., masses, overall appearance, symmetry, tracheal position, crepitus) • Examination of thyroid (e.g., enlargement, tenderness, mass)
Respiratory	• Assessment of respiratory effort (e.g., intercostal retractions, use of accessory muscles, diaphragmatic movement) • Auscultation of lungs (e.g., breath sounds, adventitious sounds, rubs)
Cardiovascular	• Auscultation of heart with notation of abnormal sounds and murmurs • Examination of peripheral vascular system by observation (e.g., swelling, varicosities) and palpation (e.g., pulses, temperature, edema, tenderness)
Chest (Breasts)	[See genitourinary (female)]
Gastrointestinal (Abdomen)	• Examination of abdomen with notation of presence of masses or tenderness • Examination for presence or absence of hernia • Examination of liver and spleen • Obtain stool sample for occult blood test when indicated
Genitourinary	**MALE:** • Inspection of anus and perineum Examination (with or without specimen collection for smears and cultures) of genitalia including: • Scrotum (e.g., lesions, cysts, rashes) • Epididymides (e.g., size, symmetry, masses)

- Testes (e.g., size, symmetry, masses)
- Urethral meatus (e.g., size, location, lesions, discharge)
- Penis (e.g., lesions, presence or absence of foreskin, foreskin retractability, plaque, masses, scarring, deformities)

Digital rectal examination including:
- Prostate gland (e.g., size, symmetry, nodularity, tenderness)
- Seminal vesicles (e.g., symmetry, tenderness, masses, enlargement)
- Sphincter tone, presence of hemorrhoids, rectal masses

FEMALE:
Includes **at least seven of the following eleven** elements identified by bullets:
- Inspection and palpation of breasts (e.g., masses or lumps, tenderness, symmetry, nipple discharge)
- Digital rectal examination including sphincter tone, presence of hemorrhoids, rectal masses

Pelvic examination (with or without specimen collection for smears and cultures) including:
- External genitalia (e.g., general appearance, hair distribution, lesions)
- Urethral meatus (e.g., size, location, lesions, prolapse)
- Urethra (e.g., masses, tenderness, scarring)
- Bladder (e.g., fullness, masses, tenderness)
- Vagina (e.g., general appearance, estrogen effect, discharge, lesions, pelvic support, cystocele, rectocele)
- Cervix (e.g., general appearance, lesions, discharge)
- Uterus (e.g., size, contour, position, mobility, tenderness, consistency, descent or support)
- Adnexa/parametria (e.g., masses, tenderness, organomegaly, nodularity)
- Anus and perineum

Lymphatic	• Palpation of lymph nodes in neck, axillae, groin and/or other location
Musculoskeletal	
Extremities	
Skin	• Inspection and/or palpation of skin and subcutaneous tissue (e.g., rashes, lesions, ulcers)
Neurological/ Psychiatric	Brief assessment of mental status including • Orientation (e.g., time, place, and person) and • Mood and affect (e.g., depression, anxiety, agitation)

Content and Documentation Requirements

Level of Exam	Perform and Document:
Problem-Focused	**One to five** elements identified by a bullet.
Expanded Problem-Focused	**At least six** elements identified by a bullet.
Detailed	**At least twelve** elements identified by a bullet.
Comprehensive	Perform **all** elements identified by a bullet; document every element in each box with a shaded border and at least one element in each box with an unshaded border.

HEMATOLOGIC/LYMPHATIC/IMMUNOLOGIC EXAMINATION

System/Body Area	Elements of Examination
Constitutional	• Measurement of **any three of the following seven** vital signs: 1) sitting or standing blood pressure, 2) supine blood pressure, 3) pulse rate and regularity, 4) respiration, 5) temperature, 6) height, 7) weight (May be measured and recorded by ancillary staff) • General appearance of patient (e.g., development, nutrition, body habitus, deformities, attention to grooming)
Head and Face	• Palpation and/or percussion of face with notation of presence or absence of sinus tenderness
Eyes	• Inspection of conjunctivae and lids
Ears, Nose, Mouth, and Throat	• Otoscopic examination of external auditory canals and tympanic membranes • Inspection of nasal mucosa, septum and turbinates • Inspection of teeth and gums • Examination of oropharynx (e.g., oral mucosa, hard and soft palates, tongue, tonsils, posterior pharynx)
Neck	• Examination of neck (e.g., masses, overall appearance, symmetry, tracheal position, crepitus) • Examination of thyroid (e.g., enlargement, tenderness, mass)
Respiratory	• Assessment of respiratory effort (e.g., intercostal retractions, use of accessory muscles, diaphragmatic movement) • Auscultation of lungs (e.g., breath sounds, adventitious sounds, rubs)
Cardiovascular	• Auscultation of heart with notation of abnormal sounds and murmurs • Examination of peripheral vascular system by observation (e.g., swelling, varicosities) and palpation (e.g., pulses, temperature, edema, tenderness)
Chest (Breasts)	
Gastrointestinal (Abdomen)	• Examination of abdomen with notation of presence of masses or tenderness • Examination of liver and spleen
Genitourinary	
Lymphatic	• Palpation of lymph nodes in neck, axillae, groin, and/or other location
Musculoskeletal	
Extremities	• Inspection and palpation of digits and nails (e.g., clubbing, cyanosis, inflammation, petechiae, ischemia, infections, nodes)
Skin	• Inspection and/or palpation of skin and subcutaneous tissue (e.g., rashes, lesions, ulcers, ecchymoses, bruises)
Neurological/ Psychiatric	Brief assessment of mental status including • Orientation to time, place, and person • Mood and affect (e.g., depression, anxiety, agitation)

Content and Documentation Requirements

Level of Exam	Perform and Document:
Problem-Focused	**One to five** elements identified by a bullet.
Expanded Problem-Focused	**At least six** elements identified by a bullet.
Detailed	**At least twelve** elements identified by a bullet.
Comprehensive	Perform **all** elements identified by a bullet; document every element in each box with a shaded border and at least one element in each box with an unshaded border.

MUSCULOSKELETAL EXAMINATION

System/Body Area	Elements of Examination
Constitutional	• Measurement of **any three of the following seven** vital signs: 1) sitting or standing blood pressure, 2) supine blood pressure, 3) pulse rate and regularity, 4) respiration, 5) temperature, 6) height, 7) weight (May be measured and recorded by ancillary staff) • General appearance of patient (e.g., development, nutrition, body habitus, deformities, attention to grooming)
Head and Face	
Eyes	
Ears, Nose, Mouth, and Throat	
Neck	
Respiratory	
Cardiovascular	• Examination of peripheral vascular system by observation (e.g., swelling, varicosities) and palpation (e.g., pulses, temperature, edema, tenderness)
Chest (Breasts)	
Gastrointestinal (Abdomen)	
Genitourinary	
Lymphatic	• Palpation of lymph nodes in neck, axillae, groin and/or other location
Musculoskeletal	• Examination of gait and station

Examination of joint(s), bone(s) and muscle(s)/tendon(s) of **four of the following six** areas: 1) head and neck; 2) spine, ribs, and pelvis; 3) right upper extremity; 4) left upper extremity; 5) right lower extremity; and 6) left lower extremity. The examination of a given area includes:

• Inspection, percussion and/or palpation with notation of any misalignment, asymmetry, crepitation, defects, tenderness, masses, or effusions
• Assessment of range of motion with notation of any pain (e.g., straight leg raising), crepitation, or contracture
• Assessment of stability with notation of any dislocation (luxation), subluxation, or laxity
• Assessment of muscle strength and tone (e.g., flaccid, cog wheel, spastic) with notation of any atrophy or abnormal movements

(continued)

MUSCULOSKELETAL EXAMINATION (*CONTINUED*)

System/Body Area	Elements of Examination
	NOTE: For the comprehensive level of examination, all four of the elements identified by a bullet must be performed and documented for each of four anatomic areas. For the three lower levels of examination, each element is counted separately for each body area. For example, assessing range of motion in two extremities constitutes two elements.
Extremities	[See musculoskeletal and skin]
Skin	• Inspection and/or palpation of skin and subcutaneous tissue (e.g., scars, rashes, lesions, cafe-au-lait spots, ulcers) in **four of the following six** areas: 1) head and neck; 2) trunk; 3) right upper extremity; 4) left upper extremity; 5) right lower extremity; and 6) left lower extremity. NOTE: For the comprehensive level, the examination of all four anatomic areas must be performed and documented. For the three lower levels of examination, each body area is counted separately. For example, inspection and/or palpation of the skin and subcutaneous tissue of two extremities constitutes two elements.
Neurological/ Psychiatric	• Test coordination (e.g., finger/nose, heel/knee/shin, rapid alternating movements in the upper and lower extremities, evaluation of fine motor coordination in young children) • Examination of deep tendon reflexes and/or nerve stretch test with notation of pathological reflexes (e.g., Babinski) • Examination of sensation (e.g., by touch, pin, vibration, proprioception) Brief assessment of mental status including • Orientation to time, place, and person • Mood and affect (e.g., depression, anxiety, agitation)

Content and Documentation Requirements

Level of Exam	Perform and Document:
Problem-Focused	**One to five** elements identified by a bullet.
Expanded Problem-Focused	**At least six** elements identified by a bullet.
Detailed	**At least twelve** elements identified by a bullet.
Comprehensive	Perform **all** elements identified by a bullet; document every element in each box with a shaded border and at least one element in each box with an unshaded border.

NEUROLOGICAL EXAMINATION

System/Body Area	Elements of Examination
Constitutional	• Measurement of **any three of the following seven** vital signs: 1) sitting or standing blood pressure, 2) supine blood pressure, 3) pulse rate and regularity, 4) respiration, 5) temperature, 6) height, 7) weight (May be measured and recorded by ancillary staff) • General appearance of patient (e.g., development, nutrition, body habitus, deformities, attention to grooming)

Head and Face

Eyes
- Ophthalmoscopic examination of optic discs (e.g., size, C/D ratio, appearance) and posterior segments (e.g., vessel changes, exudates, hemorrhages)

Ears, Nose, Mouth, and Throat

Neck

Respiratory

Cardiovascular
- Examination of carotid arteries (e.g., pulse amplitude, bruits)
- Auscultation of heart with notation of abnormal sounds and murmurs
- Examination of peripheral vascular system by observation (e.g., swelling, varicosities) and palpation (e.g., pulses, temperature, edema, tenderness)

Chest (Breasts)

Gastrointestinal (Abdomen)

Genitourinary

Lymphatic

Musculoskeletal
- Examination of gait and station

Assessment of motor function including:
- Muscle strength in upper and lower extremities
- Muscle tone in upper and lower extremities (e.g., flaccid, cog wheel, spastic) with notation of any atrophy or abnormal movements (e.g., fasciculation, tardive dyskinesia)

Extremities   [See musculoskeletal]

Skin

Neurological

Evaluation of higher integrative functions including:
- Orientation to time, place, and person
- Recent and remote memory
- Attention span and concentration
- Language (e.g., naming objects, repeating phrases, spontaneous speech)
- Fund of knowledge (e.g., awareness of current events, past history, vocabulary)

Test the following cranial nerves:
- 2nd cranial nerve (e.g., visual acuity, visual fields, fundi)
- 3rd, 4th, and 6th cranial nerves (e.g., pupils, eye movements)
- 5th cranial nerve (e.g., facial sensation, corneal reflexes)
- 7th cranial nerve (e.g., facial symmetry, strength)
- 8th cranial nerve (e.g., hearing with tuning fork, whispered voice and/or finger rub)
- 9th cranial nerve (e.g., spontaneous or reflex palate movement)
- 11th cranial nerve (e.g., shoulder shrug strength)
- 12th cranial nerve (e.g., tongue protrusion)
- Examination of sensation (e.g., by touch, pin, vibration, proprioception)
- Examination of deep tendon reflexes in upper and lower extremities with notation of pathological reflexes (e.g., Babinski)
- Test coordination (e.g., finger/nose, heel/knee/shin, rapid alternating movements in the upper and lower extremities, evaluation of fine motor coordination in young children)

Psychiatric

Content and Documentation Requirements

Level of Exam	*Perform and Document:*
Problem-Focused	**One to five** elements identified by a bullet.
Expanded Problem-Focused	**At least six** elements identified by a bullet.
Detailed	**At least twelve** elements identified by a bullet.
Comprehensive	Perform **all** elements identified by a bullet; document every element in each box with a shaded border and at least one element in each box with an unshaded border.

PSYCHIATRIC EXAMINATION

System/Body Area	Elements of Examination
Constitutional	• Measurement of **any three of the following seven** vital signs: 1) sitting or standing blood pressure, 2) supine blood pressure, 3) pulse rate and regularity, 4) respiration, 5) temperature, 6) height, 7) weight (May be measured and recorded by ancillary staff) • General appearance of patient (e.g., development, nutrition, body habitus, deformities, attention to grooming)
Head and Face	
Eyes	
Ears, Nose, Mouth, and Throat	
Neck	
Respiratory	
Cardiovascular	
Chest (Breasts)	
Gastrointestinal (Abdomen)	
Genitourinary	
Lymphatic	
Musculoskeletal	• Assessment of muscle strength and tone (e.g., flaccid, cog wheel, spastic) with notation of any atrophy and abnormal movements • Examination of gait and station
Extremities	
Skin	
Neurological	
Psychiatric	• Description of speech including: rate; volume; articulation; coherence; and spontaneity with notation of abnormalities (e.g., perseveration, paucity of language) • Description of thought processes including: rate of thoughts; content of thoughts (e.g., logical vs. illogical, tangential); abstract reasoning; and computation • Description of associations (e.g., loose, tangential, circumstantial, intact)

- Description of abnormal or psychotic thoughts including: hallucinations; delusions; preoccupation with violence; homicidal or suicidal ideation; and obsessions
- Description of the patient's judgment (e.g., concerning everyday activities and social situations) and insight (e.g., concerning psychiatric condition)

Complete mental status examination including
- Orientation to time, place, and person
- Recent and remote memory
- Attention span and concentration
- Language (e.g., naming objects, repeating phrases)
- Fund of knowledge (e.g., awareness of current events, past history, vocabulary)
- Mood and affect (e.g., depression, anxiety, agitation, hypomania, lability)

Content and Documentation Requirements

Level of Exam	Perform and Document:
Problem-Focused	**One to five** elements identified by a bullet.
Expanded Problem-Focused	**At least six** elements identified by a bullet.
Detailed	**At least nine** elements identified by a bullet.
Comprehensive	Perform **all** elements identified by a bullet; document every element in each box with a shaded border and at least one element in each box with an unshaded border.

RESPIRATORY EXAMINATION

System/Body Area	Elements of Examination
Constitutional	• Measurement of **any three of the following seven** vital signs: 1) sitting or standing blood pressure, 2) supine blood pressure, 3) pulse rate and regularity, 4) respiration, 5) temperature, 6) height, 7) weight (May be measured and recorded by ancillary staff) • General appearance of patient (e.g., development, nutrition, body habitus, deformities, attention to grooming)
Head and Face	
Eyes	
Ears, Nose, Mouth, and Throat	• Inspection of nasal mucosa, septum and turbinates • Inspection of teeth and gums • Examination of oropharynx (e.g., oral mucosa, hard and soft palates, tongue, tonsils, and posterior pharynx)
Neck	• Examination of neck (e.g., masses, overall appearance, symmetry, tracheal position, crepitus) • Examination of thyroid (e.g., enlargement, tenderness, mass) • Examination of jugular veins (e.g., distension; a, v or cannon a waves)
Respiratory	• Inspection of chest with notation of symmetry and expansion • Assessment of respiratory effort (e.g., intercostal retractions, use of accessory muscles, diaphragmatic movement)

(continued)

RESPIRATORY EXAMINATION (*CONTINUED*)

System/Body Area	Elements of Examination
	• Percussion of chest (e.g., dullness, flatness, hyperresonance)
	• Palpation of chest (e.g., tactile fremitus)
	• Auscultation of lungs (e.g., breath sounds, adventitious sounds, rubs)
Cardiovascular	• Auscultation of heart including sounds, abnormal sounds and murmurs
	• Examination of peripheral vascular system by observation (e.g., swelling, varicosities) and palpation (e.g., pulses, temperature, edema, tenderness)
Chest (Breasts)	
Gastrointestinal (Abdomen)	• Examination of abdomen with notation of presence of masses or tenderness
	• Examination of liver and spleen
Genitourinary	
Lymphatic	• Palpation of lymph nodes in neck, axillae, groin and/or other location
Musculoskeletal	• Assessment of muscle strength and tone (e.g., flaccid, cog wheel, spastic) with notation of any atrophy and abnormal movements
	• Examination of gait and station
Extremities	• Inspection and palpation of digits and nails (e.g., clubbing, cyanosis, inflammation, petechiae, ischemia, infections, nodes)
Skin	• Inspection and/or palpation of skin and subcutaneous tissue (e.g., rashes, lesions, ulcers)
Neurological/ Psychiatric	Brief assessment of mental status including
	• Orientation to time, place, and person
	• Mood and affect (e.g., depression, anxiety, agitation)

Content and Documentation Requirements

Level of Exam	*Perform and Document:*
Problem-Focused	**One to five** elements identified by a bullet.
Expanded Problem-Focused	**At least six** elements identified by a bullet.
Detailed	**At least twelve** elements identified by a bullet.
Comprehensive	Perform **all** elements identified by a bullet; document every element in each box with a shaded border and at least one element in each box with an unshaded border.

SKIN EXAMINATION

System/Body Area	Elements of Examination
Constitutional	• Measurement of any **three of the following seven** vital signs: 1) sitting or standing blood pressure, 2) supine blood pressure, 3) pulse rate and regularity, 4) respiration, 5) temperature, 6) height, 7) weight (May be measured and recorded by ancillary staff)

	• General appearance of patient (e.g., development, nutrition, body habitus, deformities, attention to grooming)
Head and Face	
Eyes	• Inspection of conjunctivae and lids
Ears, Nose, Mouth, and Throat	• Inspection of lips, teeth, and gums • Examination of oropharynx (e.g., oral mucosa, hard and soft palates, tongue, tonsils, posterior pharynx)
Neck	• Examination of thyroid (e.g., enlargement, tenderness, mass)
Respiratory	
Cardiovascular	• Examination of peripheral vascular system by observation (e.g., swelling, varicosities) and palpation (e.g., pulses, temperature, edema, tenderness)
Chest (Breasts)	
Gastrointestinal (Abdomen)	• Examination of liver and spleen • Examination of anus for condyloma and other lesions
Genitourinary	
Lymphatic	• Palpation of lymph nodes in neck, axillae, groin and/or other location
Musculoskeletal	
Extremities	• Inspection and palpation of digits and nails (e.g., clubbing, cyanosis, inflammation, petechiae, ischemia, infections, nodes)
Skin	• Palpation of scalp and inspection of hair of scalp, eyebrows, face, chest, pubic area (when indicated), and extremities • Inspection and/or palpation of skin and subcutaneous tissue (e.g., rashes, lesions, ulcers, susceptibility to and presence of photo damage) in **eight of the following ten** areas:

   - Head, including the face and neck
   - Chest, including breasts and axillae
   - Abdomen
   - Genitalia, groin, buttocks
   - Back
   - Right upper extremity
   - Left upper extremity
   - Right lower extremity
   - Left lower extremity

NOTE: For the comprehensive level, the examination of at least eight anatomic areas must be performed and documented. For the three lower levels of examination, each body area is counted separately. For example, inspection and/or palpation of the skin and subcutaneous tissue of the right upper extremity and the left upper extremity constitutes two elements.

• Inspection of eccrine and apocrine glands of skin and subcutaneous tissue with identification and location of any hyperhidrosis, chromhidroses or bromhidrosis

Neurological/ Psychiatric	Brief assessment of mental status including • Orientation to time, place, and person • Mood and affect (e.g., depression, anxiety, agitation)

Content and Documentation Requirements

Level of Exam	*Perform and Document:*
Problem-Focused	**One to five** elements identified by a bullet.
Expanded Problem-Focused	**At least six** elements identified by a bullet.
Detailed	**At least twelve** elements identified by a bullet.
Comprehensive	Perform **all** elements identified by a bullet; document every element in each box with a shaded border and at least one element in each box with an unshaded border.

C. Documentation of the Complexity of Medical Decision Making

The levels of E/M services recognize four types of medical decision making (straightforward, low complexity, moderate complexity and high complexity). Medical decision making refers to the complexity of establishing a diagnosis and/or selecting a management option as measured by:

- the number of possible diagnoses and/or the number of management options that must be considered;
- the amount and/or complexity of medical records, diagnostic tests, and/or other information that must be obtained, reviewed and analyzed; and
- the risk of significant complications, morbidity and/or mortality, as well as comorbidities, associated with the patient's presenting problem(s), the diagnostic procedure(s), and/or the possible management options.

The chart below shows the progression of the elements required for each level of medical decision making. To qualify for a given type of decision making, **two of the three elements in the table must be either met or exceeded.**

Number of Diagnoses or Management Options	Amount and/or Complexity of Data to be Reviewed	Risk of Complications and/or Morbidity or Mortality	Type of Decision Making
Minimal	Minimal or None	Minimal	*Straightforward*
Limited	Limited	Low	*Low Complexity*
Multiple	Moderate	Moderate	*Moderate Complexity*
Extensive	Extensive	High	*High Complexity*

Each of the elements of medical decision making is described below.

Number of Diagnoses or Management Options

The number of possible diagnoses and/or the number of management options that must be considered is based on the number and types of problems addressed during the encounter, the complexity of establishing a diagnosis, and the management decisions that are made by the physician.

Generally, decision making with respect to a diagnosed problem is easier than that for an identified but undiagnosed problem. The number and type of diagnostic tests employed may be an indicator of the number of possible diagnoses. Problems which are improving or resolving are less complex than those which are worsening or failing to change as expected. The need to seek advice from others is another indicator of complexity of diagnostic or management problems.

- *DG: For each encounter, an assessment, clinical impression, or diagnosis should be documented. It may be explicitly stated or implied in documented decisions regarding management plans and/or further evaluation.*

- *For a presenting problem with an established diagnosis the record should reflect whether the problem is: a) improved, well controlled, resolving or resolved; or, b) inadequately controlled, worsening, or failing to change as expected.*
- *For a presenting problem without an established diagnosis, the assessment or clinical impression may be stated in the form of differential diagnoses or as a "possible," "probable," or "rule out" (R/O) diagnosis.*
- *DG: The initiation of, or changes in, treatment should be documented. Treatment includes a wide range of management options including patient instructions, nursing instructions, therapies, and medications.*
- *DG: If referrals are made, consultations requested or advice sought, the record should indicate to whom or where the referral or consultation is made or from whom the advice is requested.*

Amount and/or Complexity of Data to Be Reviewed

The amount and complexity of data to be reviewed is based on the types of diagnostic testing ordered or reviewed. A decision to obtain and review old medical records and/or obtain history from sources other than the patient increases the amount and complexity of data to be reviewed.

Discussion of contradictory or unexpected test results with the physician who performed or interpreted the test is an indication of the complexity of data being reviewed. On occasion the physician who ordered a test may personally review the image, tracing, or specimen to supplement information from the physician who prepared the test report or interpretation; this is another indication of the complexity of data being reviewed.

- *DG: If a diagnostic service (test or procedure) is ordered, planned, scheduled, or performed at the time of the E/M encounter, the type of service, e.g., lab or X-ray, should be documented.*
- *DG: The review of lab, radiology, and/or other diagnostic tests should be documented. A simple notation such as "WBC elevated" or "chest X-ray unremarkable" is acceptable. Alternatively, the review may be documented by initialing and dating the report containing the test results.*
- *DG: A decision to obtain old records or decision to obtain additional history from the family, caretaker, or other source to supplement that obtained from the patient should be documented.*
- *DG: Relevant findings from the review of old records, and/or the receipt of additional history from the family, caretaker, or other source to supplement that obtained from the patient should be documented. If there is no relevant information beyond that already obtained, that fact should be documented. A notation of "Old records reviewed" or "additional history obtained from family" without elaboration is insufficient.*
- *DG: The results of discussion of laboratory, radiology, or other diagnostic tests with the physician who performed or interpreted the study should be documented.*
- *DG: The direct visualization and independent interpretation of an image, tracing, or specimen previously or subsequently interpreted by another physician should be documented.*

Risk of Significant Complications, Morbidity, and/or Mortality

The risk of significant complications, morbidity, and/or mortality is based on the risks associated with the presenting problem(s), the diagnostic procedure(s), and the possible management options.

- *DG: Comorbidities/underlying diseases or other factors that increase the complexity of medical decision making by increasing the risk of complications, morbidity, and/or mortality should be documented.*
- *DG: If a surgical or invasive diagnostic procedure is ordered, planned, or scheduled at the time of the E/M encounter, the type of procedure, e.g., laparoscopy, should be documented.*
- *DG: If a surgical or invasive diagnostic procedure is performed at the time of the E/M encounter, the specific procedure should be documented.*
- *DG: The referral for or decision to perform a surgical or invasive diagnostic procedure on an urgent basis should be documented or implied.*

The following table may be used to help determine whether the risk of significant complications, morbidity, and/or mortality is *minimal, low, moderate,* or *high.* Because the determination of risk is complex and not readily quantifiable, the table includes common clinical examples rather than absolute measures of risk. The assessment of risk of the presenting problem(s) is based on the risk related to the disease process anticipated between the present encounter and the next one. The assessment of risk of selecting diagnostic procedures and management options is based on the risk during and immediately following any procedures or treatment. **The highest level of risk in any one category (presenting problem(s), diagnostic procedure(s), or management options) determines the overall risk.**

TABLE OF RISK

Level of Risk	Presenting Problem(s)	Diagnostic Procedure(s) Ordered	Management Options Selected
Minimal	• One-self limited or minor problem, e.g., cold, insect bite, tinea corporis	• Laboratory tests requiring venipuncture • Chest X-rays • EKG/EEG • Urinalysis • Ultrasound, e.g., echocardiography • KOH prep	• Rest • Gargles • Elastic bandages • Superficial dressings
Low	• Two or more self-limited or minor problems • One stable chronic illness, e.g., well controlled hypertension, non-insulin dependent diabetes, cataract, BPH • Acute uncomplicated illness or injury, e.g., cystitis, allergic rhinitis, simple sprain	• Physiologic tests not under stress, e.g., pulmonary function tests • Non-cardiovascular imaging studies with contrast, e.g., barium enema • Superficial needle biopsies • Clinical laboratory tests requiring arterial puncture • Skin biopsies	• Over-the-counter drugs • Minor surgery with no identified risk factors • Physical therapy • Occupational therapy • IV fluids without additives
Moderate	• One or more chronic illnesses with mild exacerbation, progression, or side effects of treatment • Two or more stable chronic illnesses • Undiagnosed new problem with uncertain prognosis, e.g., lump in breast • Acute illness with systemic symptoms, e.g., pyelonephritis, pneumonitis, colitis	• Physiologic tests under stress, e.g., cardiac stress test, fetal contraction stress test • Diagnostic endoscopies with no identified risk factors • Deep needle or incisional biopsy • Cardiovascular imaging studies with contrast and no identified risk factors, e.g., arteriogram, cardiac catheterization	• Minor surgery with identified risk factors • Elective major surgery (open, percutaneous or endoscopic) with no identified risk factors • Prescription drug management • Therapeutic nuclear medicine • IV fluids with additives

High

- Acute complicated injury, e.g., head injury with brief loss of consciousness
- One or more chronic illnesses with severe exacerbation, progression, or side effects of treatment
- Acute or chronic illnesses or injuries that pose a threat to life or bodily function, e.g., multiple trauma, acute MI, pulmonary embolus, severe respiratory distress, progressive severe rheumatoid arthritis, psychiatric illness with potential threat to self or others, peritonitis, acute renal failure
- An abrupt change in neurologic status, e.g., seizure, TIA, weakness, sensory loss

- Obtain fluid from body cavity, e.g., lumbar puncture, thoracentesis, culdocentesis
- Cardiovascular imaging studies with contrast with identified risk factors
- Cardiac electrophysiological tests
- Diagnostic endoscopies with identified risk factors
- Discography

- Closed treatment of fracture or dislocation without manipulation
- Elective major surgery (open, percutaneous or endoscopic) with identified risk factors
- Emergency major surgery (open, percutaneous or endoscopic)
- Parenteral controlled substances
- Drug therapy requiring intensive monitoring for toxicity
- Decision not to resuscitate or to de-escalate care because of poor prognosis

D. Documentation of an Encounter Dominated by Counseling or Coordination of Care

In the case where counseling and/or coordination of care dominates (more than 50% of) the physician/patient and/or family encounter (face-to-face time in the office or other outpatient setting, floor/unit time in the hospital or nursing facility), time is considered the key or controlling factor to qualify for a particular level of E/M services.

- *DG: If the physician elects to report the level of service based on counseling and/or coordination of care, the total length of time of the encounter (face-to-face or floor time, as appropriate) should be documented and the record should describe the counseling and/or activities to coordinate care.*

NDCMedisoft™ Advanced—
Version 9—Issues and Answers

SET-UP INSTRUCTIONS

Individual Student Files on One Computer Station

The first time you use NDCMedisoft Advanced on a specific computer terminal, you will need to copy your work onto a removable media source, such as a floppy disk or writeable CD-ROM.

Each subsequent time you work at a terminal, you will need to restore your own data onto the hard drive. Then, when a particular work session is done, you will need to resave and back up your work on your personal removable disk. This routine will prevent another student from taking advantage of your work.

For example:

Class 1: Sally logs in and enters data into NDCMedisoft Advanced working from Chapter 11 and other class assignments. When she is done for this session, she will need to save a back-up file onto a floppy disk or rewriteable CD-ROM.

Class 2: Sally logs in and opens NDCMedisoft Advanced. The first thing that she will do, once the software opens, is to restore data from her floppy disk to the computer. When Sally is done working for this class session, she will need to resave a back-up file onto her floppy disk or rewriteable CD-ROM.

Class 3 through the end of term: Sally will repeat what she did on the second day, beginning each class or work session by restoring the data from her floppy disk and ending each session by saving a new back-up file onto her floppy disk.

You should get in the habit of making back-up files after each work session, so this will be your established norm behavior once you get into the workforce. You, or your school, will need to supply one blank floppy disk or rewriteable CD-ROM (if the school's computer has a CD burner).

Making a Back-Up File

After the first, and each subsequent, work session in NDCMedisoft Advanced,

1. Go to the FILE Menu and choose EXIT, or click on the EXIT button on the toolbar.
2. The Back-Up Reminder dialog box will appear on the screen. This dialog box has three buttons along its bottom border: Back-Up Data Now; Exit Program; Cancel.
3. Insert a personal removable data disk (floppy disk or rewriteable CD-ROM) into its appropriate drive.
4. Click on the Back-Up Data Now button on the bottom of the Back-Up Reminder dialog box.

---

*Please contact your McGraw-Hill Higher Education sales representative for a Medisoft demo disk.

5. The Back-Up dialog box appears. The Destination File Path and Name field of the Back-Up dialog box should show c:\medidata\fda. If not, you can key this in. Note—these are back slashes (above your right-hand Enter key), not forward slashes (next to your right-hand shift key). The computer should automatically complete the Source Path field requiring the location of the database files. NDCMedisoft Advanced will copy the latest database files to the disk in Drive A (Drive A is the typical designation for the floppy disk drive. If using a rewriteable CD-ROM in a CD burner, make certain that drive is shown). Click on the Start Back-up button.

6. An information dialog box will appear, notifying you that the back up is complete. Click OK to continue.

7. The Back-Up dialog box will disappear, NDCMedisoft Advanced will close, and your screen should return to your main desktop. Remove the floppy disk from the drive. Be certain to write your name on the floppy disk!

Restoring the Working File

At the beginning of the second, and each subsequent, work session in NDCMedisoft Advanced,

1. Start NDCMedisoft Advanced, Version 9, either by double-clicking on the desktop icon or by clicking on the START Menu, and choosing NDCMedisoft Advanced.

2. Make certain the blue title bar, across the top of the screen, says Family Doctors Associates, the health care facility you created in the beginning of Chapter 11.

3. Insert the floppy disk, on which you saved your last working session in NDCMedisoft, in Drive A (the floppy disk drive) of your computer.

4. Go to the FILE Menu and choose Restore Data.

5. A warning box will appear so you can confirm that you chose this on purpose. Click OK.

6. The Restore dialog box will appear. The Back-up File Path and Name, Existing Back-up Files, and the Destination Path fields should be completed automatically. Click on the Start Restore button.

7. A warning box will appear again, so you can confirm that you chose this on purpose. Click OK.

8. When the restoration of the files has been successfully copied from the floppy disk to the computer, an Information box will appear. Click OK.

9. The Restore dialog box will disappear, and you can begin work in NDCMedisoft Advanced.

10. REMEMBER to back up your files when you are done with this session!

Setting the Program Options

Go to the FILE Menu and choose Program Options.

General Tab

1. Make certain that the Remind to Back-up on Program Exit is checked ☑.
2. Check off Show Hints, Show Shortcuts, and Enforce Accept Assignment ☑.

Data Entry Tab

1. Check off Use Enter to move between fields ☑. This will permit you to use either the Tab key or the Enter key to move from field to field.
2. Check off Use zip code to enter city and state ☑. This will save time and errors by enabling you to key in the zip code and, after the first time, NDCMedisoft Advanced will complete the city and state for you.
3. Check off Auto format Soc. Sec. # ☑. This will save time and effort so you can enter Social Security numbers as nine straight digits. NDCMedisoft Advanced will insert the dashes for you.

Payment Application Tab

1. Check off Mark Paid Charges Complete ☑. This will help you track those charges for which payment has been received.
2. Check off Mark Complete Claims Done ☑. This will help you track those claims submitted and for which payment has been received.

Aging Reports Tab

The items on this tab relate to accounting reports regarding the length of time a patient or third-party payer owes your office money and has not yet paid.

HIPAA Tab

The items on this tab relate to security and privacy standards as mandated by HIPAA.

Color Coding Tab

1. Use this screen to mark different entries with colors. This will help you identify various items, such as assorted types of payments. Also, you can use color flags for patient identification, such as those with one particular attending physician versus another.

ISSUES AND ANSWERS

New Patient Screen or New Case Screen

Issue: Screen disappears and you are, all of a sudden, back at the Patient List screen.

Answer: You probably clicked on the SAVE button accidentally. Simply click once on the patient's name or on the case name. Then click on the EDIT PATIENT or EDIT CASE button. This will reopen the screen and you can continue working from where you left off.

Issue: The field will not accept the diagnosis code or insurance company you are trying to key in.

Answer: This means that the code or insurance company you are attempting to enter is not in the master list. You will have to save and close this screen and the patient list screen. Go to the LISTS Menu and choose Diagnosis Codes or Insurance Carriers. Click on the New button at the bottom of the List screen. Enter the appropriate information and save. Then, you can return to the case and the information will be available to you in the Diagnosis Code field or the Insurance Carrier field.

Issue: You are entering the information from the chapter and, after entering a date, you get a confirm box that says, "You have entered a future date. Do you want to change it?"

Answer: This dialog box is confirming that you have entered a date that is in the future on purpose and not by accident. Simply click on the NO button. You do not want to change it. The computer will accept the date and let you continue.

Issue: You mistakenly enter the same patient twice.

Answer: First, confirm that they are the same patient and not two patients with the same name or similar names. Once you are certain this is a duplicate entry, click once on the second listing of the name in the Patient List. With that name highlighted, click on the DELETE PATIENT button at the bottom of the Patient List dialog box, to the right side. The computer will ask you to confirm that you want to delete this file. Click YES. Then, you will see the second listing disappear.

Issue: *You mistakenly enter the same case twice.*

Answer: Click once on the second listing of the case in the Case List for that patient. With that case highlighted, click on the DELETE CASE button at the bottom of the Patient List dialog box, to the right side. The computer will ask you to confirm that you want to delete this file. Click YES. Then, you will see the second listing disappear.

Transaction Entry Screen

Issue: *The patient's insurance policy is not showing in the upper right of the screen.*

Answer: This means that no insurance policy was entered on the Policy 1 tab of the New Case screen. Close the Transaction Entry screen. Go to the LISTS Menu and open the Patient/Guarantors and Cases screen. Click once on the patient's name on the Patient List. Click once on the case name. Click on the EDIT CASE button on the lower left of the screen. Click on the Policy 1 tab. Choose the insurance carrier from the drop-down list. Click the SAVE button on the upper right-hand side of the screen. Go to the Activities Menu and open Transaction Entry (Enter Transactions). Choose the patient's file. The insurance carrier should show in the upper right corner of the screen.

NOTE: After entering new information in a List dialog box (e.g., New Patient, New Case, New Diagnosis Code, New Procedure Code, New Insurance Carrier, etc.), save that screen and close the dialog box. This must happen before the information will be available to you in a drop-down menu in any other dialog box (such as Transaction Entry). It is a good idea to get in the habit of closing the dialog box you are in before opening another. This habit will save you time and frustration.

Issue: *The field will not accept the procedure code or pay/adj code you are trying to key in.*

Answer: This means that the code you are attempting to enter is not in the master list. You will have to save and close this screen. Go to the LISTS Menu and choose Procedure/Payment/Adjustment Codes. Click on the NEW button at the bottom of the List screen. Enter the appropriate information and save. Then, you can return to the Transaction Entry dialog box, and the information will be available to you in the Procedure Code field or the Pay/Adj Code field.

Issue: *You try to print a receipt for a patient and get an information box that says, "There is no data available for this report." But you have just entered the procedure codes and the payment.*

Answer: Most frequently, the receipt cannot be created because the range of dates on the screen immediately prior to the appearance of the information box does not match the date(s) entered in the Transaction Entry dialog box to indicate when the procedures were performed or the payment made. Click OK on the information box and try the sequence again to create the receipt. This time, pay close attention that the dates entered in the range box match exactly the dates entered alongside the procedure codes and payments in the Transaction Entry dialog box.

Issue: *When you click on the PRINT CLAIM button on the bottom of the Transaction Entry dialog box, you get an information box that says, "All of the eligible displayed charge transactions have been placed on a previous claim."*

Answer: This means that all of the procedures entered on this patient's record have already been billed to the insurance carrier. If you are trying to print out a second copy of a claim already created, you will need to do that from the ACTIVITIES Menu by choosing Claim Management. In the Claim Management dialog box, click once on the claim you want to reprint; then click on the REPRINT CLAIM button at the bottom of the box.

If you are trying to recreate a claim because you made corrections to certain data, you will need to delete the first claim by going to the ACTIVITIES Menu and choosing Claim Management. In the Claim Management dialog box, click once on the claim you want to delete. Then click on the DELETE CLAIM button at the bottom of the box. Then, click on the CREATE CLAIM button at the bottom of the box and enter the information to create the new version of the claim. Remember, NDCMedisoft Advanced does not update after you have made corrections or changes to information contained in an existing claim. You have to delete the old claim and create a new one.

Claims Management

Issue: *You are trying to create a new claim for a patient, and you get an information box that says,*

"No new claims were created. If you expected some to be created, check the following items:

1. *The patient's case needs at least one insurance carrier,*
2. *The filter used to select transactions for claim creation may be excluding all transactions that are eligible to be placed on a claim,*
3. *The transaction needs at least one insurance carrier that is responsible for payment."*

Answer: There are several things you can do.

1. Close this box and go back to the Patient List. Open the case for this patient and double-check that the Policy 1 tab is completed correctly.
2. If that is not the problem, open the Transaction Entry screen for this patient and confirm the dates entered for each of the procedure codes. Then, close that screen, reopen the Claims Management screen, and try to create the claim again. This time, be very careful as you enter the transaction dates in the Create Claims dialog box.
3. If this still does not solve the problem, check to make certain that these procedures have not already been placed on a previous claim form.

Issue: *You have created a claim form, clicked on it once, and clicked the Print/Send button. You have checked Paper on the first dialog box and entered the patient's name. However, then you get an information box that says, "There are no claims to be printed using the filters specified." How can you get this claim to print?*

Answer: The first thing you need to do is check the Media 1 column on the Claims Management dialog box. If this claim is indicating a Media 1 listing that says EDI or EMC, rather than Paper, NDCMedisoft Advanced will not let you print out this claim on paper. Go to the Lists Menu and choose Insurance Carriers. Click on the name of the insurance carrier for this patient and click the EDIT button at the bottom of the List screen. Click on the Options tab and change the Default Billing Method entry at the bottom of this screen from Electronic to Paper. Click Save. Then, you can return to the Claims Management dialog box, delete the old claim, and create a new one. Now, you should be able to print the claim form without any problem.

Issue: *You created a claim form and printed it yesterday. How can you get this claim to print again?*

Answer: This time, instead of clicking on the Print/Send button, click on the Reprint Claim button.

Patient Statement

Issue: You have tried to create a patient statement but you get an information box that says, "There are no statements to be printed using the filters specified."

Answer: In the Patient Statement: Data Selection Questions dialog box, where you will enter the chart number range for the patient for whom you want to create a statement, you will see that the fifth or bottom line asks for the Statement Total Range. NDCMedisoft Advanced will automatically complete these fields to show 0.01 to 999999.99. This means that the software is instructed to create statements only when the balance of the patient's account is between 1¢ and $999,999.99. This means that, if your patient's account is now at zero, because zero is outside of the 0.01 to 999999.99 range, the statement will not be created. Simply change the 0.01 to a 0.00 and the statement should be created without further problem.

If your statement will still not format, close this dialog box and go to the Activities Menu and choose Enter Transactions. Open the transaction entry screen for the patient and check the balance of the patient's account in the upper right-hand corner. You might find that this patient has a negative balance (an error in payment entries, perhaps?). When you try to create a statement again, make certain that the first number in the Statement Total Range matches the balance shown in the Transaction Entry dialog box, and there should be no further problems with this issue.

Glossary

A

abstracting Pulling out the key words needed to code; finding the key words in the physician's notes.

accept assignment The process whereby a policyholder gives permission to the insurer to pay benefits directly to the provider; when Medicare is the insurer, this also means that the provider agrees to accept the allowed amount as payment in full.

adverse reaction Harm or danger to an individual caused by interaction with a drug or chemical.

allowed amount The maximum payment for service or treatment from an insurance carrier.

Alphabetic Index to Diseases The portion of the ICD-9-CM book listed in alphabetical order from *A* to *Z*.

anatomical site The place in the body in which a condition occurs, such as knee or heart.

anesthesia Services for administering anesthetics.

attending provider The physician who has been assigned to a patient.

B

balance billing The invoicing of a patient for the difference between the allowed amount and the physician's charge.

bilateral edit An ICD-9-CM procedure notation that indicates approval for a code to be listed twice on the same claim form to indicate that the same procedure was performed on both of the same bilateral joints.

birthday rule The rule used to establish the primary insurance policy for a child by determining which parent has a birthday closest to January 1.

C

capitation A predetermined monthly payment from a managed care organization to a health care provider for the care of each of that plan's members assigned to that provider.

carcinoma Any of a variety of types of malignant neoplasms.

case In NDCMedisoft Advanced, the file created with details pertaining to a patient's specific chief complaint or diagnosis.

causal condition One disease that affects or encourages another condition. Also referred to as an underlying disease.

CCI A computerized system used by Medicare to prevent overpayment for procedures.

Centers for Medicare & Medicaid Services (CMS) The agency under the Department of Health and Human Services (DHHS) in charge of regulation and control over benefits for individuals covered by Medicare and Medicaid.

CHAMPUS (See TriCare)

CHAMPVA A federal plan that shares health care costs for the dependents of veterans with 100% service-connected disability or those who have died from service-connected disabilities.

CMS-1500 The claim form used most often by outpatient facilities.

code linkage The process of directly connecting each procedure code to at least one diagnosis code on the insurance claim form.

coding for coverage Changing a code to fit what the insurance company will pay for, rather than accurately reflecting the procedure that was actually performed.

co-insurance The portion of a charge that an insured person pays based on a percentage of the total charge.

complexity The measure of how problematic the presenting condition is.

condition The presenting situation, such as infection, fracture, or wound.

co-payment Also known as co-pay, a fixed amount of money that an individual pays for each visit to a health care provider.

Correct Coding Initiative (CCI) A computerized system used by Medicare to prevent overpayment.

covered entities Organizations that access the personal health information of patients; they include health care providers, health plans, and health care clearinghouses.

CPT Current Procedural Terminology—4th revision. A set of codes used to report services or treatments.

D

data Pieces of information.

deductible The amount of money patients must pay, out of their own pockets, before insurance benefits begin.

denied claims Claims that will not be paid because the third-party payer has identified ineligible services, those not covered by the insured's policy.

dependent An individual's spouse, child, or legal responsibility and a person covered under someone else's health insurance policy.

diagnosis A physician's determination of a patient's condition, illness, or injury.

Diagnosis Code Set A group of codes used in a health care practice to identify conditions, illnesses, or injuries.

disability compensation An insurance plan that will reimburse an individual for a percentage of his or her income that is lost as a result of being unable to work due to illness or injury; this plan does not pay physician's bills or for therapy treatments.

disclosure As defined by HIPAA, the sharing of information by health care professionals to anyone outside of their facility.

discounted FFS An extra reduction in the rate charged to an insurer for services provided by a physician to a plan's members.

double billing Sending two separate claims for one encounter.

E

E code A code that explains *how* an injury or a poisoning happened, and/or *where* it happened.

electronic data interchange (EDI) Electronic system used to send health insurance claim forms.

electronic funds transfer (EFT) Money that is moved from one bank account to another bank account via computer; no checks actually change hands.

electronic media claim (EMC) Also referred to as an electronic medical claim, a claim form submitted electronically.

electronic remittance advice (ERA) A remittance advice that is sent to the provider electronically.

eligibility confirmation The process of contacting an insurance carrier to confirm that an individual is qualified for benefits to pay for services provided by a health care professional on a given day.

employer identification number (EIN) A corporation identifier; the same as a Social Security number for an individual.

encounter form The form that documents what occurred during a meeting between a patient and a health care provider.

episodic care One flat fee paid to the provider by an insurer to cover the entire course of treatment for an individual's condition.

eponym The name of a condition derived from the name of a person, such as Epstein-Barr syndrome or Cushing's disease.

established patient A person who has received professional services from a particular provider within the past three years.

etiology The identification of the cause of a disease.

evaluation and management A physician's services to a patient that include an assessment of the condition and the determination of what action should be taken next.

Excludes An ICD-9-CM notation that identifies a condition omitted from the description of a code.

Excludes 1 An ICD-10-CM notation that identifies that one code cannot be used on the same claim form with another code.

Excludes 2 An ICD-10-CM notation that identifies a condition omitted from the description for that code.

External cause (See E code)

F

fee-for-service (FFS) A payment agreement that outlines in a written fee schedule exactly how much money the insurance carrier will pay the physician for each treatment and/or service provided.

fields (form locators) The boxes in the CMS-1500.

G

gatekeeper A physician, typically a family practitioner or an internist, who serves as the primary care physician for an individual; this physician is responsible for evaluating and determining the course of treatment or services as well as deciding whether or not a specialist should be involved in care.

group name or number A number (or combination of letters and numbers) that connects an individual policy with a specific group of insureds.

guarantor The person who will pay any money due to a health care provider that is not paid by the insurance company.

H

health care The total management of an individual's well-being by a health care professional.

health care clearinghouses Companies that process health claim forms, convert them into proper data format, and submit them to the correct insurance carrier.

health care provider Any professional who provides health care services.

health maintenance organization (HMO) A type of health insurance that uses a primary care physician, also known as a gatekeeper, to manage all health care services for an individual.

health plan Defined by HIPAA as a company whose main business focus is providing and/or paying for health care services; also a health insurance policy.

health-related risk factors Lifestyles and behaviors such as alcohol intake, cigarette smoking, and dietary issues (high fat, high cholesterol).

highest degree of certainty What is known for a fact.

HIPAA Health Insurance Portability and Accountability Act of 1996.

HIPAA's Privacy Rule Legislation that secures patients' information so it is available to those who should see it, while protecting that information from those who should not.

I

ICD-9-CM   The International Classification of Diseases—9th Revision—Clinical Modification.

ICD-10-CM   The International Classification of Diseases—10th Revision—Clinical Modification.

ICD-10-PCS   The International Classification of Diseases—10th Revision—Procedure Coding System.

ID number (policy number)   The number (or sometimes a combination of letters and numbers) that connects an individual to a specific insurance policy.

incidental use and disclosure   The accidental release of protected health information during the course of proper patient care.

inclusion   Adds specific conditions included in a code's description.

individually identifiable health information (IIHI)   Data that can be connected to a specific person.

insurance premium   The amount of money, often paid monthly, by a policyholder or insured, to an insurance company to obtain coverage.

insured   Also called the policyholder, the person who brings the health insurance policy to the family.

L

laterality   The location of the condition, such as right, left, upper, lower, anterior, and posterior; *bilateral* means "both sides."

liability insurance   A policy that covers loss or injury to a third-party caused by the insured or something belonging to that insured.

limited data set   Stripped-down protected health information for approved research and statistics.

location   The place where the health care provider met with the patient.

M

managed care   A type of health insurance coverage that controls the care of each subscriber (or insured person) by using a primary care provider as a central health care supervisor.

manifestation   A condition caused by or developed from the existence of another condition similar to a side effect.

medical care   The identification and treatment of illness and/or injury.

medical decision making   The factors involved in the physician's determination of treatment.

medical necessity/medically necessary   The use of ICD-9-CM diagnosis codes to establish a medical reason for providing the services and/or procedures claimed; also the determination that the provider was acting according to standard practices in providing a procedure for an individual with a specific diagnosis.

medical notes   (See physician's notes) The written documentation of an encounter between a provider and an individual.

medicine   A category of health care services.

minimum necessary   The caution that should be used to release only the smallest amount of information required to accomplish the task and no more.

morbidity   The study of disease and the causes of disease in a given population or society.

mortality   The proportion of deaths to the population as a whole, also known as the death rate.

mutually exclusive codes   Two or more codes that are identified in the coding book which cannot be used on the same claim form.

N

neoplasm   Abnormal tissue, also defined as a growth or tumor.

new patient   A person who has not received any professional services within the past three years from this provider, or another provider of the same specialty who belongs to the same group practice.

Non-covered Procedure   An ICD-9-CM procedure notation that means the indicated procedure is not approved by Medicare.

Non-specific OR Procedure   An ICD-9-CM procedure notation that is recognized only when all operating room procedures performed are coded Not Otherwise Specified.

O

onset   The date the patient exhibited the first symptom of the illness; the date the accident occurred that caused the injury; or, if the patient is pregnant, the date of the patient's last menstrual period (LMP).

operating room (OR)   Sterile room for performing surgery.

P

pathology and laboratory   Lab tests and analyses.

patient   The individual seeking health care services.

payee   An individual or organization that receives payment from another individual or organization.

payer (payor)   An individual or organization that sends payment to another individual or organization.

physician's notes   The written documentation of an encounter between a provider and a patient, also called provider notes and medical notes.

place of service   A two-digit code that categorizes the location where the procedure was performed.

plan/program name   The name of the health care plan, not necessarily the same name as the insurance carrier or company name.

point-of-service (POS) A type of insurance plan that allows a health maintenance organization enrollee to choose his or her own nonmember physician at a lower benefit rate, costing the patient more money out-of-pocket.

policyholder Also called the insured, the person who brings the insurance policy to the family.

practice A health care facility, such as a physician's office.

preadmission certificate Confirmation from an insurer, in advance, that a patient's treatment in a hospital is approved.

preauthorization Approval from an insurer to perform a procedure before actually providing that service to the patient.

preferred provider organization (PPO) A type of health insurance coverage in which physicians provide health care services to members of the plan at a discount.

preventive care Services given to an individual with the intention of avoiding illness or injury.

primary insurance policy The policy that names the patient as the policyholder or insured party.

privacy notices A covered entity's written policies and procedures that it will follow in order to protect its patients' protected health information.

procedure A treatment or service provided by a health care professional.

Procedure Code Set A group of codes used to identify services or treatments provided.

procedure coding system (PCS) The new version of identifying services and treatments performed in a hospital.

protected health information (PHI) Any identifiable patient health information, regardless of the form in which it is stored (for example, paper or computer file).

Provider Identification Number (PIN) An identifier assigned to a physician by an insurance carrier.

Q

query To ask.

R

radiology X-rays, nuclear medicine, and diagnostic ultrasound.

referring physician (referring provider) The health care professional who recommends that an individual see a specialist or another health care provider.

remittance Payment for services provided.

remittance advice (RA) A notification identifying exactly what benefits are being paid for by the third-party payer with reference to a specific claim or claims.

responsible party (See guarantor)

root operation The exact procedure foundation.

S

superbill An encounter form that is preprinted with the diagnoses and ICD-9-CM codes, as well as the procedures and CPT codes, most frequently used in a given practice.

supporting documentation The paperwork in a patient's file that corroborates the codes presented on the claim form for a particular encounter.

surgery Operative or surgical procedures.

T

Tabular List of Diseases The portion of the ICD-9-CM book listed in numerical order from 001 to 999.99.

third-party payer An individual or organization not directly involved in an encounter but connected to it through an obligation to pay, in full or part, for that encounter.

tracer An official request for a third-party payer to search its system for a missing health claim form; also a health claim form submitted to replace one that was lost.

treatment, payment, and/or operations (TPO) As defined by HIPAA, three situations that permit covered entities to use or disclose protected health information, when their best professional judgment deems it necessary.

TriCare A government health plan that covers medical expenses for the dependents of active-duty service members, CHAMPUS-eligible retirees and their families, and the dependents of deceased active-duty members; formerly called CHAMPUS.

type of service A one- or two-digit code that categorizes the procedure performed.

U

unbundling Coding individual parts of a specific procedure, rather than one combination code that includes all of the components.

underlying condition A disease that affects or encourages another condition.

uniformed services The U.S. military (Army, Navy, Air Force, Marines, and Coast Guard), as well as those in service in the Public Health Service, the National Oceanic and Atmospheric Administration (NOAA), and NATO.

upcoding Using a code on a claim form indicating a higher level of service than that which was actually performed.

usual, customary, and reasonable (UCR) A formula used by insurers to determine the fee to be paid for a particular treatment or service.

use As defined by HIPAA, the sharing of information between people working in the same health care facility for purposes of caring for a patient.

V

V code A code used to describe an encounter between a provider and an individual without a specific current health concern.

verification Contacting an insurance carrier to confirm that an individual has current, valid health insurance coverage.

W

workers' compensation An insurance program that covers medical care for those who are injured or become ill as a consequence of their employment.

workforce As defined by HIPAA, those involved with a covered entity, whether or not they are full-time and whether or not they get paid.

Index

Note: Page numbers followed by f indicate illustrations; those followed by b indicate boxed material; and those followed by t indicate tables.